THE WASHINGTON MANUAL™

Nephrology   Subspecialty Consult

Third Edition

Editors

Steven Cheng, MD

Assistant Professor of Medicine
Department of Internal Medicine
Renal Division
Washington University School of Medicine
St. Louis, Missouri

Anitha Vijayan, MD

Associate Professor of Medicine
Department of Internal Medicine
Renal Division
Washington University School of Medicine
St. Louis, Missouri

Series Editors

Katherine E. Henderson, MD

Assistant Professor of Clinical Medicine
Department of Medicine
Division of Medical Education
Washington University School of Medicine
Barnes-Jewish Hospital
St. Louis, Missouri

Thomas M. De Fer, MD

Associate Professor of Internal Medicine
Washington University School of Medicine
St. Louis, Missouri

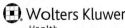 Wolters Kluwer | Lippincott Williams & Wilkins
Health
Philadelphia • Baltimore • New York • London
Buenos Aires • Hong Kong • Sydney • Tokyo

Acquisitions Editor: Sonya Seigafuse
Product Manager: Kerry Barrett
Vendor Manager: Bridgett Dougherty
Marketing Manager: Kimberly Schonberger
Manufacturing Manager: Ben Rivera
Design Coordinator: Stephen Druding
Editorial Coordinator: Katie Sharp
Production Service: Aptara, Inc.

© **2012 by Department of Medicine, Washington University School of Medicine**

Printed in China

Library of Congress Cataloging-in-Publication Data

The Washington manual nephrology subspecialty consult. — 3rd ed. / editors, Steven Cheng, Anitha Vijayan.
    p. ; cm. — (Washington manual subspecialty consult series)
    Nephrology subspecialty consult
    Includes bibliographical references and index.
    ISBN 978-1-4511-1425-6 (alk. paper) — ISBN 1-4511-1425-7 (alk. paper)
    I. Cheng, Steven. II. Vijayan, Anitha. III. Title: Nephrology subspecialty consult. IV. Series:
Washington manual subspecialty consult series.
    [DNLM: 1. Kidney Diseases—diagnosis—Handbooks. 2. Kidney Diseases—therapy—Handbooks.
3. Nephrology—methods—Handbooks. WJ 39]

    616.6′1—dc23

                             2011050022

To purchase additional copies of this book, call our customer service department at (800) 638-3030 or fax orders to (301) 223-2320. International customers should call (301) 223-2300.

Visit Lippincott Williams & Wilkins on the Internet: at LWW.com. Lippincott Williams & Wilkins customer service representatives are available from 8:30 am to 6 pm, EST.

10 9 8 7 6 5 4 3 2 1

Contributing Authors

Raghavender Boothpur, MD
Clinical Fellow
Department of Internal Medicine
Renal Division
Washington University School of Medicine
St. Louis, Missouri

Lyndsey Bowman, PharmD
Clinical Pharmacist
Abdominal Organ Transplant
Barnes-Jewish Hospital
St. Louis, Missouri

Ying Chen, MD
Instructor
Department of Internal Medicine
Renal Division
Washington University School of Medicine
St. Louis, Missouri

Steven Cheng, MD
Assistant Professor of Medicine
Department of Internal Medicine
Renal Division
Washington University School of Medicine
St. Louis, Missouri

Sindhu Garg, MD
Clinical Fellow
Department of Internal Medicine
Renal Division
Washington University School of Medicine
St. Louis, Missouri

Yekaterina Gincherman, MD
Clinical Fellow
Department of Internal Medicine
Renal Division
Washington University School of Medicine
St. Louis, Missouri

Seth Goldberg, MD
Assistant Professor of Medicine
Department of Internal Medicine
Renal Division
Washington University School of Medicine
St. Louis, Missouri

Ethan Hoerschgen, MD
Clinical Fellow
Department of Internal Medicine
Renal Division
Washington University School of Medicine
St. Louis, Missouri

Jennifer Iuppa, PharmD
Clinical Pharmacist
Lung Transplant
Barnes-Jewish Hospital
St. Louis, Missouri

Judy L. Jang, MD
Clinical Fellow
Department of Internal Medicine
Renal Division
Washington University School of Medicine
St. Louis, Missouri

Peter J. Juran, MD
Clinical Fellow
Department of Internal Medicine
Renal Division
Washington University School of Medicine
St. Louis, Missouri

Syed A. Khalid, MD
Clinical Fellow
Department of Internal Medicine
Renal Division
Washington University School of Medicine
St. Louis, Missouri

Christina L. Klein, MD
Assistant Professor of Medicine
Department of Internal Medicine
Renal Division
Washington University School of Medicine
St. Louis, Missouri

Tingting Li, MD
Assistant Professor of Medicine
Department of Internal Medicine
Renal Division
Washington University School of Medicine
St. Louis, Missouri

Biju Marath, MD
Clinical Fellow
Department of Internal Medicine
Renal Division
Washington University School of Medicine
St. Louis, Missouri

Imran A. Memon, MD
Clinical Fellow
Department of Internal Medicine
Renal Division
Washington University School of Medicine
St. Louis, Missouri

Georges Saab, MD
Assistant Professor of Medicine
Department of Internal Medicine
Renal Division
Washington University School of Medicine
St. Louis, Missouri

Sadashiv Santosh, MD
Clinical Fellow
Department of Internal Medicine
Renal Division
Washington University School of Medicine
St. Louis, Missouri

Andrew Siedlecki, MD
Instructor
Department of Internal Medicine
Renal Division
Washington University School of Medicine
St. Louis, Missouri

Nicholas Taraska, MD
Clinical Fellow
Department of Internal Medicine
Renal Division
Washington University School of Medicine
St. Louis, Missouri

Ahsan Usman, MD
Clinical Fellow
Department of Internal Medicine
Renal Division
Washington University School of Medicine
St. Louis, Missouri

Anitha Vijayan, MD
Associate Professor of Medicine
Department of Internal Medicine
Renal Division
Washington University School of Medicine
St. Louis, Missouri

Chairman's Note

I t is a pleasure to present the new edition of *The Washington Manual*® Subspecialty Consult Series: *Nephrology Subspecialty Consult*. This pocket-size book continues to be a primary reference for medical students, interns, residents, and other practitioners who need ready access to practical clinical information to diagnose and treat patients with a wide variety of disorders. Medical knowledge continues to increase at an astounding rate, which creates a challenge for physicians to keep up with the biomedical discoveries, genetic and genomic information, and novel therapeutics that can positively impact patient outcomes. The *Washington Manual* Subspecialty Series addresses this challenge by concisely and practically providing current scientific information for clinicians to aid them in the diagnosis, investigation, and treatment of common medical conditions.

I want to personally thank the authors, which include house officers, fellows, and attendings at Washington University School of Medicine and Barnes-Jewish Hospital. Their commitment to patient care and education is unsurpassed, and their efforts and skill in compiling this manual are evident in the quality of the final product. In particular, I would like to acknowledge our editors, Drs. Steven Cheng and Anitha Vijayan, and the series editors, Drs. Katherine Henderson and Tom De Fer, who have worked tirelessly to produce another outstanding edition of this manual. I would also like to thank Dr. Melvin Blanchard, Chief of the Division of Medical Education in the Department of Medicine at Washington University School of Medicine, for his advice and guidance. I believe this Subspecialty Manual will meet its desired goal of providing practical knowledge that can be directly applied at the bedside and in outpatient settings to improve patient care.

Victoria J. Fraser, MD
Dr. J. William Campbell Professor
Interim Chairman of Medicine
Co-Director of the Infectious Disease Division
Washington University School of Medicine

Preface

The first and second editions of *The Washington Manual Nephrology Subspecialty Consult* achieved the goal of the "subspecialty" series because they were well written, well organized, and served as an efficient bedside resource for residents and students. The hope of this and future editions is to build on that success by updating content with new developments while maintaining the original high standards.

The field of nephrology is changing rapidly, as new advances change the management of acute kidney injury (AKI), chronic kidney disease, and renal transplantation. AKI continues to be a life-threatening problem for the hospitalized patient, and new clinical trials have addressed the role of intensive renal replacement therapy in AKI. Glomerulonephritides generate significant challenges to the nephrologist as we strive to treat the patient effectively but at the same time try to minimize side effects from the treatment regimen. Newer agents have been added as induction therapies to decrease rejection rates after renal transplantation. Early initiation of hemodialysis has recently been proven to be not beneficial in patients with chronic kidney disease.

The field of nephrology remains a fascinating, challenging, and exciting area of internal medicine. Electrolyte and acid–base problems will always pose an interesting and thought-provoking dilemma to the trainee and the attending alike. The thrill of working up a patient with hyponatremia or narrowing down the differential diagnoses to get to the underlying etiology of hypokalemia never changes with time, and we hope to transfer our passion of nephrology to medical students and residents and inspire them to pursue a career in nephrology.

We would like to acknowledge and thank the authors for all the time and effort vested in this publication. We also would like to extend our gratitude to Katherine Henderson, MD, who gave us invaluable guidance and feedback. We hope the readers will find this publication to be a relevant, informative, and useful tool in their day-to-day clinical practice.

Last, but not least, we would like to thank our families—Vichu, Maya, Dev, and our parents for their love and support.

—AV and SC

Contents

PART III. ACUTE KIDNEY INJURY AND CONTINUOUS RENAL REPLACEMENT

PART IV. CAUSES OF KIDNEY DISEASE

PART V. PREGNANCY AND NEPHROLITHIASIS

Art and Science of Urinalysis

Biju Marath and Steven Cheng

GENERAL PRINCIPLES

- Urinalysis is the physical, chemical, and microscopic examination of urine, and is a key aspect in the evaluation of renal and urinary tract disease.

DIAGNOSIS

- When used properly, the urinalysis can offer innumerable insights into a broad variety of diagnoses. **Proper examination of the urine consists of two parts: (a) the urine dipstick test and (b) the sediment evaluation by light microscopy.** The presence or absence of features on urinalysis can be useful in narrowing diagnostic possibilities.[1–5]
  - ○ The **urine dipstick** test gives insight into the physical and chemical parameters of the urine. These properties can be invaluable in the assessment of infections, inflammation, glucose control, acid–base balance, hematuria, proteinuria, and intravascular volume status, to name but a few conditions.
  - ○ **Microscopic analysis** allows for sediment evaluation. Since the characteristics of urinary sediment vary depending on the site of injury, this assessment is helpful in localizing the injury in renal parenchymal disease.

Specimen Collection

- Urine should **ideally be examined immediately** or no longer than 2 hours after collection.
- Prolonged standing causes urine to become progressively more alkaline (urea is broken down, generating ammonia). The higher pH dissolves casts and promotes cell lysis.
- If delay is inevitable, **urine can be preserved for up to 6 hours if refrigerated at +2 to +8°C.** Refrigeration may result in precipitation of phosphates or crystals.
  - ○ Preservatives such as formaldehyde, glutaraldehyde, "cellFIX," and tubes containing lyophilized borate-formate sorbitol powder have been used to maintain the formed elements of the urine samples.
- The method for preparing a urine sample is given in Table 1-1.

Physical Properties

Visual inspection and notation of other general physical characteristics of a urine sample can yield important diagnostic information. The main physical properties to be determined include color, clarity, odor, and specific gravity.

TABLE 1-1	PROCEDURE FOR URINE SPECIMEN COLLECTION, DIPSTICK TESTING, AND MICROSCOPIC ANALYSIS

Collect midstream urine catch of first or second morning urine specimen in clean container.

- Bladder catheterization may be used (risk of hematuria).
- Suprapubic catheterization is also acceptable, though rarely used.
- Avoid collecting urine from the Foley bag (may collect fresh specimen from Foley catheter itself).

Perform dipstick testing and record results.
Centrifuge 10 mL aliquot at 1500–3000 rpm (400–450 g) for 5–10 min.
Remove 9.5 mL of supernatant urine.
Gently resuspend the sediment using pipette in remaining 0.5 mL of supernatant.
Using pipette, apply one drop of resuspended urine onto clean slide and cover with coverslip.
Examine urine under phase-contrast light microscopy at ×160 and ×400.

- Polarized light may help with lipids and crystal examination.

Color

- **Normal urine is pale to yellow in color.** Dilute urine appears lighter and concentrated urine attains a darker yellow to amber shade.
- **Red urine** may be noted with hematuria.
  - Positive dipstick test result for blood without evidence of red blood cells (RBCs) on microscopy is a clue to the presence of free hemoglobin or myoglobin in the urine, suggestive of conditions such as sickle-cell anemia, ABO incompatible blood transfusion, or rhabdomyolysis.
  - Red urine can also result from the ingestion of large amounts of food with red pigments (e.g., beets, rhubarb, blackberries), the presence of excess urates, certain drugs (e.g., phenytoin, rifampin), and porphyria.
- **Green or blue urine** can be seen with Pseudomonas urinary tract infection (UTI), biliverdinuria, as well as exposure to amitriptyline, IV cimetidine, IV promethazine, methylene blue, and triamterene.
- **Orange urine** is typically seen with rifampin, phenothiazines and phenazopyridine.
- Urine that **turns black on standing** is classically described in homogentisic acid oxidase deficiency (alkaptonuria).
- **Brown or black urine** is also seen in conditions such as copper or phenol poisoning, excessive L-dopa excretion, and with excess melanin excretion in melanoma.

Clarity

- **Normal urine is typically clear.**
- **Increased turbidity** is most commonly noted with UTIs (pyuria).
- Other causes include heavy hematuria, contamination from genital secretions, presence of phosphate crystals in an alkaline urine, chyluria, lipiduria, hyperoxaluria, and hyperuricosuria.

Odor
- **Normal urine typically does not have a strong odor.**
- Bacterial UTIs may be associated with a **pungent odor**.
- Diabetic ketoacidosis can cause urine to have a **fruity or sweet odor**.
- Other conditions associated with unusual odors include maple syrup urine disease (maple syrup odor), phenylketonuria (musty odor), gastrointestinal–bladder fistulas (fecal odor), and cystine decomposition (sulfuric odor).
- Different medications (e.g., penicillin) and diet (e.g., asparagus coffee) can also cause distinct odors.

Specific Gravity
- Specific gravity is the most common method used to assess the relative density of urine, although this is **best determined by measuring osmolality**.
  - Though commonly used, ion exchange strips typically provide falsely low results with urine pH values >6.5 and falsely high results with protein levels of >7 g/L.
- **Values ≤1.010 indicate a dilute urine.**
  - This generally suggests a state of relative hydration.
  - Very low specific gravity (≤1.005) may be indicative of diabetes insipidus or water intoxication.
- **Values ≥1.020 indicate a more concentrated urine.**
  - This generally suggests dehydration and volume contraction.
  - Very high specific gravity (≥1.032) may be suggestive of glucosuria, and even higher values may indicate the presence of an extrinsic osmotic agent such as contrast.

Chemical Properties

Urine pH
- Urine pH can be measured very accurately and is quite reproducible.
- **Normal urine pH is in the range of 4.5 to 7.8.**
- **Low urine pH** can be observed in patients with large protein consumption, metabolic acidosis, and volume depletion.
- **High urine pH** may be seen in renal tubular acidosis (especially distal) and in persons consuming vegetarian diets. Other causes include prolonged storage of urine (allowing generation of ammonia from urea) and infection with urea-splitting organisms (e.g., Proteus).

Hemoglobin
- Presence of hemoglobin noted by the dipstick test may be indicative of hematuria or point to other pathology such as intravascular hemolysis or rhabdomyolysis. A discussion of hematuria and hemoglobinuria can be found in Chapter 5.

Glucose
- Urine glucose measurement is sensitive but not specific enough for quantification by usual methods. Most laboratories give out a semiquantitative readout (e.g., + for present to ++++ for present in large amounts), but correlation with blood glucose levels is approximate and varies with the concentration of the urine.

- Glucose in the urine may be seen in diabetes, pancreatic and liver disease, Cushing syndrome, and Fanconi syndrome.
- **In individuals with normal renal function, glucose is generally not seen in the urine unless plasma levels exceed 180 to 200 mg/dL.** Glucosuria in the context of normal plasma glucose should raise suspicion of a proximal tubule defect impairing glucose reabsorption.
- **False-negative** results may be seen with the presence of ascorbic acid, uric acid, and bacteria.
- **False-positive** results can be observed in the presence of levodopa, oxidizing detergents, and hydrochloric acid.

Protein

- Proteinuria is an important marker of kidney disease and can be checked using a dipstick test. Details of the methodology and more quantitative methods are found in Chapter 4.

Leukocyte Esterase and Urine Nitrite

- These two tests are often used together in the diagnosis of a UTI.
- **A positive leukocyte esterase (LE) is suggestive of granulocyte activity in the urine.**
  - Detection of LE is dependent on esterases released from lysed granulocytes in urine reacting with the reagent strip.
  - Esterase produced from granulocyte lysis in long-standing urine or contaminating vaginal cells may give false-positive results.
  - False-negative results occur when the esterase reaction with granulocytes is inhibited, such as with hyperglycemia, albuminuria, tetracycline, cephalosporins, and oxaluria.
  - A positive LE can be found independent of a UTI. Sterile pyuria is commonly associated with nephrolithiasis, interstitial nephritis, and renal tuberculosis.
- The **presence of nitrites in the urine depends on the ability of bacteria to convert nitrate into nitrite**, which then reacts with the reagent test strip. This reaction is inhibited by ascorbic acid and high specific gravity.
  - Low levels of urinary nitrate secondary to diet, degradation of nitrites secondary to prolonged storage, and inadequate conversion of nitrates to nitrites due to rapid transit in the bladder may contribute to false-negative results despite the presence of urinary infection.
  - Certain bacteria (e.g., *Streptococcus faecalis*, *Neisseria gonorrhoeae*, and *Mycobacterium tuberculosis*) do not convert nitrate to nitrite.
  - Specificity for infection is best when both LE and nitrites are positive. However, even if both tests are negative, infection cannot be completely ruled out, and the clinical context must be considered.[6]

Ketones

- **Routine dipstick test detects only acetoacetic acid and not beta-hydroxybutyrate.**
- Ketones are mainly seen in diabetic and alcoholic ketoacidosis, but can also be observed in pregnancy, carbohydrate-free diets, starvation, vomiting, and strenuous exercise.
- The presence of free sulfhydryl groups, levodopa metabolites, or highly pigmented urine can give false-positive results.

Microscopic Exam

Urine microscopic examination of the sediment is a very important and an underutilized tool to evaluate renal pathology.[7,8] The urine sediment can contain cells, casts, crystals, bacteria, fungi, and contaminants.

Cells
- **RBCs:**
  - **More than two RBCs per high-power field are abnormal** and suggest bleeding from some point in the genitourinary system.
  - RBCs are typically 4 to 7 μm in diameter and have a characteristic red pigment with central opacity and smooth borders.
  - **Dysmorphic RBCs** are associated with glomerular disease and are best seen on phase-contrast microscopy.
  - **Swollen (ghost) cells or shrunken (crenated) cells** are normal RBCs that have been altered by osmolality of the urine. Crenated cells (5 μm in diameter) have spiked borders and can be mistaken for small, granulated cells. Ghost cells often require phase-contrast microscopy for viewing.
- **White blood cells:**
  - **White blood cells** (WBCs) are characterized by their cytoplasmic granulation.
  - They are distinguished from crenated RBCs by their lack of pigment and their large size (10 to 12 μm in diameter). Brownian motion of the granules in WBCs can be seen in phase-contrast microscopy.
  - **WBCs in the urine are associated with infection and inflammation.**
  - **Eosinophils** in urine, although thought of as a marker for allergic interstitial nephritis, are now considered a nonsensitive and a nonspecific marker. It can be seen in cholesterol embolism, glomerulonephritis, prostatitis, chronic pyelonephritis, and urinary schistosomiasis.
  - Urine eosinophils are not easily identified unless special staining (Hansel or Wright) is used.
- **Epithelial cells:**
  - Four major epithelial cell groups must be distinguished:
    - **Squamous epithelial cells:** They are large, flat, with an irregular cytoplasm of 30- to 50-μm diameter and a nucleus-to-cytoplasm ratio of 1:6. They are present in the urine because of shedding from the distal genital tract and essentially are contaminants.
    - **Transitional epithelial cells:** They are 20 to 30 μm in diameter, are pear or tadpole shaped, and have a nucleus-to-cytoplasm ratio of 1:3. They are usually seen intermittently with bladder catheterization or irrigation. Occasionally, they may be associated with malignancy, especially if irregular nuclei are noted.
    - **Renal tubular epithelial cells:** They are slightly larger than leukocytes and have a large, eccentrically placed round nucleus that takes up half the area of the cytoplasm. Their presence in significant numbers (>15 cells in 10 high-power fields) may be seen with tubular injury. Tubular epithelial cells from the proximal tubule tend to be very granulated.
    - **Oval fat bodies:** They are renal epithelial cells that are filled with lipids. They also appear granulated but are distinguished by characteristic "Maltese crosses" seen under polarized light, reflecting their cholesterol content. Oval fat bodies are typically seen in nephrotic syndrome and indicate lipiduria.

Casts

Casts are formed when proteins secreted in the lumen of renal tubules (typically the Tamm–Horsfall protein) trap cells, fat, bacteria, or other inclusions at the time of amalgamation and then are excreted in the urine. Thus, a cast provides a snapshot of the milieu of the tubule at the time of this amalgamation.[9]

- **Hyaline casts:**
  - Renal tubules secrete a protein called Tamm–Horsfall protein (uromodulin). Under certain circumstances, the protein amalgamates on its own without any other tubular inclusions, forming hyaline casts.
  - They are better seen with phase-contrast microscopy.
  - They are seen in concentrated, acidic urine.
  - They are not associated with proteinuria and can be seen with various physiologic states, such as strenuous exercise or dehydration.
- **Granular casts:**
  - They are made of Tamm–Horsfall protein filled with breakdown debris of cells and plasma proteins that appear as granules.
  - They are nonspecific and appear with many glomerular or tubular diseases.
  - Large numbers of "muddy brown" granular casts are typically seen in acute tubular necrosis.
  - They have also been reported after vigorous exercise.
- **Waxy casts:**
  - They represent the last stage in degeneration of hyaline, granular, and cellular casts.
  - They have smooth, blunt ends.
  - They are usually seen with chronic kidney disease rather than acute processes.
  - Polarized light should be used to distinguish waxy casts from artifacts, which tend to polarize unlike true casts.
- **Fatty casts:**
  - They contain lipid droplets that are very refractile.
  - They may be confused with cellular casts, but polarized light demonstrates the characteristic Maltese cross appearance.
  - They are associated with nephrotic syndrome, mercury poisoning, and ethylene glycol poisoning.
- **Red cell casts:**
  - They are identified by their orange–red color on bright-field microscopy and well-defined cellular elements.
  - They are best seen in fresh urine. At times, they may appear fractured.
  - Red cell casts signify glomerular hematuria and are an important finding, suggesting potentially serious glomerular disease. Detection of red cell casts should trigger further rigorous evaluation of the patient.
- **White cell casts:**
  - They contain WBCs trapped in tubular proteins.
  - Sometimes WBCs appear in the urine in clumps, and it is important not to confuse them with casts. Phase-contrast microscopy is useful to demonstrate protein matrix of the cast, which is not seen in white cell clumps or pseudocasts.
  - They are associated with interstitial inflammatory processes, such as pyelonephritis.

- **Epithelial cell casts:**
  - They are characterized by epithelial cells of various shapes, haphazardly arranged in a protein matrix representing desquamation from different portions of the renal tubules.

Crystals

- Cooling of urine allows many normally dissolved substances to precipitate at room temperature. Thus, most crystals are present as artifacts and may be present in the urine without an underlying disease.
- The formation of crystals also depends on urinary pH.
  - Crystals that precipitate in acidic urine are as follows: uric acid, monosodium urate, amorphous urates, and calcium oxalate.
  - Crystals that precipitate in alkaline urine are as follows: triple phosphate, ammonium biurate, calcium phosphate, calcium oxalate, and calcium carbonate.
- **Calcium-based crystals** are among the most commonly encountered.
  - **Calcium oxalate crystals** appear in characteristic octahedral "envelope" shapes. They may also take rectangular, dumbbell, and ovoid shapes (may be confused with RBCs).
  - **Triple phosphate crystals** are usually three- to six-sided prisms in "coffin-lid" form but may present as flat, fern leaf-like sheets.
  - **Calcium phosphate crystals** are usually small rosettes.
  - **Calcium carbonate** usually presents as tiny spheres in pairs or crosses.
- Crystals produced from pathologic excess of metabolic products (e.g., cystine, tyrosine, leucine, bilirubin, and cholesterol) are seen more frequently in acidic urine.
- **Drug-associated crystals** (e.g., acyclovir, indinavir, sulfonamides, and ampicillin) are seen in more acidic concentrated urine.
- **Uric acid crystals** come in various forms, including rhomboid, rosettes, lemon shaped, and four-sided "whetstones." Other urate forms are very tiny crystals, spheres, or needles that are hard to distinguish.
- **Ammonium biurate,** which is usually seen in aged urine, is usually a dark, yellow sphere with a "thorn apple" shape.
- **Cystine crystals** are hexagons that can polarize and are confused with uric acid crystals.
- **Tyrosine and leucine crystals** usually occur together. The former forms fine needles arranged in rosettes, whereas the latter forms spheres with concentric striations like the core of a tree.
- **Bilirubin crystals** occur in many shapes but are usually distinguished by the bilirubin color.
- **Cholesterol crystals** are usually flat with a corner notch and are sometimes confused with crystals of contrast medium, which also have a corner notch.
- **Sulfonamide crystals** appear as spheres or needles. Ampicillin crystals usually take a long, slender needle shape. Acyclovir crystals have a similar needle-like shape but display negative birefringence under polarized light.

Organisms

- **Bacteria:**
  - They are frequently seen in urine specimens, given the fact that urine is typically collected under nonsterile conditions.
  - Gram-negative organisms such as *Escherichia coli* tend to predominate in uncomplicated UTI, followed by *Staphylococcus saprophyticus*, and occasionally

by Proteus, Klebsiella, Enterococci, Group B Streptococci, *Pseudomonas aeruginosa*, and Citrobacter species.

○ Complicated UTI may be caused by a myriad of organisms. Identification and susceptibilities of these organisms typically require high-powered magnification, staining, culture, and *in vitro* testing against antibiotics.

- **Fungal:**
  ○ Presence of **Candida** in urine is typically thought to be a contaminant from genital secretions or, in the presence of a long, indwelling bladder catheter, colonization.
  ○ Candida UTIs can cause similar symptoms to that seen with a bacterial infection.
  ○ Candida species are the most frequent cause of fungal UTIs, with *C. albicans* as the most common, followed by *C. glabrata* and *C. tropicalis.*
  ○ Candida may have the appearance of yeast (spherical cells), budding yeast, and pseudohyphae depending on reproductive cycle.
  ○ Other infectious fungal agents, including Aspergillus, Cryptococcus, and Histoplasmosis, can be seen in the chronically ill or immunocompromised patients.

- **Parasites:**
  ○ Presence of *Trichomonas vaginalis* and *Enterobius vermicularis* in urine are typically thought of as contaminants stemming from genital secretions.
  ○ **Trichomonads** are single-celled, flagellated protozoans characterized by their "corkscrew" motility, which can cause a sexually transmitted disease, with white vaginal discharge and itching as part of its symptoms.
  ○ *Enterobius vermicularis* (human pinworm) do not typically reside in the urinary tract, but may occasionally be found in the vagina leading to urine contamination.
  ○ Painful hematuria with exposure to fresh river waters in endemic areas is characteristic of **Schistosoma haematobium.** The large, abundant ova can be detected in a fresh urine sample, with the urine tending to be dark in color.

REFERENCES

1. Fogazzi G, Pirovano B. Urinalysis. In: Feehally J, Floege J, Johnson RJ, eds. *Comprehensive Clinical Nephrology.* 3rd ed. Philadelphia, PA: Mosby Elsevier; 2007:35–50.
2. Lorincz AE, Kelly DR, Dobbins GC. Urinalysis: current status and prospects for the future. *Ann Clin Lab Sci.* 1999;29:169.
3. Becker GJ, Fairley KF. Urinalysis. In: Massry SG, Glassock RJ, eds. *Textbook of Nephrology.* 4th ed. Philadelphia, PA: Lippincott Williams and Wilkins; 2001:1765–1783.
4. Rose BD, ed. Clinical assessment of renal function. In: *Pathophysiology of Renal Disease.* 2nd ed. New York, NY: McGraw-Hill; 1987:1–40.
5. Misdraji J, Nguyen PL. Urinalysis. When—and when not—to order. *Postgrad Med.* 1996;100:173.
6. Van Nostrand JD, Junkins AD, Bartholdi RK. Poor predictive ability of urinalysis and microscopic examination to detect urinary tract infection. *Am J Clin Pathol.* 2000;113:709.
7. Rasoulpour M, Banco L, Laut JM, et al. Inability of community-based laboratories to identify pathologic casts in urine samples. *Arch Pediatr Adolesc Med.* 1996;150:1201.
8. Ringsrud KM, Linne JJ. *Urinalysis and Body Fluids: A Color Text and Atlas.* St. Louis, MO: Mosby; 1995.
9. Simerville JA, Maxted WC, Pahira JJ. Urinalysis: a comprehensive review. *Am Fam Physician.* 2005;71:1153–1162.

Assessment of Kidney Function

2

Imran A. Memon

GENERAL PRINCIPLES

- Assessing kidney function is a critical step in the recognition and monitoring of acute and chronic kidney diseases (CKD).
- Creatinine measurement has become the preferred method for routine clinical monitoring of renal function.
- Clinicians need to understand the assumptions and pitfalls regarding the various measurements of kidney function, in order to use and interpret them appropriately.

Pathophysiology

- Kidney function is best reflected by the **glomerular filtration rate (GFR)**.
  - GFR is defined as the sum of the filtration rates of all functional nephrons.
  - The normal GFR is ~125 mL/min/1.73 m^2 in men and 100 mL/min/1.73 m^2 in women.
  - A decline in nephron numbers may not necessarily result in a decline of GFR, as the remaining nephrons can increase filtration rate to compensate.
    - For example, one might expect a 50% reduction in GFR after the donation of a kidney. However, the measured GFR is often at 80% of prenephrectomy levels because of compensatory hyperfiltration in the remaining kidney.
  - Changes in GFR parallel changes in overall filtering capacity of the kidney.
    - An increase in GFR, as seen in early diabetic nephropathy, can reflect glomerular hyperfiltration, whereas a fall in GFR can reflect kidney injury and disease.
    - The Kidney Disease Outcomes Quality Initiative guidelines separate CKD into **five stages of progressive decline** (Table 2-1).
  - The **classification into CKD stage can be misleading**.
    - A GFR of 30 mL/min/1.73 m^2 has half of the renal function as a GFR of 60 mL/min/1.73 m^2, even though they are both classified as stage III CKD.
    - A GFR of 29 mL/min/1.73 m^2 has virtually the same renal function as a GFR of 30 mL/min/1.73 m^2, even though one is classified as stage IV and the other is classified as stage III.
    - Damage to specific components of the nephron may initially manifest in other ways, without a prominent fall in GFR.
- Damage to the glomerular architecture may initially present with proteinuria only.
  - Damage to the tubules may result in solute wasting or concentration defects.

TABLE 2-1	CKD STAGES	
	GFR (mL/min/ 1.73 m^2)	Description
CKD stage 1	≥90	Normal kidney function, but urine findings or structural abnormalities or genetic trait point to kidney disease
CKD stage 2	60–89	Mildly reduced kidney function, and other findings (as for stage 1) point to kidney disease
CKD stage 3	30–59	Moderately reduced kidney function
CKD stage 4	15–29	Severely reduced kidney function
CKD stage 5	<15 (or dialysis)	Very severe or end-stage kidney failure (sometimes called *established renal failure*)

○ Structural diseases, such as polycystic kidney disease, can be detected on ultrasound prior to any changes in GFR.

DIAGNOSIS

Diagnostic Testing

Creatinine

- Creatinine is a metabolic product of creatine derived mainly from skeletal muscle cells and dietary meat.
  ○ The typical daily production rates are 20 to 25 mg/kg/d in men and 15 to 20 mg/kg/d in women.
    ■ Persons with larger muscle mass have a higher creatinine production and level than those with a smaller muscle mass.
    ■ The normal range for creatinine is reported between 0.4 and 1.5 mg/dL.
- The kidney eliminates creatinine by glomerular filtration and, to a lesser extent, by proximal tubular secretion.
  ○ In persons with normal kidney function, glomerular filtration accounts for >90% of creatinine elimination.
  ○ Creatinine is not reabsorbed or metabolized to any significant degree in the kidney.
- Creatinine is clinically used to track kidney function, as it accumulates when renal elimination is compromised.
  ○ An upward trend in creatinine suggests a reduction in GFR.
  ○ A downward trend in creatinine suggests an improvement in GFR.
  ○ It is important to realize that **a change in plasma creatinine does not correlate with a decline in renal function in a linear fashion** (Fig. 2-1).
    ■ A small increase in creatinine at a lower creatinine level signals a greater decline in renal function, as compared to the same increase in creatinine when the baseline creatinine levels are high.
    ■ For example, a change of 1.0 to 1.4 mg/dL represents a greater decline in kidney function than a change of 3.0 to 3.4 mg/dL.

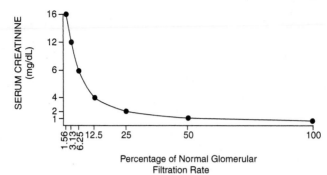

FIGURE 2-1. The nonlinear relationship between rise in plasma creatinine and fall in the glomerular filtration rate. (Adapted from Lazarus JM, Brenner BM, eds. *Acute Renal Failure.* 3rd ed. New York, NY: Churchill Livingstone; 1993:133.)

- ○ **Creatinine is not a perfect marker because of the variable contribution of tubular secretion.**
  - ▪ As renal function declines, tubular secretion of creatinine increases. Therefore, creatinine-based estimations of GFR can overestimate renal function because of the increasing proportion of creatinine eliminated by tubular secretion in renal failure.
  - ▪ The measurement of creatinine can also be subject to intra-laboratory variation.

Urea

- • The elimination of urea by the kidney is more complex than creatinine, which renders the blood urea nitrogen (BUN) a less useful marker of kidney function when evaluated in isolation.
- • BUN can be increased by a number of nonrenal etiologies, including gastrointestinal bleeding, steroid use, and parenteral nutrition.
- • BUN can be reduced by malnutrition and liver disease, which reduce urea generation rates.
- • For practical purposes, **BUN is most informative when the ratio of BUN: Cr exceeds 20:1, which is suggestive of a prerenal state.**

Clearance

- • Clearance describes the quantity of fluid which is completely cleared of a marker over a definite period of time.
  - ○ It is usually expressed in mL per minute.
  - ○ The ideal marker should be biologically inert, freely and completely filtered by the glomerulus, neither secreted nor absorbed by tubules, and not degraded by the kidney.
  - ○ With an ideal marker, GFR can be calculated from the measurements of the marker's clearance.
- • **GFR = $(U_{\text{Marker}} \times$ volume of urine/$P_{\text{Marker}})/1440$**
  - ○ Where, U_{Marker} is the concentration of the marker in the urine.
  - ○ Volume of urine is the volume produced over 24 hours (in mL).
  - ○ P_{Marker} is concentration of the marker in the plasma.

○ The value 1440 is used to convert the units to mL per minute (1440 minutes in 24 hours).
- Inulin was the classic gold standard marker for such measurements, but has been superceded by other substances such as iothalamate, diethylenetriamine pentaacetic acid, ethylenediamine tetraacetic acid, and iohexal.
  ○ Although these methods are useful in obtaining a very accurate GFR measurement, they are inconvenient for most purposes and are used only in specific situations that require more precision than estimates from creatinine clearance (CrCl).
  ○ Although creatinine is not a perfect marker because of the contribution of tubular secretion, it is easily measurable and is clinically used to estimate GFR.
- **CrCl** can be estimated through equation-based estimations or by a 24-hour urine collection.
  ○ Creatinine-based equations: There are two widely used equations used to estimate kidney function in adults based on their serum creatinine levels in conjunction with basic patient characteristics.
  ○ **Cockcroft–Gault equation:**
    Estimated CrCl = (140–age) × weight (in kg)
    × 0.85 (if female)/72 × plasma creatinine

    - The Cockcroft–Gault equation was originally developed in a male inpatient population but has been found to be reasonably accurate in other populations.[1]
    - The **main pitfalls of this estimate are determining the patient's actual lean body weight and overestimation of true GFR by CrCl with lower levels of kidney function.**
  ○ **MDRD equation:**
    Estimated GFR = $170 \times (P_{cr})^{-0.999} \times (age)^{-0.175} \times 0.762$ (if female)
    $\times 1.180$ (if African American) $\times (BUN)^{-0.170} \times (Alb)^{+0.318}$

  ○ **Abbreviated MDRD equation:**
    Estimated GFR (mL/min/1.73 m^2) = $186 \times (S_{cr})^{-1.154} \times (age)^{-0.203}$
    $\times 0.742$ (if female) $\times 1.21$
    (if African American)

    - The MDRD equation was developed in established outpatient CKD patients using ^{125}I-iothalamate renal clearance as a reference.[2]
    - In CKD patients with measured GFR <60 mL/min/1.73 m^2, the MDRD equation correlates well. It has not been well validated in other patient populations.[3] For instance, it is **not useful in persons with normal renal function**, and was not validated in persons aged >70 years or in hospitalized or malnourished patients.[4] It is also **does not measure true GFR in patients with advanced kidney disease.**[5]
    - The MDRD equation has an adjustment factor for African American populations,[6] but not for Hispanic or Asian populations.[7,8]
  ○ **Limitations of equation-based CrCl.**
    - In renal transplant donors, both the MDRD and the Cockcroft–Gault equation significantly underestimate the measured GFR by as much as 9% to 29%.[9]

- MDRD study equation was derived from predominantly white subjects who had nondiabetic kidney disease.
- MDRD equation is reasonably accurate in nonhospitalized patients known to have CKD, regardless of diagnosis.
- The MDRD study equation and the Cockcroft–Gault equation may not be accurate in obese individuals.
- The MDRD equation and the Cockcroft–Gault equation may not be accurate in different age groups; they provided higher estimates at younger ages and lower estimates at older ages.[10]
- The MDRD study and the Cockcroft–Gault equation are less accurate in populations with normal or near-normal GFR.[11]
- Among recipients of renal allograft, these equations have variable accuracy in predicted true GFR.[12]
- These equations may be less accurate in a population of different ethnicities outside the United States.[13,14]

- **The 24-hour CrCl.**
  - The 24-hour urine collection has been used as a semi-gold standard to evaluate kidney function in the clinical setting, particularly when equations may not be sufficiently accurate (Table 2-2).
  - CrCl can be measured by collecting a 24-hour urine sample and using the following formula:

$$\text{GFR} = (U_{\text{Creatinine}} \times \text{volume of urine} / P_{\text{Creatinine}})/1440$$

  - Where $U_{\text{Creatinine}}$ is the concentration of creatinine in the urine.
  - Volume of urine is the volume produced over 24 hours (in mL).
  - $P_{\text{Creatinine}}$ is concentration of creatinine in the plasma.
  - The value 1440 is used to convert the units to mL per minute (1440 minutes in 24 hours).
  - In the intensive care unit setting, shorter-timed collection (e.g., 8 or 12 hours) can also be done to decrease collection errors.[15]
  - Increased creatinine excretion occurs as GFR falls, resulting in a normal estimation of **CrCl** in 25% to 50% of the patients with true GFR of 51 to 70 mL/min.

TABLE 2-2	SITUATIONS IN WHICH A 24-HOUR URINE COLLECTION IS MORE ACCURATE THAN MDRD EQUATION

1. GFR >60 mL/min/1.73 m^2
2. Age <18 or >70
3. Extreme body size
4. Severe malnutrition
5. Pregnancy
6. Skeletal muscle disease
7. Paraplegia or quadriplegia
8. Vegetarian
9. Rapid changing renal function

TABLE 2-3	PROPER STEPS IN 24-HOUR URINE COLLECTION

1. After waking up in the morning, empty the bladder completely and discard urine
2. Save all subsequent urine samples during the rest of the day and through the night
3. The next morning, save the first urine sample

Differential Diagnosis

- An estimation of GFR using any of these techniques should give clinicians a fairly accurate impression of overall kidney function. However, there are pitfalls that an astute clinician must be aware of.
- **Factors affecting serum creatinine.**
  - *Trimethoprim* and *cimetidine* block proximal tubular secretion of creatinine. They can increase plasma creatinine level up to as much as 0.5 mg/dL. This effect is more pronounced in CKD when baseline creatinine is already elevated.[16,17]
  - *Cefoxitin* and *flucytosine* interfere with the creatinine assay, giving a false elevation of plasma creatinine levels.[18,19]
  - *Acetoacetate* in diabetic ketoacidosis can be falsely recognized by the colorimetric assay as creatinine and may elevate creatinine by as much as 0.5 to 2 mg/dL.[20]
  - *Hypothyroidism* increases plasma creatinine levels and *hyperthyroidism* decreases plasma creatinine levels.[21,22]
- **Factors affecting CrCl.**
  - The limitations of equation-based calculations are listed above.
  - **Two major factors** that can limit the accuracy of the 24-hour urine collections are **incomplete urine collection** and **increasing creatinine secretion.**[23]
    - Meticulous volume collection is important to prevent over collection (thus overestimating CrCl) or under collection (thus underestimating CrCl). Table 2-3 lists the steps needed for collecting a 24-hour urine sample.
    - Completeness of urine collection can be assessed by calculating the total creatinine excretion per kg of body weight. It should be ~20 to 25 mg/kg of lean body weight for men and 15 to 20 mg/kg for women.
    - Measurement of **CrCl** at two separate occasions can also help in improving accuracy.

SPECIAL CONSIDERATIONS: FUTURE DIRECTIONS IN TESTING METHODOLOGIES

- There is an active ongoing search for newer markers that will accurately predict GFR and detect early loss of renal function.
- **Cystatin C** holds promise, as it has a constant daily production and is excreted by the kidney.[24]
  - Cystatin C is a low molecular weight protein that is a member of cystatin superfamily of cysteine protease inhibitors. It is thought to be produced by all nucleated cells and its rate of production is thought to be constant.[25]

○ Cystatin C is filtered at the glomerulus and not reabsorbed, but is metabolized in the tubules, limiting its utility in measuring clearance directly.[26]

○ Recently, it has been reported that many factors affect the cystatin C levels,[27] but despite these findings cystatin C may correlate more closely to GFR than creatinine, and it has been proposed that cystatin C-based equations may be more accurate[28] in populations with lower creatinine production such as the elderly, children, renal transplant recipients, and patients with cirrhosis.[29]

○ Despite the potential accuracy of cystatin C in assessment of GFR, it is unclear whether measurement of cystatin C will improve patient care.

REFERENCES

1. Cockcroft DW, Gault MH. Prediction of creatinine clearance from serum creatinine. *Nephron.* 1976;16:31–41.

2. Levey AS, Bosch JP, Lewis JB, et al. A more accurate method to estimate glomerular filtration rate from serum creatinine: a new prediction equation. Modification of Diet in Renal Disease Study Group. *Ann Intern Med.* 1999;130(6):461–470.

3. Poggio ED, Wang X, Greene T, et al. Performance of the modification of diet in renal disease and Cockcroft-Gault equations in the estimation of GFR in health and in chronic kidney disease. *J Am Soc Nephrol.* 2005;16(2):459–466.

4. Gonwa TA, Jennings L, Mai ML, et al. Estimation of glomerular filtration rates before and after orthotopic liver transplantation: evaluation of current equations. *Liver Transpl.* 2004;10:301–309.

5. Beddhu S, Samore MH, Roberts MS, et al. Creatinine production, nutrition, and glomerular filtration rate estimation. *J Am Soc Nephrol.* 2003;14:1000–1005.

6. Lewis J, Agodoa L, Cheek D, et al. Comparison of cross-sectional renal function measurements in African Americans with hypertensive nephrosclerosis and of primary formulas to estimate glomerular filtration rate. *Am J Kidney Dis.* 2001;38(4):744–753.

7. Horio M, Imai E, Yasuda Y, et al. Modification of the CKD epidemiology collaboration (CKD-EPI) equation for Japanese: accuracy and use for population estimates. *Am J Kidney Dis.* 2010;56(1):32–38.

8. Imai E, Horio M, Nitta K, et al. Modification of the Modification of Diet in Renal Disease (MDRD) Study equation for Japan. *Am J Kidney Dis.* 2007;50(6):927–937.

9. Gera M, Slezak JM, Rule AD, et al. Assessment of changes in kidney allograft function using creatinine-based estimates of glomerular filtration rate. *Am J Transplant.* 2007;7(4):880–887.

10. Froissart M, Rossert J, Jacquot C, et al. Predictive performance of the modification of diet in renal disease and Cockcroft-Gault equations for estimating renal function. *J Am Soc Nephrol.* 2005;16(3):763–773.

11. Lin J, Knight EL, Hogan ML, et al. A comparison of prediction equations for estimating glomerular filtration rate in adults without kidney disease. *J Am Soc Nephrol.* 2003;14:2573–2580.

12. Mariat C, Alamartine E, Barthelemy JC, et al. Assessing renal graft function in clinical trials: can tests predicting glomerular filtration rate substitute for a reference method? *Kidney Int.* 2004;65:289–297.

13. Mahajan S, Mukhiya GK, Singh R, et al. Assessing glomerular filtration rate in healthy Indian adults: a comparison of various prediction equations. *J Nephrol.* 2005;18:257–261.

14. Matsuo S, Imai E, Horio M, et al. Revised equations for estimated GFR from serum creatinine in Japan. *Am J Kidney Dis.* 2009;53(6):982–992.

15. Baumann TJ, Staddon JE, Horst HM, et al. Minimum urine collection periods for accurate determination of creatinine clearance in critically ill patients. *Clin Pharm.* 1987;6:393–398.

16. van Acker BA, Koomen GC, Koopman MG, et al. Creatinine clearance during cimetidine administration for measurement of glomerular filtration rate. *Lancet.* 1992;340(8831):1326–1329.

17. Berg KJ, Gjellestad A, Nordby G, et al. Renal effects of trimethoprim in ciclosporin- and azathioprine-treated kidney-allografted patients. *Nephron.* 1989;53:218–222.

18. Mitchell EK. Flucytosine and false elevation of serum creatinine level. *Ann Intern Med.* 1984;101:278.

19. Saah AJ, Koch TR, Drusano GL. Cefoxitin falsely elevates creatinine levels. *JAMA.* 1982;247:205–206.

20. Molitch ME, Rodman E, Hirsch CA, et al. Spurious serum creatinine elevations in ketoacidosis. *Ann Intern Med.* 1980;93:280–281.

21. Verhelst J, Berwaerts J, Marescau B, et al. Serum creatine, creatinine, and other guanidino compounds in patients with thyroid dysfunction. *Metabolism.* 1997;46(9):1063–1067.

22. Kreisman SH, Hennessey JV. Consistent reversible elevations of serum creatinine levels in severe hypothyroidism. *Arch Intern Med.* 1999;159:79–82.

23. Markantonis SL, Agathokleous-Kioupaki E. Can two-, four- or eight-hour urine collections after voluntary voiding be used instead of twenty-four-hour collections for the estimation of creatinine clearance in healthy subjects? *Pharm World Sci.* 1998;20:258–263.

24. Coll E, Botey A, Alvarez L, et al. Serum cystatin C as a new marker for noninvasive estimation of glomerular filtration rate and as a marker for early renal impairment. *Am J Kidney Dis.* 2000;36(1):29–34.

25. Newman DJ, Thakkar H, Edwards RG, et al. Serum cystatin C measured by automated immunoassay: a more sensitive marker of changes in GFR than serum creatinine. *Kidney Int.* 1995;47:312–318.

26. Knight EL, Verhave JC, Spiegelman D, et al. Factors influencing serum cystatin C levels other than renal function and the impact on renal function measurement. *Kidney Int.* 2004;65:1416–1421.

27. Macdonald J, Marcora S, Jibani M, et al. GFR estimation using cystatin C is not independent of body composition. *Am J Kidney Dis.* 2006;48(5):712–719.

28. White C, Akbari A, Hussain N, et al. Estimating glomerular filtration rate in kidney transplantation: a comparison between serum creatinine and cystatin C-based methods. *J Am Soc Nephrol.* 2005;16(12):3763–3770.

29. Fliser D, Ritz E. Serum cystatin C concentration as a marker of renal dysfunction in the elderly. *Am J Kidney Dis.* 2001;37(1):79–83.

Renal Biopsy

3

Imran A. Memon

GENERAL PRINCIPLES

- Diagnosis of many kidney diseases depends on histologic evaluation of tissue.
- Early biopsy methods were done with manual needle systems and without the benefit of imaging, resulting in higher complication rates and poor tissue yield.[1,2]
- Modern techniques now use accurate ultrasound imaging and semiautomatic needle biopsy devices to obtain samples of renal cortex for histopathologic exam to aid in the specific diagnosis of renal diseases.

DIAGNOSIS

- The tissue obtained from renal biopsy is invaluable to the diagnosis of many forms of kidney diseases. It provides crucial information about the localization of kidney injury, the basic underlying mechanisms, and the patterns of injury, which, along with a clinical correlate, can make an appropriate diagnosis.[3]
  - Localization:
    - A tissue diagnosis allows one to appreciate which segments of the kidney are most affected by the injury.
    - Generally, these areas are categorized as glomerular, tubular, interstitial, or vascular components of the kidney.
  - Mechanisms:
    - The presence of certain types of infiltrative cells can be extremely helpful in making a diagnosis.
    - For example, a dense infiltration of lymphocytes and monocytes in the interstitium points toward acute interstitial nephritis.
  - Patterns of injury:
    - Certain patterns of injury characterize many of the forms of kidney injury, particularly in the glomerulus.
    - For example, focal segmental glomerulosclerosis describes a pattern of injury in which there is a "segmental" injury (discrete areas of sclerosis without involving the entire glomerular tuft) to a "focal" subset of glomeruli (some, but not all, glomeruli exhibit this pattern).
- Generally, patients who benefit most from renal biopsy and subsequent pathologic diagnosis have nephrotic syndrome, a nephritic presentation, acute renal failure, proteinuria and hematuria, or renal allograft dysfunction (Table 3-1).
  - Several studies have shown that ~40% of patients subjected to renal biopsy will have a change of diagnosis or management based on the results of the biopsy. [4]
  - Adult patients with **nephrotic syndrome** generally require a kidney biopsy because treatment algorithms vary for the disorders depending on the pathology.

TABLE 3-1	COMMON CURRENT INDICATIONS FOR RENAL BIOPSY

Major

Acute renal failure—diagnosis not apparent by clinical data
Nephrotic syndrome
Nephritic syndrome of unclear etiology
RPGN
Acute or chronic renal allograft dysfunction

Relative Indications Depending on Other Clinical Features

Asymptomatic hematuria
Asymptomatic proteinuria

RPGN, rapidly progressive glomerulonephritis.

- Patients with **acute renal failure** without clear etiology need to be evaluated for interstitial nephritis, acute nephritic syndromes, or systemic disorders, such as systemic lupus eythematosus or small-vessel vasculitis.
- The management of **proteinuria or hematuria** of unclear etiology can be affected by biopsy results, although the decision process is more complex depending on other clinical features.
- In the **evaluation of renal allograft dysfunction,** renal transplant biopsy is invaluable in diagnosing acute rejection or acute tubular necrosis in the immediate posttransplant period. Deterioration in previously stable renal function can also be evaluated when distinguishing acute or chronic rejection from cyclosporine nephrotoxicity or infection.

DIAGNOSTIC TESTING

Preprocedural Evaluation

- Planning a biopsy requires assessing risks with a good history and physical, laboratory assessment, and imaging (Table 3-2).

TABLE 3-2	PREBIOPSY CHECKLIST

History and physical

Laboratory data
  Complete blood count with platelets
  Basic chemistry panel
  Coagulation assessment (INR, aPTT, platelet function)
  Urinalysis and/or urine culture

Baseline kidney ultrasound

Hold antiplatelet and antithrombotic agents at least 1 to 2 weeks prior to biopsy

INR, international normalized ratio.

- **Renal imaging** should be performed to ensure that the patient has two kidneys of normal size and shape.
  - ○ **Native kidney biopsy is relatively contraindicated for atrophic kidneys <9 cm in size,** as the risk of capsular hemorrhage increases in fibrotic kidneys (so does the risk of a low-yield biopsy result).
  - ○ **Renal biopsy of a solitary native kidney should be undertaken only when absolutely necessary** to preserve renal function, as there is a risk of marked bleeding leading to nephrectomy.
  - ○ It has been suggested that surgically performed open renal biopsy should be the procedure of choice in this setting, but the risk of percutaneous biopsy is so low that it may be lower than the risk of general anesthesia and surgery.
- **Blood pressure (BP)** should be optimally controlled, with diastolic BP <95 mm Hg, to minimize bleeding complications.
- **Urine culture** should be sterile before a biopsy attempt.
- **Blood coagulation parameters** should be normalized as much as possible before renal biopsy.
  - ○ Systemic anticoagulants, including antiplatelet therapy, aspirin, and nonsteroidal antiinflammatory drugs, should be discontinued ≥5 days before renal biopsy.
  - ○ Prothrombin Time (PT) should be <1.2 times control; activated partial thromboplastin time (aPTT) should be <1.2 times control.
  - ○ The role for bleeding time or other functional platelet testing procedures remains unclear, but is usually done to screen for unsuspected aspirin use or other platelet disorders.
  - ○ In a patient with renal insufficiency and elevated blood urea nitrogen levels with a prolonged bleeding time, DDAVP, 0.4 mcg/kg IV for 2 to 3 hours, is usually given before biopsy.
  - ○ The diagnostic and therapeutic utility of a renal biopsy in patients needing chronic anticoagulation should be carefully considered and balanced with the risk of reversal of anticoagulation and of postbiopsy bleeding. Consultation with cardiologists and hematologists may be needed.
    - One approach is to allow the international normalized ratio (INR) to decline to 1.5 over several days or to reverse the anticoagulation with vitamin K, depending on the urgency of the biopsy.
    - Intravenous or subcutaneous unfractionated heparin should be stopped at least 6 hours prior to the procedure and should not be resumed until at least 18 to 24 hours after the procedure.
- **Informed consent** should be obtained from the patient by the physician(s) performing the biopsy.
  - ○ Risks, benefits, possible complications, and alternatives to the procedure should always be discussed in detail with the patient.
  - ○ Difficult or high-risk biopsies (e.g., single kidney, morbid obesity, requirement for ongoing systemic anticoagulation) should be given careful consideration as to whether risks outweigh benefits. The main contraindications for renal biopsy are given in Table 3-3.
  - ○ Consideration may be given to computed-tomography-guided biopsy, transjugular biopsy, or open biopsy, depending on local center expertise.

TABLE 3-3	CONTRAINDICATIONS FOR RENAL BIOPSY

Absolute Contraindications

Uncooperative patient
Bleeding diathesis or anticoagulation
Uncontrolled hypertension

Relative Contraindications

Small kidneys (9 cm)
Multiple, bilateral cysts or a renal tumor
Hydronephrosis
Active renal infection
Medium-to-large–vessel vasculitis with multiple intrarenal aneurysms
Anatomical abnormalities of the kidneys (e.g., horseshoe kidney)
Pregnancy

Procedure for Native Kidney Biopsy

- **Patient position** is the most critical step in performing a successful kidney biopsy.
  - The patient should lie prone on the examination table, with or without a support under the upper abdomen.
  - If the patient is **pregnant** or **very obese**, biopsy can be performed in the seated or lateral decubitus position.
  - The decision to perform biopsy on the left or right kidney depends on imaging quality, presence of cysts, and operator preference.
- **Ultrasound guidance** should be used to localize the lower pole of the kidney and mark the overlying skin site.
  - Particular attention should be given to the depth and angle of the renal cortex in relation to the skin entry site of the biopsy needle (this will minimize the risk of puncturing a major vessel).
  - The amount and direction of movement of the kidney in relation to inspiration and expiration should be carefully noted, especially if real-time ultrasound is not used during the actual biopsy.
- **Sterile technique** should be followed to prepare the skin entry site with Betadine and to drape the field with sterile towels.
- **Local anesthetic** (e.g., 1% lidocaine + bicarbonate) should be injected with a small-gauge needle to raise a skin wheal and then infiltrated down to the capsule of the kidney along the anticipated biopsy tract with a larger needle.
- **Needle insertion:**
  - A scalpel should be used to make a small stab incision at the skin site.
  - A variety of biopsy needles are commercially available.
    - Most commonly, 16- or 18-gauge needles are used, as sample size is poor with smaller needle gauges.
    - The incidence of major bleeding complications is lower with a spring-loaded needle under ultrasound guidance compared with manual needles.
  - The biopsy needle should be advanced (either with or without real-time ultrasound guidance with a sterile probe) just short of the depth of the renal capsule. The patient may breathe normally during this phase.

- Since the kidney normally moves up and down with the respiratory cycle, the patient should be asked to hold his or her breath as the biopsy needle is slowly advanced through the capsule.
  - Once the biopsy needle is appropriately positioned in the renal cortex, clear movement of the needle should be obvious with the patient's normal breathing.
  - The patient should again be asked to hold his or her breath while the biopsy gun is fired to obtain the core sample. The biopsy needle can then be withdrawn and the core recovered for pathologic exam.
- A **pathology technician** is invaluable for examining the core of tissue under an operating microscope to determine if sufficient glomeruli are present.
  - Usually, two to three cores suffice for an adequate biopsy, with one core fixed in formalin for light microscopy and the remainder divided for electron microscopy, immunofluorescence, and special studies.
  - An adequate sample is usually obtained when a total of 10 to 15 glomeruli are present.

Renal Allograft Biopsy

- Biopsy of a transplanted kidney is simplified by the superficial abdominal location of the allograft.
- Standard indications are summarized in Table 3-4.
- Biopsy can be done as an outpatient, as risk of significant bleeding is much less than with native biopsy.
- Transplant biopsies are usually done with real-time ultrasound guidance, as the kidney does not move with the respiratory cycle.
- After the core tissues are obtained, direct pressure should be applied to the biopsy site for ≥15 minutes to control local bleeding, with a sandbag placed at the site afterward.
- Patients are usually observed for 6 hours and may then go home in the absence of complications or other factors.

ROUTINE POSTBIOPSY CARE

- The major complication rate (bleeding severe enough to require transfusion or invasive procedure, septicemia, acute renal obstruction or failure, or death) is 6.4%, whereas the rate of minor complications is 6.6% (the rate of complications would likely be higher among clinicians with less experience).[5]

TABLE 3-4	COMMON INDICATIONS FOR RENAL ALLOGRAFT BIOPSY
Failure of graft function 1 week postengraftment	
Rapid deterioration after initial good function, before antirejection Rx	
Slow allograft function deterioration	
New onset of nephrotic-range proteinuria	

- **Observation of patients for ~24 hours** is usually done to avoid missing most complications.
  - Clinical recognition of a major complication occurs within 8 to 24 hours among 67% and 91% of patients, respectively. [6]
  - Typically, the patient should remain supine for 6 hours and then remain at bed rest overnight.
  - To help detect bleeding and other complications, vital signs are closely monitored and complete blood counts are obtained at various time points postbiopsy.
  - To minimize the risk of bleeding, **BP** should ideally be well controlled (goal <140/90 mm Hg).[7]
- In low-risk patients (e.g., serum creatinine concentration <2 mg/dL [177 µmol/L], **BP** <140/90 mm Hg, and no evidence of coagulopathy), a shorter observation period may be reasonable.

COMPLICATIONS

The main complications after biopsy are due to bleeding and pain (Table 3-5).

- **Hematuria** and the formation of a perinephric hematoma occur to some degree in all patients after renal biopsy, although only ~3% to 10% of patients experience gross hematuria.[8]
  - Serial examination of urine specimens for clearing of visible blood is useful in these cases. Complete blood count should be monitored every 6 hours in all patients after renal biopsy.
  - A fall in hemoglobin of ~1 g/dL is average after an uncomplicated renal biopsy.
  - **Blood loss requiring transfusion** occurs in 2.4% to 5% of renal biopsies.[5,9]
    - This will depend, in part, on prebiopsy hemoglobin and risk.
    - The most common site of significant blood loss is into the perinephric space, leading to a large perinephric hematoma.
    - **Subcapsular bleeds** usually tamponade themselves. Significant bleeding into the urinary collecting system may also occur, which manifests as gross hematuria and may lead to ureteral obstruction.
    - **Intervention to control bleeding** is required in ~0.3% of cases and **nephrectomy** may be necessary in 0.06% of cases.[10]

TABLE 3-5	POSTBIOPSY COMPLICATIONS

Bleeding
   Into collecting system—microscopic-to-gross hematuria
   Subcapsular—pressure tamponade and pain
   Perinephric space—hematoma formation and fall in hematocrit

Colicky pain due to ureteral obstruction from a blood clot from bleeding

Arteriovenous fistula

"Page Kidney"—chronic hypertension due to pressure-induced ischemia from a large subcapsular hematoma

Perinephric soft tissue infection

Puncture of other organs (i.e., liver, pancreas, or spleen)

- **Hypotension** after renal biopsy can occur in 1% to 2% of patients and is usually fluid responsive.[11]
  - ○ **Arteriovenous fistulas** can be detected radiologically in up to 18% of cases, but are rarely of clinical significance and usually resolve spontaneously.[12]
  - ○ The diagnosis is suggested by development of hypotension, high-output heart failure, or persistent hematuria, and can be confirmed by color-flow Doppler ultrasound.
- **Persistent pain** at the biopsy site may result from a subcapsular or perinephric hematoma or from renal colic as blood clots pass through the collecting system.
- **Biopsy of nonrenal tissues** (most commonly liver or spleen) can occur inadvertently during an intended renal biopsy. Serious complications are rare in these instances. Mortality rate was reported to be 0.1% in two series, but is substantially lower using modern techniques.[5,9]

REFERENCES

1. Iverson P, Brun C. Aspiration biopsy of the kidney. *Am J Med.* 1951;11:324.
2. Ball RP. Needle aspiration biopsy. *J Tenn Med Assoc.* 1934;27:203.
3. Appel GB. Renal biopsy: how effective, what technique, and how safe. *J Nephrol.* 1993;6:4.
4. Richards NT, Darby S, Howie AJ, et al. Knowledge of renal histology alters patient management in over 40% of cases. *Nephrol Dial Transplant.* 1994;9(9):1255–1259.
5. Whittier WL, Korbet SM. Timing of complications in percutaneous renal biopsy. *J Am Soc Nephrol.* 2004;15:142–147.
6. Renal Physicians Association. RPA position on optimal length of observation after percutaneous renal biopsy. *Clin Nephrol.* 2001;56:179.
7. Shidham GB, Siddiqi N, Beres JA, et al. Clinical risk factors associated with bleeding after native kidney biopsy. *Nephrology.* 2005;10(3):305–310.
8. Parrish AE. Complications of percutaneous renal biopsy: a review of 37 years' experience. *Clin Nephrol.* 1992;38:135.
9. Gonzalez-Michaca L, Chew-Wong A, Soletero L, et al. Percutaneous kidney biopsy, analysis of 26 years: complication rate and risk factors. *Rev Invest Clin.* 2000;52(2):125–131.
10. Korbet SM. Percutaneous renal biopsy. *Semin Nephrol.* 2002;22:254.
11. Manno C, Strippoli GF, Arnesano L, et al. Predictors of bleeding complications in percutaneous ultrasound-guided renal biopsy. *Kidney Int.* 2004;66:1570–1577.
12. Harrison KL, Nghiem HV, Coldwell DM, et al. Renal dysfunction due to an arteriovenous fistula in a transplant recipient. *J Am Soc Nephrol.* 1994;5(6):1300–1306.

Approach to Proteinuria

4

Peter J. Juran

GENERAL PRINCIPLES

Definition and Background

- Increased protein in the urine is a common sign of kidney disease. Typically, urinary protein is described in terms of total protein or total albumin.
- Normal individuals excrete <150 mg of total protein and <30 mg of albumin in urine every 24 hours. Other proteins found in the urine are either secreted by tubules (Tamm–Horsfall protein) or are small filtered proteins that have escaped reabsorption or degradation by renal tubule cells.
- **Any level of protein excretion in the urine >150 mg per 24 hours is abnormal** and merits further evaluation.
- The urine dipstick is the most common initial screening test for proteinuria, but is only sensitive for protein concentrations >20 mg/dL (roughly equivalent to 300 mg per 24 hours).
- **Nephrotic syndrome** is defined as a urine protein excretion >3.5 g per 24 hours, associated with hypoalbuminemia, hyperlipidemia, and edema. The same level of proteinuria without the other features is referred to as nephrotic range proteinuria.
- The approach to the patient with proteinuria is determined by the degree of proteinuria, other renal manifestations, and the overall clinical picture.

Why Test for Proteinuria?

- Even relatively small increases in protein or albumin in the urine can be early signs of kidney disease and often precede a detectable change in glomerular filtration rate (GFR).
- Persistently high levels of proteinuria may cause further kidney damage and result in accelerated progression of kidney disease.
- Proteinuria is a strong and independent risk factor for cardiovascular disease and death, mostly in patients with advanced age, diabetes, hypertension, and chronic kidney disease.[1–3]
- Interventions that reduce the amount of proteinuria may retard the progression of kidney disease and improve the prognosis of cardiovascular disease.

Pathophysiology

- Proteinuria can occur due to glomerular or tubular dysfunction.[4]
- **Glomerular proteinuria** results from a disruption of the glomerular filtration barrier, leading to increased filtration of plasma proteins in amounts that exceed tubular reabsorptive capacity. If the amount of protein in 24 hours exceeds 2 g, a glomerular disease is usually present.

- **Tubular proteinuria** is a consequence of inadequate reabsorption of filtered low-molecular-weight proteins (e.g., $beta_2$-microglobulin or lysozyme), which then appear in the urine. Tubular proteinuria can coexist with glomerular proteinuria or be an isolated finding in the setting of defective proximal tubule function. Typically, tubular proteinuria is <2 g per 24 hours.
- **Overflow proteinuria** occurs when there is excessive systemic production of abnormal proteins of small molecular weight that exceeds the capacity of the tubule for reabsorption. A prime example is the increased urinary excretion of light chains in myeloma. Occasionally, lysozymuria appears in acute monocytic leukemia.
- **Tissue proteinuria** is associated with an inflammatory or neoplastic process within the urinary tract.

Classification of Proteinuria

- **Transient proteinuria:**
  ○ Transient proteinuria is primarily seen in children and adolescents who are healthy and asymptomatic, and who have normal urinary sediment.[5-7] It is believed to result from alterations in renal hemodynamics.
  ○ Transient proteinuria **disappears on repeat testing and requires no further evaluation.** Some individuals have recurrent episodes of transient proteinuria that often goes into permanent remission within a few years.
  ○ Some studies of this patient population have reported a histological association and progression toward renal insufficiency and hypertension.[8] It is therefore recommended to monitor this subgroup yearly.
  ○ Transient proteinuria can occur reversibly in hyperadrenergic states like fever, exercise, congestive heart failure, seizures, use of vasopressors, pregnancy, and obstructive sleep apnea. A 10% incidence of functional proteinuria has been reported among ER admissions, with the most common causes being congestive heart failure, seizures, and fever. Pathogenesis is believed to be secondary to increased glomerular permeability and decreased tubular reabsorption of proteins, possibly due to angiotensin II or norepinephrine.[9]
- **Orthostatic proteinuria:**
  ○ This syndrome is characterized by the excretion of abnormal quantities of protein in the upright position, with normal levels of protein excretion while in supine position.
  ○ Orthostatic proteinuria is present in up to 3% to 5% of adolescents and young men, aged mostly <30 years.
  ○ Most patients have rates of protein excretion <2 g per 24 hours in the upright position, although higher rates have been reported.[10]
  ○ Diagnosis can be made with 24-hour split urine collections in the supine and upright positions. The 24-hour collection is divided into a 16-hour daytime portion and an 8-hour overnight portion.
  ○ Long-term follow-up of these patients shows no deterioration in renal function and spontaneous resolution in 50% of patients 10 years after diagnosis.[11]
- **Persistent proteinuria**
  ○ Persistent proteinuria is present regardless of position, activity level, or functional status. It is established by confirming proteinuria on subsequent testing a week or two after the first positive test.

○ It may result from an isolated kidney disease or may be part of a multisystem process with renal involvement.

○ Patients with persistent proteinuria are typically classified as having nephrotic or nonnephrotic range proteinuria, and by the presence or absence of features of the nephrotic syndrome.

DIAGNOSIS

Semi-Quantitative Methods

• **Routine urine dipstick:**

○ The simplest and least expensive method of detecting proteinuria is by routine dipstick. This dye-impregnated paper uses tetrabromophenol blue as a pH indicator. Urine albumin binds to the reagent and changes its pH, which then results in a spectrum of color changes depending on the degree of pH change. A typical scale for a positive test is shown in Table 4-1.

○ The lower threshold concentration for detection of protein by the routine dipstick is ~15 to 20 mg/dL. This is roughly equivalent to a 24-hour urine protein of 300 to 500 mg.

○ False-positive and false-negative results may occur because these semi-quantitative estimates of proteinuria are concentration dependent and are therefore influenced by the degree of urinary concentration.

  ▪ Highly concentrated urine may show an abnormal result even when the absolute daily protein excretion is normal.

  ▪ Highly dilute urine may show normal or only modestly elevated results for protein concentration even when elevated amounts of protein are excreted. Even with 30 mg/dL of protein, the dipstick can be negative up to 50% of the time.

○ The dipstick **will not detect nonalbumin proteins,** such as immunoglobulins, and thus false-negative results may be seen in diseases such as multiple myeloma.

○ **False-positive results** can occur in patients who receive contrast up to 24 hours before the test. Also, false-positive results may occur when highly alkaline urine overwhelms the dye's buffer.

• **Sulfosalicylic acid (SSA) test:**

○ Unlike routine dipstick, which detects only albumin, the SSA test **detects all proteins.**

TABLE 4-1	SCALE FOR DETECTING PROTEINURIA ON ROUTINE URINE DIPSTICK

Negative
Trace: 15–30 mg/dL
1+: 30–100 mg/dL
2+: 100–300 mg/dL
3+: 300–1000 mg/dL
4+: >1000 mg/dL

○ A positive SSA test in the context of a negative dipstick is indicative of nonalbumin proteinuria, such as immunoglobulin light chains. Results of the SSA test are recorded on a scale from 0 to 4+, similar to routine dipstick.[12]

- **Albumin sensitive tests:**
  ○ Test strips that are more sensitive to albumin are also available (Albustix).
  ○ Dye-impregnated strips and special immunoassays can detect albumin concentrations as low as 30 mg/d, which is far below the 300 mg per 24 hours threshold of the standard dipstick.
  ○ These strips **can be used to screen for microalbuminuria,** and their sensitivity and specificity range from 80% to 97% and 33% to 80%, respectively.
- **Implications of a positive dipstick:**
  ○ Detection of proteinuria should **prompt an examination of urinary sediment.** Any evidence of hematuria, red blood cell casts, or lipiduria should be noted and may be a sign of underlying pathology.

Quantitative Methods

- **Spot urine protein-to-creatinine ratio:**
  ○ The degree of urinary dilution will directly affect protein concentration. The concentration of creatinine in the urine serves as an internal control for urine dilution. The ratio of protein to creatinine is therefore independent of urine concentration.
  ○ As the rate of creatinine excretion remains fairly constant, the ratio of protein to creatinine on a random specimen is a good estimate of the amount of protein excreted.
  ○ The **protein-to-creatinine ratio in a normal person is <0.2** and is roughly equivalent to an excretion of <0.2 g per 24 hours per 1.73 m^2.[13] For instance, a ratio of 2 roughly translates to a 24-hour urinary protein excretion of 2 g.
  ○ The accuracy of the total protein-to-creatinine ratio is related to the assumption that daily creatinine excretion is only slightly >1000 mg per 24 hours per 1.73 m^2.
- The accuracy of the ratio is diminished when creatinine excretion is either markedly increased, as in a muscular man (the ratio will underestimate proteinuria), or markedly reduced, as in a cachectic patient (the ratio will overestimate proteinuria).
- **Microalbumin-to-creatinine ratio:**
  ○ The presence of increased amounts of urinary albumin is an important marker for early kidney disease and cardiovascular risk. Validation of this concept is strongest in early diabetic kidney disease, but may also apply to other forms of kidney disease.
  ○ The term microalbuminuria resulted from early studies that used more sensitive assays for albumin and detected its presence despite negative results for usual dipstick tests for protein. **Microalbuminuria** thus refers to a small amount of albuminuria and not a particular form of albumin.
  ○ The urinary albumin is most often assessed using the albumin (microalbumin)-to-creatinine ratio on an untimed or spot specimen. The microalbumin-to-creatinine ratio can be used in the same way as the urine protein-to-creatinine ratio.
  ○ A **value <30 mcg/g is considered normal,** whereas values from 30 to 300 mcg/g indicate microalbuminuria. Values >300 mcg/g are detected by the routine dipstick and fall into the category of overt proteinuria (macroalbuminuria).
  ○ The **microalbumin-to-creatinine ratio is the preferred routine screening tool for all diabetic patients for detection of early nephropathy.**[14] A single

first-morning voided specimen has a sensitivity and specificity of >90% when compared with a 24-hour collection, but this varies when the urine samples are taken at other times of the day.

○ Falsely elevated values may be obtained with hyperglycemia, vigorous exercise, infection, and ketoacidosis.

• **The 24-hour urine protein collection:**

○ The 24-hour urine collection is the **definitive method of urinary protein quantification,** but is used less often because of frequent errors in collection, patient inconvenience, and the increased use of the protein-to-creatinine ratio.

○ A 24-hour urinary protein is preferable in patients in whom urine creatinine excretion is less reliable (changing renal function, high and low muscle mass).

○ To verify proper collection, a **24-hour urine creatinine should always be measured in the same urine specimen.** Excretion of creatinine in male patients during a 24-hour period should be roughly 20 to 25 mg/kg and for female patients it should be ~15 to 20 mg/kg. If the amount of creatinine in the urine sample is quite different from the expected range, an error in the collection of the sample should be suspected.

CLINICAL APPROACH TO PROTEINURIA

• Once proteinuria has been detected on a dipstick, the next step is to **confirm the abnormal result by repeat measurement after several weeks with a freshly voided specimen.**

• No confirmatory test is needed if the proteinuria is heavy on dipstick.

• Once proteinuria is confirmed, the next step is to **quantify protein excretion by a protein-to-creatine ratio, albumin-to-creatinine ratio, or a 24-hour urine collection.**

• The **history and physical examination** should include a search for symptoms and signs attributable to kidney disease and identify risk factors for kidney disease. Key issues to be addressed are:

○ The presence and duration of common causes of kidney disease such as diabetes and hypertension.

○ Features suggestive of a connective tissue disorder such as arthralgias, arthritis, skin rashes, and constitutional symptoms.

○ Clinical features of malignancy should be sought. For example, solid organ malignancies have been associated with membranous nephropathy, whereas lymphomas have been associated with minimal change disease.

○ Features suggestive of infections such as hepatitis, endocarditis, syphilis, or human immunodeficiency virus should be explored. These disorders can lead to many different forms of glomerular disease.

○ A complete drug history detailing all prescription, illicit, herbal/alternative, and over-the-counter medications should be taken. For example, nonsteroidal antiinflammatory drugs can cause nephrotic syndrome.

○ A family history of kidney disease should be noted, such as hereditary nephritis, nail–patella syndrome, or polycystic kidney disease.

• Additional testing is determined by the clinical context. In all cases, a urine sediment, GFR estimation, complete blood count, basic metabolic profile, and serum albumin are appropriate. Urine protein electrophoresis and serum protein electrophoresis should be ordered if there is suspicion of an overflow proteinuria from myeloma, amyloidosis, or other immunoglobulin diseases. Dysmorphic red blood cells in the sediment or nephrotic range proteinuria would likely prompt a kidney biopsy. An evaluation of the anatomy of the urinary tract is usually not needed unless there is significant hematuria or history of recurrent urinary tract infection (Fig. 4-1).

○ Therapy for proteinuria will depend on the specific etiology determined.

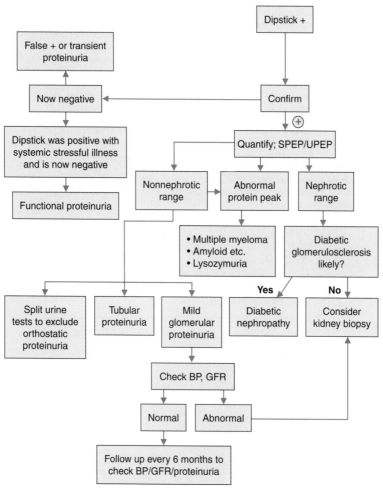

FIGURE 4-1. Evaluation of proteinuria. ⊕, positive; BP, blood pressure; GFR, glomerular filtration rate; SPEP, serum protein electrophoresis; UPEP, urine protein electrophoresis.

REFERENCES

1. Damsgaard EM, Froland A, Jorgensen OD, et al. Microalbuminuria as predictor of increased mortality in elderly people. *BMJ.* 1990;300:297–300.
2. Grimm RH, Svendsen KH, Kasiske B, et al. Proteinuria is a risk factor for mortality over 10 years follow up. *Kidney Int.* 1997;52:10–14.
3. Wagner DK, Harris T, Madans JH. Proteinuria as a biomarker risk of subsequent morbidity and mortality. *Environ Res.* 1994;66:160–172.
4. Wingo CS, Clapp WL. Proteinuria: potential causes and approach to evaluation. *Am J Med Sci.* 2000;320:188–194.
5. Larrsson SO, Thysell H. Four years' follow up of asymptomatic isolated proteinuria diagnosed in general health survey. *Acta Med Scand.* 1969;186:375–381.
6. Wagner MD, Smith FG, Tinglof BO, et al. Epidemiology of proteinuria: a study of 4807 school children. *J Pediatr.* 1968;73:825–832.
7. Wolman IJ. The incidence, causes and intermittency of proteinuria in young men. *Am J Med Sci.* 1945;210:86–100.
8. Muth RG. Asymptomatic mild proteinuria. *Arch Intern Med.* 1965;115:569–574.
9. Robinson RR. Isolated proteinuria in asymptomatic patients. *Kidney Int.* 1980;18:395–406.
10. Springberg PD, Garrett LE, Thompson AL, et al. Fixed and reproducible orthostatic proteinuria: results of a 20-year follow up study. *Ann Intern Med.* 1982;97:516–519.
11. Rytand DA, Spreiter S. Prognosis in postural (orthostatic) proteinuria: forty to fifty-year follow up of six patients after diagnosis by Thomas Addis. *N Engl J Med.* 1981;305:618–621.
12. Rose, BD. *Pathophysiology of Renal Disease,* 2nd ed. New York, NY: McGraw-Hill, 1987.
13. Lemann J, Doumas BT. Proteinuria in health and disease assessed by measuring the urinary protein/creatinine ratio. *Clin Chem.* 1987;33:297–299.
14. Gross JL, de Azevedo MJ, Silveiro SP, et al. Diabetic nephropathy: diagnosis, prevention, and treatment. *Diabetes Care.* 2005;28:164–176.

Approach to Hematuria

5

Peter J. Juran

GENERAL PRINCIPLES

Definition

- Hematuria, or blood in the urine, can be a sign of serious underlying pathology of the kidney or urinary tract. Therefore, it is important to identify and, if necessary, treat the underlying disease at an early stage.
- Hematuria can be either gross or microscopic:
  - ○ **Gross hematuria** is blood in the urine that is grossly visible to the eye.
  - ○ The American Urological Association (AUA) has defined **microscopic hematuria** as three or more red blood cells (RBCs) per high-power field (HPF) on microscopic examination of urinary sediment from two out of three properly collected urine specimens in average- or low-risk patients, and from one out of three specimens in high-risk patients (defined below).[1]

Epidemiology

- Gross hematuria is estimated to have a community prevalence of 2.5%.
- According to population-based studies, the prevalence of microscopic hematuria varies widely depending on the age and sex distribution of the populations at hand and on the method of detection that is utilized. The prevalence in the general population ranges from 0.18% to 16.1%.[2] It is unclear whether there is a higher prevalence with increasing age.

Etiology

- Hematuria can be **glomerular or nonglomerular** in origin.
- **Nonglomerular hematuria** can be **further divided into upper and lower urinary tract.**
- In persons <50 years of age, the most common glomerular causes are IgA nephropathy and thin basement membrane disease, whereas nephrolithiasis, pyelonephritis, cystitis, prostatitis, and urethritis are the most common nonglomerular causes in that age group.
- In persons >50 years of age, renal, prostate, and transitional cell cancers (bladder/ ureteral) are common nonglomerular sources of bleeding, whereas IgA nephropathy continues to be the leading cause of glomerular hematuria.
- The various etiologies of hematuria are listed in Table 5-1.

Screening

- Hematuria is usually an incidental finding on urinalysis (UA) dipstick testing, and screening for asymptomatic microscopic hematuria is generally not recommended.
- The **presence of a positive dipstick result demands microscopic analysis of the urine sediment for RBCs,** as dipstick testing cannot differentiate between RBCs, myoglobin, and hemoglobin.

TABLE 5-1 CAUSES OF MICROSCOPIC HEMATURIA

Origin		Causes
Glomerular		IgA nephropathy
		Thin basement membrane disease (benign familial hematuria)
		Hereditary nephritis (Alport syndrome)
		Loin pain hematuria syndrome (may also have gross hematuria)
		Glomerulonephritis due to other causes (see Chaps. 17 and 18)
Nonglomerular	*Upper urinary tract (renal, vascular, and ureteral)*	Nephrolithiasis
		Pyelonephritis
		Renal cell cancer
		Polycystic kidney disease
		Medullary sponge kidney
		Hypercalciuria, hyperuricosuria, or both, without documented stones
		Renal pelvis or ureteral transitional cell cancer
		Renal trauma
		Papillary necrosis
		Renal infarction/arteriovenous malformation/renal vein thrombosis/Nutcracker syndrome
		Ureteral stricture and hydronephrosis
		Sickle cell trait or disease
		Renal tuberculosis
	Lower urinary tract (bladder, prostate, and urethra)	Cystitis, prostatitis, urethritis
		Bladder cancer
		Prostate cancer/benign prostatic hypertrophy
		Benign bladder and ureteral polyps and tumors
		Urethral and meatal strictures
		Schistosoma haematobium in North Africans
		Trauma (catheterization/blunt urethral or bladder trauma)
Uncertain		Exercise hematuria
		Menstrual contamination
		Over anticoagulation (usually with warfarin)
		Sexual intercourse
		"Benign hematuria" (unexplained microscopic hematuria)

- Further investigation may be warranted depending on the clinical scenario and risk for serious underlying disease.

DIAGNOSIS AND EVALUATION

Clinical Presentation

There is no consensus as to a standard protocol to be followed when performing a hematuria workup. In 2001, the AUA published recommendations on evaluating hematuria, and these recommendations are partly incorporated into the algorithm shown in Figure 5-1.

- **Detection of hematuria:**
  - In gross hematuria, urine may appear red, cola-colored, or brown. In microscopic hematuria, it will appear clear and the diagnosis is usually made by dipstick test.
  - The **urine collection should be a freshly voided, clean-catch, midstream urine specimen.**
  - **Dipstick testing:**
    - It is highly sensitive (91% to 100%) but less specific (65% to 99%).[3]
    - **False-negative results** can be due to ingestion of large amounts of ascorbic acid or other reducing agents, low pH, or the presence of formaldehyde.
    - **False-positive results** can be due to semen, high pH, presence of oxidizing agents, and myoglobinuria.
    - When positive, the urine sample should be centrifuged and the sediment examined microscopically to count the number of RBCs per HPF (see Chap. 1 about urine centrifugation).
  - **Microscopic analysis:**
    - It allows for examination of RBC morphology and the detection of RBC casts.
    - **Dysmorphic RBCs and RBC casts** are indicative of a glomerular pathology and a renal cause for hematuria.
    - Dysmorphic urinary RBCs are best seen by phase-contrast microscopy and are variable in size and shape, having irregular borders compared with the normal, doughnut-shaped RBCs.
    - If >80% of urinary RBCs are dysmorphic, hematuria is more likely due to a glomerular cause. If >80% of urinary RBCs are normal, this indicates a lower urinary tract source of bleeding.
    - Dysmorphic RBCs may be seen in hematuria of nonglomerular origin and isomorphic (normal morphology) RBCs can be seen in hematuria of glomerular origin. The relative proportion of each type of RBC remains the key to determining the origin of hematuria.
    - **Acanthocytes,** or doughnut-shaped RBCs with membrane blebs, have also been used as a marker for glomerular bleeding, whereas **crenated RBCs** (with spicules) are not usually relevant and indicate concentrated urine.

History
- **Medications** should be carefully reviewed as certain commonly prescribed drugs can cause hematuria (nonsteroidal anti-inflammatory drugs, busulfan, aspirin, oral contraceptives, and warfarin).
  - Over anticoagulation with warfarin may cause hematuria, but such a presentation still warrants further investigation as underlying pathology may be unmasked.[4]

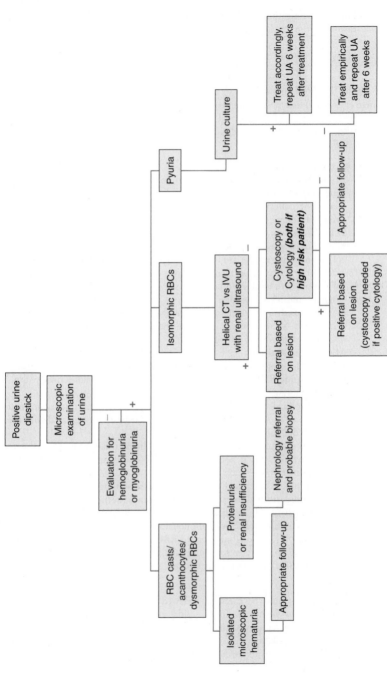

FIGURE 5-1. Algorithm for microscopic hematuria evaluation. IVU, intravenous urography; RBC, red blood cell; CT, computed tomography.

TABLE 5-2	RISK FACTORS FOR SIGNIFICANT UROLOGIC PATHOLOGY IN PATIENTS WITH MICROSCOPIC HEMATURIA

Age >40 years
History of smoking
History of gross hematuria
Occupational exposure to chemicals or dyes (benzenes or aromatic amines)
Recurrent urinary tract infections
Irritative voiding symptoms
History of high-dose cyclophosphamide
Pelvic irradiation
Analgesic abuse

- Certain **risk factors** for significant disease should also prompt further evaluation of hematuria: increased age (>40 years), cigarette smoking, occupational exposure to chemicals, and high doses of cyclophosphamide all increase the risk of transitional cell cancers of the bladder and the urinary tract.
  - Gross hematuria is four times more likely than microscopic hematuria to be associated with urothelial cancers, and is by itself considered a risk factor for serious pathology. Table 5-2 lists the various risk factors for significant urologic disease.
- Patients should also be checked for signs of a glomerular etiology or systemic disease and be examined for edema, purpura, and skin rashes.
- Fever, dysuria, and flank pain are suggestive of pyelonephritis or a complicated urinary tract infection.
- **Travel history** may uncover a risk for schistosomiasis.
- A **family history** of hematuria can be significant in Alport syndrome and thin basement membrane disease.

Physical Examination
- Physical examination should include measurement of blood pressure, pulse, and volume status.
- Hypertension could be a manifestation of glomerulonephritis.
- Edema may be a sign of proteinuria.
- Fever, costovertebral angle tenderness, and suprapubic tenderness are suggestive of an infectious etiology.
- A nonblanching purpuric rash may be evidence of vasculitis.
- Cardiovascular exam may reveal atrial fibrillation or murmurs due to endocarditis—both sources for renal emboli.
- Abdominal exam may reveal a mass, enlarged bladder, or polycystic kidneys.
- A detailed genitourinary exam should be performed to look for local sources of bleeding and to exclude rectal or vaginal bleeding.
- If a careful history and examination are suggestive of a benign source of hematuria, urinalysis should be repeated 48 hours after cessation of the precipitating cause (e.g., menstruation, vigorous exercise, sexual activity, or trauma). If the hematuria has resolved, no further workup is necessary.

Diagnostic Testing

Laboratory Evaluation

- Laboratory evaluation should **begin with urine dipstick testing and microscopic examination** of the urine sediment.
- If pyuria or bacteriuria is present, **urine culture** should be obtained to look for infection. If urine culture is positive, appropriate treatment with antibiotics should be given and urine dipstick test and microscopy examination repeated 6 weeks later to ensure resolution of hematuria.
- If the hematuria has resolved, no further evaluation is needed.
- If dipstick result is positive for protein, **quantification of the proteinuria** is necessary. A ratio of urinary protein to urinary creatinine in a spot urine specimen of >0.3 or a 24-hour urinary protein excretion of >300 mg suggests a renal source of bleeding and warrants evaluation by a nephrologist.
- **Serum creatinine** should be checked and an abnormal value should prompt a workup for renal disease. **Complete blood count, electrolytes, and blood urea nitrogen** should also be obtained.
- Dysmorphic RBCs, RBC casts, or acanthocytes in the urine suggest glomerular bleeding and should be followed by a glomerulonephritis workup, including measurement of antinuclear antibody, antineutrophil cytoplasmic antibody, anti-glomerular basement membrane antibodies, complement levels, cryoglobulins, serology for hepatitis B and C viruses, and human immunodeficiency virus antibody test. A renal biopsy would often be indicated at this point.
- **Urine cytology** is indicated in those at risk for bladder cancer (Table 5-2). This test has only ~66% to 79% sensitivity but very high specificity (95% to 100%). Sensitivity is improved if the urine is collected on three consecutive days from the first void sample in the morning. Sensitivity is higher for carcinoma *in situ* and high-grade bladder cancer than for cancers of low histologic grade. Urine cytology remains insensitive for renal cell cancer.

Imaging

- If infection and a glomerular source of bleeding are ruled out, imaging of the upper urinary tract should be obtained to evaluate for renal cell cancer, transitional cell cancer of the ureter or renal pelvis, nephrolithiasis, cystic disease, or obstructive lesions.
- Computed tomography (CT) is being used more frequently now as the initial study, although traditionally intravenous urography (IVU) had been recommended as the modality of choice.
- **Computed tomography:**
  - This is the best modality for the detection of stones (94% to 98% sensitivity) and solid masses of the urinary tract, as well as renal and perirenal infections or abscesses.
  - If possible, a noncontrast helical CT should be done first to evaluate for stones. If this is negative or if the patient has risk factors for renal or transitional cell cancer, CT urography should then be obtained.
  - Although CT is more expensive than either IVU or ultrasound, these tests are often followed by additional cross sectional imaging, resulting in even greater expense.
  - CT detects masses <3 cm in size that can be missed by IVU or ultrasound. High detection rates for transitional cell carcinoma have also been reported for CT.

- ○ Disadvantages of CT include expense, risk of contrast nephropathy (which can also occur with IVU), and availability. Note that in pregnancy ultrasound is the preferred imaging modality.
- **Intravenous urography:**
  - ○ Traditionally, IVU has been the initial modality of choice for imaging of the upper urinary tract, but has now been largely replaced by CT.
  - ○ IVU is more sensitive than ultrasound for detection of transitional cell cancer in the kidney or the ureter, but it cannot differentiate between solid and cystic components. Thus, it is often followed by further imaging such as ultrasound or CT.[5]
  - ○ IVU is less costly than CT, but still carries the risk of contrast nephropathy, and may miss upper tract lesions <3 cm in size.[6]
- **Ultrasound:**
  - ○ Ultrasound is excellent for characterizing solid versus cystic components, but can miss lesions <3 cm (82% sensitivity for masses between 2 and 3 cm).
  - ○ It is the preferred initial test in pregnancy, as it causes no harm to the fetus.
  - ○ Its use is becoming more limited in the evaluation of hematuria since the advent of CT.

Diagnostic Procedures
- **Cystoscopy:**
  - ○ It is recommended that cystoscopy be performed as part of the initial evaluation of microscopic hematuria in all adults older than 40 years of age and in all those at risk for bladder cancer (Table 5-2).
  - ○ Cystoscopy has a lower yield in patients younger than 40 years and in those with no risk factors for malignancy. It can be deferred in these cases but urinary cytology should be performed instead.
  - ○ Disadvantages of cystoscopy include its invasive nature, risk for iatrogenic infection, and patient discomfort.
- **Ureterorenoscopy:**
  - ○ Once the above radiologic tests are performed and are negative, fiber optic imaging of the upper urinary tract and the kidney may be performed.
  - ○ Ureterorenoscopy is mostly done in patients who have recurrent macroscopic hematuria with negative radiologic/laboratory workup or hematuria that localizes to one side of the bladder on cystoscopy.[7]
  - ○ Renal calculi or upper tract transitional cell carcinomas are found in 5% to 10% of patients.
  - ○ Discrete vascular lesions like arteriovenous malformations or hemangiomas can be fulgurated and are found in 0.50% of cases.
  - ○ Biopsies of lesions suspicious for neoplasm can be taken in the ureters or the kidneys, with partial nephrectomy performed for those with high suspicion of renal cell cancer.
  - ○ Vascular lesions can be successfully treated with the holmium: yttrium–aluminum–garnet laser.
  - ○ Calculi can be extracted.

MONITORING/FOLLOW-UP

- Some patients, who initially have a negative workup for microscopic hematuria, eventually develop significant disease (although most do not).

- Microscopic hematuria can precede bladder cancer and certain glomerulone-phritides by years, despite a negative initial evaluation. For this reason, patient follow-up is recommended.
- **Repeating urinalysis and urine cytology at 6, 12, 24, and 36 months in high-risk patients is recommended.** In addition, in such high-risk patients, repeat imaging or cystoscopy may be considered at 1 year.
- Low-risk patients may be followed with periodic urinalysis and urine cytology.
- In patients who develop worrisome signs such as irritative voiding symptoms or gross hematuria, further evaluation with imaging and cystoscopy is war-ranted.
- **Positive cytology** should naturally be **followed by cystoscopy and possibly imaging.**
- Immediate **referral to a nephrologist** should be done if proteinuria, hyperten-sion, or renal insufficiency were to develop during follow-up, as they may be indicative of glomerular disease.
- In cases of isolated microscopic hematuria that is persistent, renal biopsy is controversial as available data does not suggest that identification of the disease may alter management or outcome (e.g., IgA or thin basement membrane disease).

REFERENCES

1. Grossfield G, Wolf JS, Litwin M, et al. Asymptomatic microscopic hematuria in adults: summary of the AUA best practice policy recommendations. *Am Fam Physician.* 2001;63:1145–1154.
2. Cohen RA, Brown RS. Microscopic hematuria. *New Eng J Med.* 2003;348:2330–2338.
3. McDonald MM, Swagerty D, Wetzel L, et al. Assessment of microscopic hematuria in adults. *Am Fam Physician.* 2006;73:1748–1754.
4. Van Savage JG, Fried FA. Anticoagulant-associated hematuria: a prospective study. *J Urol.* 1995;153:1594–1596.
5. Jaffe JS, Ginsberg PC, Harkaway RC, et al. A new diagnostic algorithm for the evaluation of microscopic hematuria. *Urology.* 2001;57:889–894.
6. Khadra MH, Pickard RS, Charlton M, et al. A prospective analysis of 1,930 patients with hematuria to evaluate current diagnostic practice. *J Urol.* 2000;163:524–527.
7. Dooley RE, Pietrow PK. Ureteroscopy for benign hematuria. *Urol Clin North Am.* 2004;31:137–143.

Disorders of Water Balance

6

Georges Saab

GENERAL PRINCIPLES

- Disorders of sodium (hypo- or hypernatremia) reflect abnormalities in water homeostasis.[1,2]
- Both hypo- and hypernatremia are associated with increased morbidity and mortality in a number of clinical syndromes and disease states.[3–6]
- Rapid correction of hypo- and hypernatremia additionally contributes to these adverse outcomes.[7]
- Antidiuretic hormone (ADH), also known as '*arginine vasopressin*,' is the main determinant of renal water regulation and free water balance. ADH is secreted in response to an increase in plasma osmolarity, decreased effective circulatory volume, and other factors such as pain, nausea, and certain medications.
- Disruption in ADH release or signaling, along with alterations in water intake, all contribute to the development of hypo- or hypernatremia.
- Plasma sodium is governed by the sum of the total body exchangeable electrolytes divided by total body water (TBW).
  - Plasma sodium = $(Na_E + K_E)/TBW$ (**Eq. 1**)[8]
- Urinary electrolyte-free water clearance (C_{H20}) is a measure of free water excreted sans electrolytes for a particular urine volume V.
  - $C_{H20} = V(1 - (U_{Na} + U_K)/P_{Na})$, where U_{Na} and U_K are urinary sodium and potassium, respectively, and P_{Na} is plasma sodium (**Eq. 2**)[9]
- TBW is 50% and 60% of body weight (kg) for females and males, respectively. In dehydrated patients, these estimates decrease by ~10% (i.e., 40% and 50%, respectively).

Definition: Hyponatremia

- Hyponatremia is defined as a serum or plasma sodium concentration <135 mmol/L.
- Acute hyponatremia is defined as a fall in sodium over a period of <48 hours.

Classification

- Pseudohyponatremia (isotonic hyponatremia) has classically been caused by severe elevations of plasma lipids or proteins. Flame photometers measure the sodium concentration in whole plasma, and assume that the plasma water concentration is 93% of the plasma. Since sodium is restricted to serum water, a marked increase in plasma lipids or plasma proteins essentially "dilutes" the sodium concentration, as measured by flame photometry.[1] Alternate methods, using ion-specific electrodes, only measure the concentration in the aqueous portion of plasma and will provide a more accurate measure.[10] Pseudohyponatremia is of no clinical relevance save the recognition of this phenomenon and avoiding unnecessary interventions that could potentially be harmful.

- Hypertonic hyponatremia occurs when the extracellular plasma osmolarity is increased. Here, the osmolarity of the extracellular space is increased, drawing water movement from the intracellular to the extracellular space. The increase in the aqueous fraction of plasma thereby lowers the serum sodium concentration causing a true hyponatremia.[1]
- Hypotonic hyponatremia occurs when the extracellular plasma osmolarity is decreased and is the most common form encountered in clinical practice. This is primarily due to increased water intake and/or impaired water excretion.[1]

Epidemiology

- Hyponatremia is the most common electrolyte abnormality among hospital inpatients and is present on admission in 15% to 30% of patients.[6,11]
- When present, hyponatremia is an independent predictor of mortality, even at mildly reduced levels, both in short and long terms.[6]
- As expected, the prevalence of hyponatremia is lower in the general ambulatory population (2% to 5%),[5,11] but is still associated with poor outcomes.[5]

Etiology

- Isotonic hyponatremia:
  - Pseudohyponatremia from elevated lipids or proteins
  - Mannitol solution (5%)[12] used as irrigant during surgical procedure
    - The solution is relatively isotonic, but does not contain sodium, and thus hyponatremia occurs if large quantities are absorbed.
- Hypertonic hyponatremia:
  - Hyperglycemia lowers [Na^+] by 2.4 mmol/L for every 100 mg/dL increase in the plasma glucose.[13] Osmotic diuresis can cause water loss, which may ultimately result in converting hyponatremia to hypernatremia.
  - Intake of ethylene glycol, ethanol, and methanol
- Hypotonic hyponatremia:
  - Low urine osmolality (<100 mOsm/kg): Primary polydipsia, severe malnutrition, and beer potomania
  - High urine osmolality (>100 mOsm/kg):
    - Volume excess: Congestive heart failure, nephrotic syndrome, renal failure, and cirrhosis
    - Volume depletion
    - Euvolemia
      - Syndrome of inappropriate ADH (SIADH)[14] (**see Table 6-1**)
      - Hypothyroidism
      - Adrenal insufficiency (sometimes)
      - Glycine (1.5%)[15] or sorbitol (3%)[1] solution used as irrigant during surgical procedure
        - As opposed to mannitol, these agents are hypotonic to plasma and thus a hypotonic hyponatremia occurs when large volumes are absorbed.
        - Reduction in serum sodium is often initially out of proportion to reduction in plasma osmolarity because of the fact that these agents are

TABLE 6-1	COMMON CAUSES OF SIADH
CNS disorders	Hemorrhage, psychosis, infection, alcohol withdrawal
Malignancy (ectopic ADH)	Small-cell lung carcinoma (most commonly implicated), CNS disease, leukemia, Hodgkin's disease, duodenal cancer, pancreatic cancer
Pulmonary	Infection, acute respiratory failure, mechanical ventilation
Miscellaneous	Pain, nausea (powerful stimulator of ADH), HIV (multifactorial), general postoperation state
Pharmacologic agents (either mimic or enhance ADH)	Cyclophosphamide, vincristine, vinblastine, NSAIDs, tricyclics and related agents, selective serotonin reuptake inhibitors, chlorpropamide, nicotine, bromocriptine, oxytocin, DDAVP

ADH, antidiuretic hormone; CNS, central nervous system; HIV, human immunodeficiency virus; NSAID, nonsteroidal antiinflammatory drug.

effective osmoles and facilitate water transfer from the intra- to extracellular space. However, glycine slowly diffuses into cells and sorbitol is rapidly metabolized, and thus plasma osmolarity will slowly decrease to the level expected by serum sodium.

Pathophysiology

- As plasma sodium and tonicity drops, cells in the brain must readjust intracellular osmolality by lowering the osmotic content. If changes occur rapidly or in the face of severe hyponatremia, this adaptation fails, leading to cerebral edema, altered mental status, and seizures.[1] Hyponatremia can be fatal should brainstem herniation result.
- Patients with underlying metabolic disorders, such as cirrhosis[16] or preexisting neurologic disease, as well as children and young women,[17] may be at particular risk of severe complications without rapid reversal of acute hyponatremia.
- *Central pontine myelinolysis* (osmotic demyelination)[7,18,19] is thought to be due to rapid correction of chronic hyponatremia. Alcoholic patients and those with severe malnutrition appear to be at particular risk for osmotic demyelination due to rapid sodium correction.[1] Cognitive, behavioral, and movement disorders due to the occurrence of osmotic demyelination may not be apparent for days after the correction of hyponatremia, and visible changes on magnetic resonance imaging scan may take weeks to appear. This does not appear to be a major concern in the correction of acute hyponatremia.

RISK FACTORS

- Comorbid conditions: Congestive heart failure, cirrhosis, nephrotic syndrome, renal failure, alcoholism, and malignancy (SIADH)
- Medications:
  - Impairing water excretion: Thiazide
  - SIADH: Antidepressants, antipsychotics[14]
  - Volume depletion: Diuretics[20]
- Psychiatric illness (polydipsia)[21]

DIAGNOSIS

Clinical Presentation

- It is usually asymptomatic until serum sodium <125 mmol/L, but fatalities have been reported with an extremely rapid decrease from a normal [Na⁺] to the 120- to 128-mmol/L range.
- Symptoms include central nervous system (CNS) effects, such as confusion, weakness, headache, obtundation, or seizures, with acute hyponatremia.[1]
- Chronic hyponatremia (developing over >48 hours) is generally fairly well tolerated. Symptoms include cognitive defects as well as nausea, vomiting, weakness, and headache.[1]

History

- A thorough *history* should include the estimated duration of inciting factors and an assessment of signs or symptoms suggesting that immediate intervention may be necessary (mental status change, lethargy, coma, seizure). Management of a patient with hyponatremia depends on whether the process is considered to be *acute* or *chronic* and the severity of symptoms.

Physical Examination

- The physical exam should be geared toward assessing the volume status of the patient. Elevated blood pressure, an S3 heart sound, or increased jugular venous pressure indicates volume excess often in the setting of early congestive heart failure. Edema in the lower extremities or presacral region or evidence of pulmonary edema indicates increased extracellular fluid volume in heart failure and kidney disease. Conversely, orthostatic hypotension, decreased skin turgor, dry mucosal membranes, and decreased jugular venous pressure suggest intravascular volume depletion.

Diagnostic Testing

- Blood tests:
  - Renal function panel, plasma osmolarity, thyroid-stimulating hormone, and cortisol level
  - Calculate osmolar gap:
    - Calculated plasma osmolarity = $2 \times [Na] + (BUN/2.8) + (glucose/18)$
    - Osmolar gap = Measured−calculated plasma osmolarity
- Urine tests:
  - Urine osmolarity, urine sodium, urine potassium, urine protein, and urine creatinine

- Imaging:
  - Head computed tomography (CT), if the patient has neurologic symptoms
  - Chest x-ray to evaluate for lung cancer

Diagnostic Criteria

- Plasma osmolarity:
  - Isotonic:
    - Pseudohyponatremia: Confirm hyponatremia via ion-specific electrodes. If unconfirmed, measure plasma lipid and protein levels.
    - Mannitol (5%): Review of medications will reveal likely etiology if hyponatremia is confirmed via ion-specific electrodes.
  - Hypotonic:
    - Examination of volume status
    - Hypovolemic: will have low urine sodium (<20 mmol/L) and high urine osmolality (>100 mOsm/kg)
    - Euvolemic:
      - SIADH: High urine sodium (>40 mmol/L) and high urine osmolality (>100 mOsm/kg)
      - Primary polydipsia\beer potomania: Low urine sodium (<20 mmol/L) and low urine osmolality (<100 mOsm/kg). Clinical history will confirm studies.
    - Hypervolemic:
      - Congestive heart failure (physical exam): Elevated jugular venous pressure, S3 gallop, peripheral edema, and crackles on lung exam. Low urine sodium (<20 mmol/L) and high urine osmolality (>100 mOsm/kg)
      - Cirrhosis (physical exam): Ascites, peripheral edema, palmar erythema, spider angiomata, jaundice, and caput medusa. Low urine sodium (<20 mmol/L)
      - Nephrotic syndrome (physical examination with edema): Periorbital and peripheral edema. Low urine sodium (<20 mmol/L) and nephrotic range proteinuria (>3 g over 24 hours)
  - Hypertonic:
    - Toxic ingestions: Elevated osmolar gap (>10 mOsm/L), elevated anion gap (>12 mmol/L), and acidosis. Measurement of toxic compound is definitive diagnosis.
    - Hyperglycemia: No osmolar gap as glucose is included in the calculated plasma osmolarity. Hyperglycemia will obviously be present.

TREATMENT

Chronic Asymptomatic Hyponatremia

- Chronic hyponatremia without acute neurologic events is best treated by fluid restriction.
  - Experts have suggested that examining the urinary electrolyte content will aid in determining the degree of fluid restriction. The ratio of (urine sodium + urine potassium)/plasma sodium can be used as a guide.[9]
    - 1: No free water.
    - 0.5 to 1.0: 500 mL.
    - 0.5: 1000 mL

○ If the ratio >1, the patient is excreting no electrolyte-free water and any water ingested will be retained. Withholding free water will allow the concentration of serum sodium to rise via insensible water losses (800 to 1000 mL/d).[9] For a ratio of 0.4, 60% of urine volume is electrolyte-free water (from **Eq. 2**). If the patient produces 2000 mL of urine that day, 1200 mL will be electrolyte-free water. Restricting fluid intake to 1000 mL will result in a net of 1000 mL − (1200 + 800 mL) = −1000 mL of free water lost per day. Accordingly, the above recommendations should be adjusted to the patient's urine output. These recommendations also assume that the urinary electrolyte loss is matched by dietary intake.

- Chronic treatment of SIADH seldom requires pharmacologic agents and these are usually reserved for cases resistant to the above interventions.
  ○ Lithium and demeclocycline both induce nephrogenic diabetes insipidus[22] and have been used to treat SIADH; however, the former is unpredictable and can have numerous side effects, whereas the latter is expensive and potentially nephrotoxic.[1] Either can cause severe hypernatremia without adequate free water intake.
  ○ Oral urea is another safe alternative for cases of refractory SIADH. Palatability is probably its biggest drawback, but doses of 30 to 60 g/d reportedly are effective in managing SIADH.[23]
  ○ New classes of agents that block vasopressin-2 receptors (aquaretics) are being evaluated for use in SIADH and other states of ADH excess. So far, they have only been approved for the short-term management of hyponatremia.[24]

Acute and/or Symptomatic Hyponatremia

- Hyponatremia—acute or chronic—presenting with significant symptoms, may necessitate emergent therapy with hypertonic saline. Loop diuretics are often used in tandem to aid in free water excretion (by lowering the U_{osm}) and to prevent volume overload.
- Severe CNS symptoms due to hyponatremia usually respond to very modest increases in serum sodium, often a <5% increase in the presenting value.[1]
- The initial rate of correction generally should be 1 to 2 mmol/L/h, unless persistent symptoms such as continued seizure activity justify a faster reversal rate.[1]
- Once symptoms have been controlled, the rate of correction is adjusted to no more than a total of 8 mmol/L in the first 24 hours, including the initial rapid correction.[1]
- Over the next 24 hours, sodium correction should probably not exceed an additional 10 mmol/L. More rapid correction increases the risk of osmotic demyelination, especially in chronic hyponatremia.
- Serum sodium should be checked frequently, every 1 to 2 hours, to avoid overcorrection.
- The human body is not a closed system and one must take into account urinary losses of electrolytes and insensible water losses when calculating replacement strategies.
- Potassium replacement can increase serum sodium concentration and may result in overcorrection.[25]

- For example, in a 70 kg male with SIADH and a sodium concentration of 110 mmol/L with mild mental status changes, urine sodium is 100 mmol/L and urine potassium is 71 mmol/L.
  - Assume that changes are due to water gain, calculate the TBW.
  - Initially, with normal serum sodium, TBW for a male is 60% of body weight in kg. In this case, 42 L.
  - Thus, using **Eq. 1**, we get $(Na_E + K_E) = 42 * 110$ mmol/L = 4620 mmol.
  - To increase serum sodium by 4 mmol/L over 2 hours, some ignore the urinary and insensible losses.
    - Suppose V = volume of 3% saline administered. Thus, the original total body exchangeable cations will increase by 513 mmol/L $\times$ V and the new TBW is increased by V.
    - Using **Eq. 1**, $(4620 + 513 \times V)/(42 + V) = 114$ and solving for V we get 420 mL or 210 mL/h.
    - Giving normal saline may be harmful in this situation. Each 1 L of normal saline contains 154 mmol of sodium. This will be excreted in 154/171 = 900 mL of urine, thus retaining 100 mL of water.
    - After loop diuretics such as furosemide, the urine is usually hypotonic to plasma and is roughly half-normal saline solution in content.[26] Thus, the sodium in 1 L of normal saline given after furosemide would therefore be excreted in 2 L of urine, creating a net loss of 1 L of free water.[26]
- However, monitoring urine output and urine electrolyte is crucial, because many may have more than one reason for hyponatremia (i.e., concomitant volume depletion) and hypertonic saline may suppress ADH release, leading to a prompt aquaresis.[27] If not accounted for, these equations may markedly over-estimate the degree of correction.
- **Calculations only provide a rough estimate to help initiate therapy and do not replace frequent monitoring and adjustment.** Accidental overcorrection may occur if vigilant monitoring is not maintained, with potentially fatal consequences. Treatment of accidental overcorrection may be of benefit, especially if symptoms suggestive of osmotic demyelination appear. Free water or ADH analogs may need to be used to reduce the sodium concentration to levels dictated by correction calculations.

DEFINITION: HYPERNATREMIA

- Any increase in the serum sodium to >145 mmol/L automatically increases hypertonicity, leading to intracellular dehydration.

Classification
- Unlike hyponatremia, all cases of hypernatremia are true hyperosmolar states.
- Although the serum sodium is elevated, intravascular volume may be low or high, depending on the etiology.

Epidemiology
- The overall incidence of hypernatremia is significantly lower than hyponatremia.
  - Hypernatremia has been reported in <2% of all admissions.[3,11]
  - Hospital-acquired hypernatremia has been reported to occur in 2% to 5% of all admissions.[3,11]

○ Patients admitted with hypernatremia were more likely to be elderly, whereas those with hospital-acquired hypernatremia had similar ages to the general hospital population.[3]

○ Similar to hyponatremia, the presence of hypernatremia is also associated with an increased risk of poor outcomes.[3]

Etiology

- Urinary concentrating deficits:
  - ○ Diuretics
  - ○ Solute diuresis:
    - ▪ Mannitol infusion
    - ▪ Hyperglycemia
    - ▪ High protein feeding
  - ○ Diabetes insipidus:
    - ▪ Central—decreased or absent ADH
- Postpituitary surgery
- Sarcoidosis
- Pregnancy—placental production of vasopressinase[28]
  - ○ Nephrogenic—renal resistance to ADH[22,29]
- Lithium toxicity
- Hypercalcemia
- Hypokalemia
- Cidofovir
- Amphotericin B
- Foscarnet
- Post acute tubular necrosis
- Amyloidosis
- Sickle-cell disease
- Congenital
- Water losses:
  - ○ Insensible
  - ○ Enteral
- Lack of free water intake

Pathophysiology

- As the sodium concentration increases, increased cellular volume loss can lead to rupture of cerebral blood vessels with associated morbidity and mortality. Just as with hyponatremia, chronic development of hypernatremia is better tolerated than an equivalent acute change.[2]
- Cerebrospinal fluid movement into the interstitial areas of brain tissue, as well as the increase in intracellular electrolyte and other effective osmoles, initially serves to protect from the effects of hypernatremia.[2]

DIAGNOSIS

Clinical Presentation

Symptoms are primarily a reflection of CNS involvement, and include lethargy, irritability, weakness, confusion, and progression to coma, but they are generally not apparent until the sodium concentration has increased to >160 mmol/L.[2]

History
- A careful history should follow similar lines to those outlined in the hyponatremia section.
- Additional history should include a careful assessment of fluid intake and output (including enteral).

Physical Examination
- Similar to the patient with hyponatremia, a careful exam should assess volume status.

Diagnostic Testing
- Blood tests:
  - Renal function panel and plasma osmolarity
- Urine tests:
  - Urine osmolarity, urine sodium, and urine potassium
  - Calculate C_{H20} (**Eq. 2**)
- Imaging
  - Head CT, if the patient has neurologic symptoms

TREATMENT

- Hypernatremia corrected too rapidly may have unintended consequences; thus, the sodium concentration should be returned to the normal range slowly and with vigilant lab and clinical monitoring. Correction at a rate of 0.5 mmol/L/h has been shown to have a low likelihood of complications.[2] Faster correction rates can prevent adequate time for intracellular adjustment of tonicity, leading to cellular swelling.
- Severe volume depletion or hemodynamic instability merits treatment with normal saline. Lesser degrees of clinical volume depletion can be treated with 0.2% or 0.45% saline solution.
- Once the volume status has been restored satisfactorily, D_5W alone should be used to correct hypernatremia. The dextrose component is metabolized as long as insulin deficiency is not present, leaving free water. Overwhelming the ability to metabolize dextrose is not a concern with the low administration rates used in the slow correction of hypernatremia.
- For example, you are asked to see a patient in the intensive care unit who has developed polyuria and hypernatremia. The patient has been receiving high protein feeding. Urine output has been 5 L. Laboratory results reveal serum sodium of 160 mmol/L, urine osmolality 1000 mOsm/kg, urine sodium 40 mmol/L, and urine potassium 40 mmol/L.
  - $C_{H20} = 5\ L \times (1 - (40 + 40)/160) = 2.5\ L$
  - Therefore, the patient has lost 2.5 L of electrolyte-free water in the urine from a solute diuresis in the setting of high protein intake (note the high urine osmolality).
- Example, an 80-year-old, 60 kg female is brought in from a nursing home with lethargy and confusion. Exam is consistent with volume depletion. Initial serum sodium is 160 mmol/L. The patient receives 2 L of normal saline in the emergency room and admitted to the floor. Calculate how much free water to give to correct sodium by 12 mmol/L (down to 148 mmol/L) over 24 hours.

- ○ Current TBW = 40% × 60 = 24 L.
- ○ Current $(Na_E + K_E) = 24$ L × 160 = 3840 mmol.
- ○ The new TBW to get sodium to 148 = 3840/148 = 26 L.
- ○ Therefore, patient should get 2 + 1 L (to replace insensible losses) = 3 L of free water over 24 hours or 125 mL/h.

- As with hyponatremia, **calculations only provide a rough estimate to help initiate therapy and do not replace frequent monitoring and adjustment.** Frequent assessment of urine output, volume status, and laboratory data is essential. Failure to do so can once again lead to undesired outcomes.

KEY POINTS TO REMEMBER

- Abnormalities of plasma [Na+] actually reflect imbalances of water homeostasis.
- Effective plasma osmolarity must always be checked in hyponatremia.
- Astute estimation of the volume state is key in making a correct diagnosis.
- Symptomatic sodium disorders need emergent therapy. All asymptomatic cases require gradual and deliberate treatment with frequent monitoring to avoid complications of overcorrection.
- It is best to methodically define treatment goals, speed of correction, and fluid type at the outset. One must be prepared to modify the plan according to ongoing changes and follow-up laboratory values.

REFERENCES

1. Adrogue HJ, Madias NE. Hyponatremia. *N Engl J Med.* 2000;342:1581–1589.
2. Adrogue HJ, Madias NE. Hypernatremia. *N Engl J Med.* 2000;342:1493–1499.
3. Palevsky PM, Bhagrath R, Greenberg A. Hypernatremia in hospitalized patients. *Ann Intern Med.* 1996;124:197–203.
4. Renneboog B, Musch W, Vandemergel X, et al. Mild chronic hyponatremia is associated with falls, unsteadiness, and attention deficits. *Am J Med.* 2006;119:71. e1–8.
5. Sajadieh A, Binici Z, Mouridsen MR, et al. Mild hyponatremia carries a poor prognosis in community subjects. *Am J Med.* 2009;122:679–686.
6. Waikar SS, Mount DB, Curhan GC. Mortality after hospitalization with mild, moderate, and severe hyponatremia. *Am J Med.* 2009;122:857–865.
7. Sterns RH, Riggs JE, Schochet SS, Jr. Osmotic demyelination syndrome following correction of hyponatremia. *N Engl J Med.* 1986;314:1535–1542.
8. Edelman IS, Leibman J, O'Meara MP, et al. Interrelations between serum sodium concentration, serum osmolarity and total exchangeable sodium, total exchangeable potassium and total body water. *J Clin Invest.* 1958;37:1236–1256.
9. Furst H, Hallows KR, Post J, et al. The urine/plasma electrolyte ratio: a predictive guide to water restriction. *Am J Med Sci.* 2000;319:240–244.
10. Nguyen MK, Ornekian V, Butch AW, et al. A new method for determining plasma water content: application in pseudohyponatremia. *Am J Physiol Renal Physiol.* 2007;292: F1652–F1656.
11. Hawkins RC. Age and gender as risk factors for hyponatremia and hypernatremia. *Clin Chim Acta.* 2003;337:169–172.
12. Phillips DR, Milim SJ, Nathanson HG, et al. Preventing hyponatremic encephalopathy: comparison of serum sodium and osmolality during operative hysteroscopy with 5.0% mannitol and 1.5% glycine distention media. *J Am Assoc Gynecol Laparosc.* 1997;4:567–576.

13. Hillier TA, Abbott RD, Barrett EJ. Hyponatremia: evaluating the correction factor for hyperglycemia. *Am J Med.* 1999;106:399–403.
14. Ellison DH, Berl T. Clinical practice. The syndrome of inappropriate antidiuresis. *N Engl J Med.* 2007;356:2064–2072.
15. Istre O, Bjoennes J, Naess R, et al. Postoperative cerebral oedema after transcervical endometrial resection and uterine irrigation with 1.5% glycine. *Lancet.* 1994;344:1187–1189.
16. Papadakis MA, Fraser CL, Arieff AI. Hyponatraemia in patients with cirrhosis. *Q J Med.* 1990;76:675–688.
17. Arieff AI. Influence of hypoxia and sex on hyponatremic encephalopathy. *Am J Med.* 2006;119:S59–S64.
18. Adams RD, Victor M, Mancall EL. Central pontine myelinolysis: a hitherto undescribed disease occurring in alcoholic and malnourished patients. *AMA Arch Neurol Psychiatry.* 1959;81:154–172.
19. Brunner JE, Redmond JM, Haggar AM, et al. Central pontine myelinolysis and pontine lesions after rapid correction of hyponatremia: a prospective magnetic resonance imaging study. *Ann Neurol.* 1990;27:61–66.
20. Sterns RH. Diuretic-induced hyponatremia. *Arch Intern Med.* 1986;146:2414–2415.
21. Goldman MB, Luchins DJ, Robertson GL. Mechanisms of altered water metabolism in psychotic patients with polydipsia and hyponatremia. *N Engl J Med.* 1988;318:397–403.
22. Garofeanu CG, Weir M, Rosas-Arellano MP, et al. Causes of reversible nephrogenic diabetes insipidus: a systematic review. *Am J Kidney Dis.* 2005;45:626–637.
23. Decaux G, Genette F. Urea for long-term treatment of syndrome of inappropriate secretion of antidiuretic hormone. *Br Med J (Clin Res Ed).* 1981;283:1081–1083.
24. Ghali JK, Koren MJ, Taylor JR, et al. Efficacy and safety of oral conivaptan: a V1A/V2 vasopressin receptor antagonist, assessed in a randomized, placebo-controlled trial in patients with euvolemic or hypervolemic hyponatremia. *J Clin Endocrinol Metab.* 2006;91:2145–2152.
25. Laragh JH. The effect of potassium chloride on hyponatremia 1. *J Clin Invest.* 1954; 33:807– 818.
26. Yee J, Parasuraman R, Narins RG. Selective review of key perioperative renal-electrolyte disturbances in chronic renal failure patients. *Chest.* 1999;115:149S–157S.
27. Mohmand HK, Issa D, Ahmad Z, et al. Hypertonic saline for hyponatremia: risk of inadvertent overcorrection. *Clin J Am Soc Nephrol.* 2007;2:1110–1117.
28. Davison JM, Sheills EA, Philips PR, et al. Metabolic clearance of vasopressin and an analogue resistant to vasopressinase in human pregnancy. *Am J Physiol.* 1993;264:F348–F353.
29. Hatch FE, Culbertson JW, Diggs LW. Nature of the renal concentrating defect in sickle cell disease. *J Clin Invest.* 1967;46:336–345.

Disorders of Potassium Balance

7

Sadashiv Santosh

GENERAL PRINCIPLES

- Normal daily potassium (K^+) intake is ~80 mEq/d. Total body potassium (K^+) is ~50 mEq/kg, 98% of which is intracellular. Intracellular concentrations (~140 mEq/L) are 35 times that normally present in the extracellular (plasma) space (~4 mEq/L); changes in plasma $[K^+]$ may not reflect total body K^+ stores.
- **Renal regulation of plasma potassium:**
  - Aldosterone plays a central role in $[K^+]$ regulation by stimulating its excretion in the cortical collecting duct of the nephron.[1-3] Decreased effective circulating volume (ECV) or an increase in plasma $[K^+]$ leads to increased aldosterone production and increased potassium secretion in exchange for sodium retention.
  - Hyperkalemia is also a direct stimulus for renal K^+ secretion. Renal secretion of K^+ is dependent on adequate tubular flow in the distal nephron. Decreased ECV leads not only to increased aldosterone production (favoring K^+ excretion) but also to decreased distal flow rate (reducing K^+ excretion), allowing plasma $[K^+]$ to remain in a relatively stable state. Conversely, increased ECV leads to not only a decrease in aldosterone production but also an increased distal flow rate, allowing plasma $[K^+]$ to again remain normal.
  - Changes in plasma $[K^+]$ can occur due to shifting of K^+ in or out of cells, independent of changes in total body K^+.

HYPOKALEMIA

GENERAL PRINCIPLES

Definition
Hypokalemia is defined as $[K^+]$ <3.5 mEq/L.

Pathophysiology
Hypokalemia may result from decreased intake, intracellular shift of K^+, or increased K^+ losses (usually renal or gastrointestinal [GI]).

- **Decreased intake:** In the setting of decreased intake, the normally functioning kidney can decrease K^+ excretion to <25 mEq/d. Thus, moderate dietary K^+ restriction should not by itself cause hypokalemia.[3]
- **Intracellular shift:** A variety of factors can cause potassium to shift into cells.
  - **Alkalosis**—if extracellular pH rises, H^+ will be driven out of cells in exchange for K^+ shifting into cells.[3]
  - **Stimulation of the Na/K-ATPase pump.** This pump maintains the high intracellular potassium concentrations and its activity can be increased by

catecholamines, particularly β_2-adrenergic stimulation and insulin.[4] The latter may also mediate hypokalemia often seen with refeeding syndrome.[5]

○ **Treatment of anemia or neutropenia** with vitamin B_{12}/folic acid or granulocyte-macrophage colony stimulating factor (GM-CSF) can cause hypokalemia because of increased uptake by hematopoietic cells.[6,7]

○ **Hypokalemic periodic paralysis,** a result of amputation of skeletal muscle dihydropyridine-sensitive calcium channels,[3] and thyrotoxic periodic paralysis, mutation of a skeletal muscle K^+ channel, cause K^+ shifting into muscle cells.[8]

○ **Hypothermia.**

• **GI losses:**

○ Normal fecal K^+ excretion is ~10 mEq/d. With normal dietary K^+ intake, if fecal losses exceed ~55 mEq/d, the kidney's ability to conserve K^+ may be exceeded and K^+ depletion will occur.

○ **Large volume stool output** of any cause, especially if coupled with decreased oral intake, may cause hypokalemia.

○ Gastric secretions normally contain very little K^+. **In the case of vomiting or large-volume nasogastric suction, hypokalemia may occur, but this is NOT due to K^+ loss in the gastric fluid.** The proton loss and volume contraction cause metabolic alkalosis (with elevated plasma bicarbonate). Although intracellular shift of K^+ from alkalemia might be expected, the major contributor to hypokalemia is increased distal nephron K^+ secretion due to bicarbonaturia- and hypovolemia-induced aldosterone release, leading to K^+ wasting.[3]

• **Renal losses:**

○ **Diuretics:** Loop and thiazide diuretics induce hypokalemia by increasing distal nephron fluid delivery as well as stimulating aldosterone secretion by inducing hypovolemia.[3,6] Bartter's and Gitelman's syndromes are loss-of-function mutations in furosemide- and thiazide-sensitive channels, respectively.[9]

○ **Syndromes of mineralocorticoid excess:**

■ **Primary hyperaldosteronism (Conn's syndrome)** due to adrenal adenoma or hyperplasia

■ **Secondary hyperaldosteronism** due to renal artery stenosis, fibromuscular dysplasia, renin-secreting tumor (rare)

■ **Apparent mineralocorticoid excess**

□ **11β-Hydroxylase deficiency**

– Cortisol is a potent mineralocorticoid, but is inactivated in the kidney by 11β-hydroxysteroid dehydrogenase. Licorice, which can be found in some tobacco and chewing gum, can inactivate this enzyme

□ **Cushing's syndrome**

– Hypokalemia results from the excess production of steroids that are normally metabolized by 11β-hydroxysteroid dehydrogenase enzyme.

■ **Liddle's syndrome,** a gain-of-function mutation of distal epithelial Na^+ channels, increases sodium reabsorption in the collecting duct and enhances the excretion of potassium.

■ **Glucocorticoid remediable hyperaldosteronism,** caused by mutation resulting in ACTH-sensitive aldosterone synthase gene. This results in increased aldosterone production, remediable by suppressing ACTH synthesis using glucorticoids.

○ **Increased distal nephron flow** from saline diuresis, salt-wasting nephropathy, and glucosuria (diabetes mellitus or Fanconi's syndrome).

○ **Nonreabsorbable anion:** The presence of a nonreabsorbable anion in the distal nephron creates negative charge in the lumen, promoting K^+ secretion. This phenomenon can be seen with bicarbonaturia (metabolic alkalosis) and urinary hippurate (glue sniffing).

○ **Tubular toxins:** Amphotericin, gentamicin, hypercalcemia, and cisplatin all cause tubular damage, impairing K^+ reabsorption.

○ **Hypomagnesemia:** It can cause renal potassium wasting. Adequate potassium retention often cannot take place until the magnesium deficit is replaced. Hypomagnesemia is often associated with alcoholism, diuretics, diarrhea, poor nutrition, aminoglycoside, and cisplatin use.

CLINICAL PRESENTATION

• Mild hypokalemia (3.0 to 3.5 mEq/L) is generally asymptomatic, although it does pose an increased risk of mortality for patients who also have cardiovascular disease or who are on digitalis.

• **Weakness and muscle pain,** usually initially involving the lower extremities, can develop as the $[K^+]$ drops below 3 mEq/L.

• Further decreases to below 2.5 mEq/L can lead to **paralysis,** including involvement of the muscles of respiration. Some patients can present with an ileus due to hypokalemic effects on smooth muscle. Rhabdomyolysis can occur with severe hypokalemia. This elevates the $[K^+]$ and prevents further decrements, but can also serve to mask the underlying etiology. Checking serum creatine phosphokinase (CPK) level may aid in the diagnosis of suspected hypokalemia-induced rhabdomyolysis.

• Hypokalemia can impair renal water reabsorption and cause a nephrogenic diabetes insipidus.

• Prolonged hypokalemia can cause irreversible interstitial nephritis, renal cysts, hypertension, and glucose intolerance. Increased renal ammonia synthesis occurs in the presence of hypokalemia and can potentially lead to hepatic coma in an individual with advanced liver disease.[10]

History

• The history should try to elicit common causes such as vomiting, diarrhea, laxative abuse, and diuretic use. A family history of hypokalemia may suggest Bartter's, Gitelman's, or Liddle's syndrome. A history of weakness after adrenergic stimuli, insulin, or high-carbohydrate meals suggests hypokalemic periodic paralysis. Concurrent hyperthyroidism may represent thyrotoxic periodic paralysis.

Physical Examination

• Physical exam findings should focus on signs of volume depletion (volume contraction may lead to metabolic alkalosis and hypokalemia) or hypertension (suggesting mineralocorticoid excess).

Diagnostic Testing

Laboratories

- **Urine potassium excretion:** Random urine [K^+] can be misleading. A low value may falsely suggest extrarenal causes of K^+ depletion if the urine is very dilute. A 24-hour urine K^+ is helpful but cumbersome. Normally, daily K^+ excretion should fall to <25 mEq/d in the setting of hypokalemia. The **transtubular K^+ gradient (TTKG)** is more easily obtained than a 24-hour collection, and can be helpful.[11] TTKG should be <3 if the kidney is appropriately conserving K^+, in which case hypokalemia is likely being caused by GI or sweat losses, or *prior* diuretic therapy.

$$TTGK = (urine\ [K^+] \times serum\ osmolality)/(serum\ [K^+] \times urine\ osmolality)$$

If urine K^+ excretion, determined as described above, is inappropriately high and the cause is not obvious from history and physical exam, then measuring **plasma renin activity and aldosterone levels** can be helpful.

- **High renin:** It usually indicates diuretic use, salt-wasting nephropathies, GI volume losses, or renovascular disease. Rarely, renin-secreting tumors may be the cause.
- **Low renin/high aldosterone:** It indicates primary hyperaldosteronism due either to adrenal adenoma or adrenal hyperplasia. Adrenal computed tomographic scan or magnetic resonance imaging can be helpful.[12]
- **Low renin/low aldosterone:** It indicates increased nonaldosterone mineralocorticoid effect, such as licorice ingestion.
- It should be emphasized that **assessment of urinary potassium and renin/aldosterone activity do not always differentiate between all specific causes of hypokalemia.** Therefore, the clinical history remains important in pinpointing the cause.
- **Acid-base status:** Hypokalemia with metabolic alkalosis is usually due to diuretics, vomiting, or mineralocorticoid excess. Hypokalemia with metabolic acidosis is less common; types I and II renal tubular acidosis (RTA), salt-wasting nephropathy, and diabetic ketoacidosis (especially after insulin administration has caused intracellular shift of K^+) are on the differential diagnosis.
- **Magnesium:** As described above, hypomagnesemia can cause urinary K^+ wasting; hence, it should be excluded as a cause of (often refractory) hypokalemia.

Electrocardiography

- **EKG changes due to hypokalemia:** Prominent U waves, diminished or inverted T waves, and ST-segment depression are observed; with extremely low [K^+] levels, the PR and QRS intervals can lengthen and lead to ventricular fibrillation. EKG changes do not correlate well with the degree of hypokalemia.[3,13]

TREATMENT

- The potassium deficit at plasma [K^+] of 3 mEq/L may be in the range of 200 to 400 mEq. As the plasma level decreases to <3 mEq/L, the deficit can be >600 mEq, but is unpredictable due to transcellular shifts. This is classically seen in hyperglycemic states in which the combination of hyperglycemia, glucosuria, ketonuria, and insulin treatment all affect the $[K^+]$, and levels can change dramatically during the course of treatment.

- **Potassium replacement should be given PO whenever possible** due to the potential for cardiac arrhythmias, vein sclerosis, and the increased cost in using intravenous (IV) administration.
  - Oral doses of 40 mEq of potassium are generally well tolerated and can be given q4 hours.
  - Potassium chloride is usually administered, as the chloride component helps correct the often-coinciding alkalosis and bicarbonaturia.
  - Potassium citrate can be given if hypokalemia associated with acidemia is present.
  - IV potassium can be administered in concentrations of 40 mEq/L via a peripheral line or 60 mEq/L via a central line.
    - The rate of infusion should generally not be >10 mEq/h unless absolutely necessary.
    - Intravenous potassium should be administered in a saline solution rather than with dextrose; insulin release in response to the dextrose can further decrease the $[K^+]$.
- **Correction of metabolic alkalosis will help prevent renal K^+ wasting that accompanies bicarbonaturia.** In cases of vomiting, H_2-blockers or proton pump inhibitors can reduce the acidity of the gastric secretions and prevent acid loss. In hypovolemic patients with a contraction alkalosis, volume repletion can be accomplished with isotonic IV fluids.
- In the **treatment of hypokalemia due to hyperaldosteronism or diuretic use** (e.g., for congestive heart failure (CHF), hypertension), potassium-sparing diuretics are useful.
  - **Spironolactone,** which reduces aldosterone synthesis, is commonly used in patients with liver disease and ascites, as well as in patients with CHF.
  - **Amiloride and triamterene** block the apical Na^+ channel in the distal nephron. Amiloride is favored over triamterene because of a significant risk of nephrolithiasis and potential renal insufficiency with the latter.[14]
- In states of aldosterone excess, doses of 20 to 40 mg/d PO of amiloride may be needed; otherwise, doses of 5 to 10 mg/d may suffice.
- Amiloride is the treatment of choice for Liddle's syndrome and Gitelman's syndrome.

HYPERKALEMIA

GENERAL PRINCIPLES

Definition
Hyperkalemia is defined as $[K^+]$ >5 mEq/L.

Pathophysiology
- **Acute hyperkalemia** may result from various **causes, typically reflecting transcellular shifting of potassium.**
  - **Pseudohyperkalemia:** It is characterized by release of potassium from cellular elements (white blood cells, platelets, hemolyzed red blood cells (RBCs)) after sample collection. Repeated fist clenching or prolonged tourniquet application during phlebotomy can also cause spurious elevations in $[K^+]$.[15]

○ **Very large oral or intravenous K⁺ loads:** With normally functioning homeostatic mechanisms, oral K⁺ loads of up to 135 to 160 mEq are reasonably well tolerated, producing rises in plasma K⁺ of <3.5 mEq/L. Potassium release from RBCs after transfusion can result in hyperkalemia,[16] which can be prevented by washing the RBCs.[17] Citrate anticoagulant used in RBC storage can cause concurrent hypocalcemia, increasing the potential for arrhythmia.

○ **Decreased cellular uptake** due to insulin deficiency or nonselective beta-blockade. Digitalis toxicity also impairs Na⁺/K⁺ ATPase activity (e.g., due to digitalis toxicity).

○ **Extracellular K⁺ release:** It is caused by trauma, tissue necrosis, rhabdomyolysis, tumor lysis syndrome, severe exercise,[18,19] depolarizing neuromuscular blockers (succinylcholine).[20]

○ **Metabolic acidosis *not* due to organic acids.** Metabolic acidosis due to organic acids (e.g., ketoacids and lactic acid) usually do NOT cause hyperkalemia. The extracellular K⁺ shift seen in, for example, diabetic ketoacidosis (DKA) and the nonketotic hyperosmolar state, is thought to be due to hyperosmolality from hyperglycemia and insulin deficiency and not metabolic acidosis.[21]

○ **Hyperkalemic periodic paralysis** (due in some cases to a mutation in the skeletal muscle Na⁺ channel).

• **Chronic hyperkalemia implies *decreased renal K⁺ excretion*,** due usually to decreased aldosterone effect or decreased flow in the distal nephron. In chronic kidney disease, decreased nephron mass is compensated for by increased K⁺ secretion per nephron.

○ Decreased aldosterone effect:
  ▪ Decreased synthesis of aldosterone.
    □ **Medications** that disrupt the renin–angiotensin–aldosterone axis (angiotensin-converting enzyme [ACE] inhibitors, angiotensin receptor blockers, and renin inhibitors) decrease the synthesis of aldosterone. Nonsteroidal antiinflammatory drugs and heparin, including low-molecular-weight heparin,[22] are also known to reduce aldosterone synthesis.
    □ A variety of **medical conditions** decrease aldosterone production. These include:
      – Adrenal insufficiency (acquired immune deficiency syndrome, and Addison's disease)
      – Diabetes mellitus
      – Type II pseudohypoaldosteronism (PHA) (Gordon's syndrome/chloride shunt)[23]

○ **Aldosterone resistance:**
  ▪ **Medications** such as aldosterone antagonists (amiloride, triamterene, spironolactone, eplerenone, and trimethoprim) and cyclosporine[24] decrease the response to aldosterone.
  ▪ **Type I PHA** is caused by loss-of-function mutation of either the mineralocorticoid receptor (renal PHA type I) or in the amiloride-sensitive epithelial Na⁺ channel (multiple target organ defect PHA type I).[23]
  ▪ **Type IV RTA** is a term used to describe the nonanion gap metabolic acidosis and hyperkalemia that occur in the setting of decreased aldosterone effect.

• **Decreased distal flow.**

• A marked reduction in distal flow can be seen with severe volume contraction, poor ECVs, or intense vasoconstriction, as seen in CHF, cirrhosis, renal artery stenosis, and hypovolemia. Ordinarily, volume contraction stimulates the secretion of aldosterone and enhances K^+ secretion. However, this homeostatic mechanism can be overwhelmed with severe reductions in distal flow and/or concurrent predisposition toward hyperkalemia (from medications such as ACE inhibitors, angiotensin receptor blockers, or aldosterone antagonists, for example).

DIAGNOSIS

Clinical Presentation

- The two principal clinical manifestations of hyperkalemia are **muscle weakness** and **cardiac conduction disturbances.** Hyperkalemia raises the resting membrane potential of muscle cells. Although muscle contraction is normally associated with membrane depolarization, persistent elevation of membrane potential inactivates Na^+ channels, resulting in muscle weakness.

History
- In hyperkalemia, the first step is to confirm true hyperkalemia by checking **whole-blood [K^+]** and **assessing the EKG for conduction abnormalities** that warrant immediate treatment (see below). Once the patient is out of danger, evaluation of the underlying cause can be undertaken.
- **Review of medications and medical history** often make the diagnosis. Diabetes mellitus may suggest hyporeninemic hypoaldosteronism (HRHA), and chronic kidney disease implies limited ability to excrete K^+. A **dietary history of high K^+ foods** (bananas, tomatoes, potatoes, oranges, melons, avocados, meats, kiwis, milk, spinach, apricots, lima beans, papayas, cucumber) or K^+-containing salt substitutes should be sought. History of trauma may indicate rhabdomyolysis (elevated CPK). Recent chemotherapy should raise the possibility of tumor lysis syndrome (hyperphosphatemia hyperuricemia). If the cause of hyperkalemia is still not obvious, then an evaluation of urinary potassium excretion should follow.

Diagnostic Testing
Laboratories
- **Pseudohyperkalemia** should be ruled out by checking whole-blood [K^+].
- **TTKG:** As with hypokalemia, spot measurements of urine K^+ may be misleading. Therefore, TTKG should be checked.
- Normal renal response to hyperkalemia is to raise TTKG to >10.
  - A TTKG <7 suggests decreased aldosterone effect. Two caveats for a valid TTKG assessment are that the urine osmolality should be greater than the plasma osmolality (to ensure that water is being reabsorbed in the collecting duct) and that the urine sodium is >25 mEq/L (to ensure that potassium excretion is not limited by decreased sodium delivery). The causes of decreased aldosterone effect are described above.
  - If the TTKG suggests hypoaldosteronism and the clinical presentation does not reveal an obvious etiology, plasma renin activity, aldosterone, and cortisol levels can be obtained from a morning sample after the patient has been ambulating for ≥3 hours or after the administration of furosemide the previous evening and again in the morning.

TABLE 7-1	RENIN AND ALDOSTERONE LEVELS WITH HYPERKALEMIA AND A LOW TRANSTUBULAR POTASSIUM GRADIENT		
Disorder		Renin	Aldosterone
Primary hypoaldosteronism		↑	↓
Aldosterone receptor blockade, pseudohypoaldosteronism type I		↑	↑
Hyporeninemic hypoaldosteronism		↓	↓

↓, decreased; ↑, increased.

○ Hyporeninemic hypoaldosteronism presents with low/low-to-normal renin and low aldosterone levels.

○ In primary adrenal insufficiency, renin is high but aldosterone and cortisol levels are low.

○ In pseudohypoaldosteronism type I (aldosterone resistance) and pharmacologic aldosterone receptor blockade (e.g., amiloride and triamterene), renin and aldosterone levels are high (see Table 7-1).

• **Acid-base status:** Nonanion gap acidosis along with low urine pH is often seen along with decreased aldosterone effect (type IV RTA). Hyperkalemic variant of type I RTA also presents with nongap acidosis, but in this disorder the urine pH will be high.

Electrocardiography

• EKG changes classically involve increased amplitude and narrowing of the T wave and shortening of the QT interval at [K^+] levels >6 mEq/L. As [K^+] increases further to >7 to 8 mEq/L, the PR interval increases, and loss of the P wave can occur along with widening of the QRS. This sine-wave pattern can degenerate rapidly to ventricular fibrillation or asystole if untreated. The level at which neuromuscular symptoms or EKG changes occur in a particular

TABLE 7-2	SYNDROMES OF APPARENT MINERALOCORTICOID EXCESS

Primary hyperaldosteronism (low renin, high aldosterone)—Adrenal adenoma, hyperplasia, carcinoma, glucocorticoid-remediable hyperaldosteronism
Secondary hyperaldosteronism (high renin, high aldosterone)—Renal artery stenosis, malignant hypertension, renin-secreting tumors, low ECV
Increased alternate mineralocorticoids (low renin, low aldosterone)—11β-HSD-2 deficiency (real licorice, chewing tobacco, genetic mutation), overwhelmed 11β-HSD-2 (Cushing syndrome, salt-sparing CAH)

CAH, congenital adrenal hyperplasia; ECV, effective circulating volume; HSD, hydroxysteroid dehydrogenase patient is highly variable. Chronic hyperkalemia is more likely to present with normal EKG. In addition, the presence of other abnormalities, such as hypocalcemia or hyponatremia, amplifies the effects of hyperkalemia on cardiac conduction.

TREATMENT

- As described previously, the treatment of hyperkalemia must be initiated in the context of the [K$^+$], and the presence or absence of neuromuscular symptoms and electrocardiography changes.
- A significant elevation in the absence of symptoms or EKG changes may be due to pseudohyperkalemia (which should be ruled out by checking whole-blood K$^+$) or chronic hyperkalemia (in which cellular adaptation has taken place).
- Correction of contributing factors such as acidemia, hypocalcemia, and hyponatremia decreases the hyperkalemic effects on the cell membrane. Other modalities involve stabilizing the cell membrane with calcium, driving potassium into the cells, and, ultimately, removing excess potassium.
- **Methods to stabilize the cell membrane or move potassium inside the cell are only temporizing measures, and potassium needs to be removed to resolve the total body excess.**
  - **Calcium IV is the first treatment in severe hyperkalemia,** because it stabilizes the myocardial membrane.
    - Calcium chloride contains 13.6 mEq (272 mg) of elemental calcium per gram, whereas calcium gluconate contains 4.7 mEq (93 mg) per gram. Therefore, 1 g of calcium chloride may be sufficient, but if calcium gluconate is given, 2 g may be required.
    - If extravasation occurs, calcium can cause tissue necrosis; administration through a central venous line is preferred to peripheral IV, especially with calcium chloride. Each gram of calcium should be given slowly (over 5 to 10 minutes).
  - **Insulin** rapidly (within minutes) lowers serum [K$^+$] by causing intracellular shift, and the effect can last up to a few hours.[4,25,26]
    - It is usually given as a dose of 10 units of regular insulin IV along with 25 to 50 g of dextrose (1 to 2 ampules of 50% dextrose).
    - A peak reduction in serum [K$^+$] of 1 to 1.5 mEq/L can be expected.
    - If the patient already has hyperglycemia, insulin can be given alone. Patients who are normoglycemic may become hypoglycemic when 10 units of regular insulin is administered with only 25 g of dextrose.
    - If glucose alone is given to nondiabetic patients, endogenous secretion of insulin will lower serum [K$^+$]. However, in insulin-dependent diabetics, glucose alone can produce hyperkalemia due to increased serum osmolality.[27]
  - **β_2-Adrenergic agents** have a similar effect on intracellular transport of potassium.[25]
    - **Albuterol** is classically given in a dose of 5 to 20 mg by nebulizer or 0.5 mg IV. With IV administration, the onset of action is similar to insulin, but the effect is slightly delayed when given by nebulizer.

- The magnitude and duration of effect is similar to that of insulin administration.
- Owing to the risk of precipitating coronary events secondary to beta-agonist–induced tachycardia, alternate agents are preferred in patients with known or suspected hyperkalemia.

○ **Renal elimination** is preferred when possible and is often the only measure necessary for mild to moderate hyperkalemia.

- Increasing delivery of sodium and poorly reabsorbed anions (e.g., bicarbonate) will increase K^+ excretion; this can be accomplished by sodium chloride, sodium bicarbonate (see below), or diuretic (especially loop diuretic) administration.
- The patient with hyperkalemia and volume depletion may respond readily to fluid administration alone.
- The euvolemic patient may be treated with simultaneous saline and loop diuretics.
- The volume overloaded patient may respond to diuresis alone.
- Patients with PHA type II respond dramatically to thiazide diuretics.
- Sodium bicarbonate, although raising extracellular pH, causes K^+ to shift into cells; the primary mechanism by which bicarbonate lowers serum $[K^+]$ is through stimulating renal excretion.[25,28]
  □ As a treatment for hyperkalemia, bicarbonate should be used with caution, after correction of hypocalcemia.[29]
  □ It is administered as 50 mEq (one ampule) IV for several minutes. Administration is often limited by the complications of sodium loading in patients with CHF or chronic kidney disease, which can be followed by a continuous IV infusion.

○ **Cation-exchange resins** like sodium polystyrene sulfonate (SPS, Kayexalate) are used to eliminate excess potassium by exchanging potassium for sodium in the GI tract.

- They can be given orally or rectally.
- Although the rectal preparation has a faster onset of action than the oral preparation, the oral route is preferable, given recent reports of intestinal necrosis, particularly in patients with recent abdominal surgery, bowel injury, or intestinal dysfunction.[30]
- The normal dose is 15 g PO q6 h or 30 to 50 g PR, as needed. Each gram removes up to 1 mEq of potassium. In exchange, 1 to 2 mEq of sodium is absorbed.
- There is no role for these agents in patients with impending dialysis treatments as it will cause them to have loose bowel movements during their treatment.

○ **Dialysis:** If hyperkalemia is severe, especially when renal and GI routes of elimination are not feasible, dialysis can be life saving.

- Peritoneal dialysis (PD) can lower $[K^+]$ as well, but not nearly as rapidly as hemodialysis (HD).
  □ If PD is chosen, several rapid exchanges (~60- to 70-minutes dwell time per exchange) may be performed conveniently using a cycler.
  □ In a patient with plasma $[K^+]$ of 6.0 mEq, four rapid exchanges can be expected to remove a total of ~25 to 30 mEq of K^+ (similar to two doses of SPS), which may be enough to get the patient out of danger.[31]

- In more severe hyperkalemia or clinical conditions in which continued K^+ influx into plasma is expected (i.e., tissue necrosis), HD may be necessary.
  - If HD is used, a dialysate $[K^+]$ of 2 mEq/L is often sufficient.
  - In severe hyperkalemia, dialysate $[K^+]$ of 1 mEq/L may be used for the first 30 to 60 min, with close monitoring of whole-blood $[K^+]$.
  - If one anticipates HD will be started in a timely manner, IV calcium may be the only treatment necessary; treatment with insulin and beta agonist will only reduce the efficacy of HD by driving K^+ into cells, where it cannot be removed by the dialyzer.
  - Similarly, use of SPS should be avoided prior to anticipated HD; SPS takes several hours to work and will only cause the patient to have diarrhea while on dialysis.
  - It is important to remember that immediate post-HD plasma $[K^+]$ represents a nadir, and intracellular K^+ will subsequently shift to the extracellular space (called "rebound"). Thus, potassium repletion for a serum $[K^+]$ that appears to have overcorrected after dialysis is seldom appropriate.
- Chronic hyperkalemia is often associated with diabetic-associated HRHA, renal failure, or CHF. The serum potassium in this setting is usually stable and ≤6 mEq/L. Many of these patients are appropriately maintained on medications to treat the underlying condition(s), such as ACE inhibitors or spironolactone. Not infrequently these medications are discontinued due to mild elevations in the $[K^+]$. In almost all cases, a moderate reduction in potassium intake, the use of diuretics as indicated, and a tolerance for stable mild to moderate hyperkalemia allows successful continuation.

REFERENCES

1. Giebisch G. Renal potassium channels: function, regulation, and structure. *Kidney Int.* 2001;60:436–445.
2. Palmer LG, Frindt G. Aldosterone and potassium secretion by the cortical collecting duct. *Kidney Int.* 2000;57:1324–1328.
3. Rose, BD. *Clinical Physiology of Acid-Base and Electrolyte Disorders.* New York, NY: McGraw-Hill, Medical Publishing Division; 2001.
4. Clausen T, Flatman JA. Effects of insulin and epinephrine on Na+-K+ and glucose transport in soleus muscle. *Am J Physiol.* 1987;252[4 Pt 1]:E492–499.
5. Crook MA, Hally V, Panteli JV. The importance of the refeeding syndrome. *Nutrition.* 2001;17:632–637.
6. Gennari FJ. Hypokalemia. *N Engl J Med.* 1998;339:451–458.
7. Viens P, Thyss A, Garnier G, et al. GM-CSF treatment and hypokalemia. *Ann Intern Med.* 1989;111(3):263.
8. Ryan DP, da Silva MR, Soong TW, et al. Mutations in potassium channel Kir2.6 cause susceptibility to thyrotoxic hypokalemic periodic paralysis. *Cell.* 2010;140:88–98.
9. Scheinman SJ, Guay-Woodford LM, Thakker RV, et al. Mechanisms of disease: genetic disorders of renal electrolyte transport. *N Engl J Med.* 1999;340:1177–1187.
10. Junco E, Perez R, Jofre R, et al. Renal ammoniagenesis in acute hypokalemia *in vivo* in the dog. *Contrib Nephrol.* 1988;63:125–131.
11. Ethier JH, Kamel KS, Magner PO, et al. The transtubular potassium concentration in patients with hypokalemia and hyperkalemia. *Am J Kidney Dis.* 1990;15(4):309–315.

12. Cely CM, Contreras G. Approach to the patient with hypertension, unexplained hypoka-lemia, and metabolic alkalosis. *Am J Kidney Dis.* 2001;37(3):E24.

13. Roden DM, Iansmith DH. Effects of low potassium or magnesium concentrations on isolated cardiac tissue. *Am J Med.* 1987;82:18–23.

14. Roy LF, Villeneuve JP, Dumont A, et al. Irreversible renal failure associated with triam-terene. *Am J Nephrol.* 1991;11:486–488.

15. Don B, Sebastian A, Cheitlin M, et al. Pseudohyperkalemia caused by fist clenching during phlebotomy. *N Engl J Med.* 1990;322:1290–1292.

16. Rutledge R, Sheldon GF, Collins ML. Massive transfusion. *Crit Care Clin.* 1986;2:791–805.

17. Knichwitz G, Zahl M, Van Aken H, et al. Intraoperative washing of long-stored packed red blood cells by using an autotransfusion device prevents hyperkalemia. *Anesth Analg.* 2002;95:324–325.

18. Bystrom S, Sjogaard G. Potassium homeostasis during and following exhaustive submaxi-mal static handgrip contractions. *Acta Physiol Scand.* 1991;142:59–66.

19. Medbo JI, Sejersted OM. Plasma potassium changes with high intensity exercise. *J Physiol.* 1990;421:105–122.

20. Markewitz BA, Elstad MR. Succinylcholine-induced hyperkalemia following prolonged pharmacologic neuromuscular blockade. *Chest.* 1997;111:248–250.

21. Perez G, Oster J, Vaamonde C. Serum potassium concentration in acidemic states. *Nephron.* 1981;27:233–243.

22. Wiggam MI, Beringer TR. Effect of low-molecular-weight heparin on serum concentra-tions of potassium. *Lancet.* 1997;349:1447.

23. Furgeson S, Linas S. Mechanisms of type I and type II pseudohypoaldosteronism. *J Am Soc Nephrol.* 2010;21(11):1842–1845.

24. Heering P, Degenhardt S, Grabensee B. Tubular dysfunction following kidney transplanta-tion. *Nephron.* 1996;74:501–511.

25. Allon M, Shanklin N. Effect of bicarbonate administration on plasma potassium in dialysis patients: interactions with insulin and albuterol. *Am J Kidney Dis.* 1996;28:508–514.

26. Ljutic D, Rumboldt Z. Should glucose be administered before, with, or after insulin, in the management of hyperkalemia? *Ren Fail.* 1993;15:73–76.

27. Viberti GC. Glucose-induced hyperkalemia: a hazard for diabetics? *Lancet.* 1978;1:690–691.

28. Gutierrez R, Schlessinger F, Oster JR, et al. Effect of hypertonic versus isotonic sodium bicarbonate on plasma potassium concentration in patients with end-stage renal disease. *Miner Electrolyte Metab.* 1991;17(5):297–302.

29. Oberleithner H, Greger R, Lang F. The effect of respiratory and metabolic acid-base changes on ionized calcium concentration: *in vivo* and *in vitro* experiments in man and rat. *Eur J Clin Invest.* 1982;12(6):451–455.

30. Watson M, Abbott KC, Yuan CM. Damned if you do, damned if you don't: potassium binding resins in hyperkalemia. *Clin J Am Soc Nephrol.* 2010;5(10):1723–1726.

31. Brown ST, Ahearn DJ, Nolph KD. Potassium removal with peritoneal dialysis. *Kidney Int.* 1973;4(1):67–69.

Disorders of Calcium Metabolism

8

Yekaterina Gincherman

GENERAL PRINCIPLES

- The average diet contains 1000 to 1200 mg of calcium, mainly from dairy products.
  - Approximately 20% to 40% is absorbed in the small intestine, whereas the remaining calcium is excreted in the stool along with a small additional amount from colonic secretions.
  - Maintenance of calcium balance involves buffering in the skeletal system and tightly controlled excretion in the kidneys, as seen in Figure 8-1.
    - In the kidney, 80% to 85% of the calcium load is reabsorbed along the proximal nephron. In the ascending loop of Henle, calcium is reabsorbed passively through the tight junction protein, paracellin-1.
    - Although a smaller percentage is reabsorbed in the distal tubule, distal calcium reabsorption is actively regulated by the actions of parathyroid hormone (PTH).[1]
- A total of 99% of elemental calcium is found in the bone, complexed as hydroxyapatite crystals. A measure of <1% of total body calcium remains in the extracellular fluid (ECF).
- In the ECF, 50% of calcium is in the ionized state, 40% is bound to albumin (and thus not filterable at the kidney), and 10% is bound to anions like citrate, sulfate, and phosphate as a filterable complex. The normal calcium range is 8.6 to 10.3 mg/dL. The ionized fraction is physiologically active and therefore tightly regulated in a narrow range (4.5 to 5.1 mg/dL) by the following mechanisms:
  - **PTH:**
    - The parathyroid gland senses the ECF-ionized calcium concentration via a calcium-sensing receptor. High levels of ECF calcium stimulate the receptor and cause a transient rise in intracellular calcium concentration that inhibits the release of PTH. Low concentrations of ECF calcium stimulate PTH production and secretion.
    - **In the kidney,** PTH enhances tubular reabsorption of calcium, decreases proximal tubular reabsorption of phosphate, and stimulates the generation of calcitriol in the proximal tubule.
    - By promoting calcitriol synthesis, PTH has an indirect effect of increasing gut absorption of calcium and phosphorus.
  - **Vitamin D** is a fat-soluble vitamin present in diet and produced in the skin in the presence of ultraviolet light. 25-Hydroxylase in the liver forms calcidiol.[2]

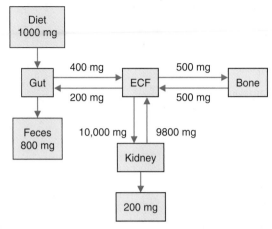

FIGURE 8-1. Daily calcium fluxes in a healthy adult in zero mineral ion balance. Values are expressed in mg/day. ECF, extracellular fluid.

○ **Calcitriol** is formed in the proximal tubule from 1-α hydroxylation of calcidiol. It can also be formed in activated macrophages and a population of lymphocytes derived from thymus.

- The main role of calcitriol is to improve the availability of calcium and phosphate.
- In the **intestine and kidney,** calcitriol stimulates **calcium absorption.**
- In the **bone,** calcitriol complements the actions of PTH, stimulating osteoclastic **bone resorption.**
- Calcitriol acts directly on the **parathyroid gland** to **inhibit** both **PTH synthesis and secretion.**
- Calcitriol is inactived by 24-hydroxylase. Activity of this enzyme is increased by calcitriol and decreased by PTH.

HYPERCALCEMIA

GENERAL PRINCIPLES

Pathophysiology

- Clinically significant hypercalcemia is invariably caused by both an increase in entry of calcium into the ECF from bone resorption or intestinal absorption and a decrease in renal clearance of calcium. Primary hyperparathyroidism (>50%) and malignancy (~40%) account for the majority (>90%) of cases (Table 8-1).[3]
- **Increased bone resorption:**
  ○ **Primary hyperparathyroidism** (sporadic, familial, MEN1, MEN2, lithium therapy) is the **most common cause of hypercalcemia in *ambulatory* patients.**
    - An adenoma of a single gland is found in 85% of cases and 15% of cases are due to hyperplasia of all four glands.

TABLE 8-1	CAUSES OF HYPERCALCEMIA

Increased Bone Resorption
Primary hyperparathyroidism
MEN1 & MEN2A
Malignancy
Postrenal transplant
Immobilization
Familial hypocalciuric hypercalcemia
Thyrotoxicosis
Paget disease
Vitamin A intoxication
Lithium
Adrenal insufficiency

Increased Intestinal Absorption
Milk-alkali syndrome
Granulomatous disease
Vitamin D intoxication

Decreased Renal Excretion
Thiazide diuretics
Acute renal failure
Volume depletion
Vasoactive intestinal polypeptide tumors (VIPoma)
Pheochromocytoma

- Parathyroid carcinoma is responsible for <1% of the cases.
- Most patients are asymptomatic, and hypercalcemia, which is usually modest, is discovered incidentally.
- These patients remain at risk for long-term consequences of hyperparathyroidism such as nephrolithiasis and osteopenia.
  - **Malignancy** is responsible for most cases of hypercalcemia among *hospitalized* patients. There are three mechanisms of malignant hypercalcemia:
    - **Osteolytic hypercalcemia** is caused by cytokines produced by the tumor cells that act locally to stimulate osteoclastic bone resorption.
      - This form of malignant hypercalcemia is responsible for the majority of malignancy-associated cases.
      - It occurs only with extensive bone involvement by tumor, most often due to breast carcinoma, non–small-cell lung cancer, myeloma, and lymphoma.
    - **Humoral hypercalcemia of malignancy** results from tumor products acting systemically to stimulate bone resorption and decrease renal calcium excretion.
      - **PTH-related peptide (PTHrP)** is an important mediator of this syndrome.
    - Humoral hypercalcemia of malignancy is caused most often by squamous carcinoma of the lung, head and neck, or esophagus, or by renal, bladder, or ovarian carcinoma.
    - **Tumoral calcitriol production** may occasionally occur in Hodgkin's and nonHodgkin's lymphomas.

- **Tertiary hyperparathyroidism:** Long-term dialysis patients may develop parathyroid hyperplasia and an autonomous secretion of PTH.
  - Persistent PTH secretion after a successful transplant may lead to hypercalcemia.[4] This is usually mild and tends to decrease over 6 to 12 months.
  - The use of calcimimetics in end-stage renal disease patients has been associated with parathyroid hyperplasia, predisposing transplant patients to hypercalcemia after transplant, which can often be severe.
- **Immobilization:** Sustained bed rest leads to an increase in bone resorption and may lead to hypercalcemia.
  - This is usually seen in patients with spinal cord injuries, those in full body casts, or in intensive care unit setting.
  - Mobilization corrects hypercalcemia.
- **Familial hypocalciuric hypercalcemia (FHH)** is an autosomal-dominant disorder in which mutation in the calcium-sensing receptor causes decreased receptor activity.
  - Patients have a mild hypercalcemia, hypophosphatemia, and normal or mildly elevated PTH levels.
  - FHH can be differentiated from primary hyperparathyroidism by the reduction in urinary calcium excretion.
  - Parathyroidectomy is not indicated.
- **Thyrotoxicosis** may stimulate osteoclastic bone resorption, causing a mild hypercalcemia. Concurrent hyperparathyroidism can also occur.
- **Vitamin A intoxication** (doses >50,000 IU/d) can be associated with hypercalcemia secondary to increased osteoclast bone resorption.
- **Increased intestinal absorption:** This is a less frequent cause of hypercalcemia, but assumes greater importance in the setting of chronic renal failure.
  - **Milk-alkali syndrome:** Ingestion of large quantities of calcium-carbonate-based antacids can lead to this condition, characterized by hypercalcemia, alkalemia, nephrocalcinosis, and renal failure.
  - **Granulomatous disease:** Sarcoidosis, tuberculosis, and leprosy cause hypercalcemia because of the conversion of calcidiol to calcitriol by the 1-α hydroxylase present in macrophages contained in the granulomas. Treatment of the underlying disease corrects the hypercalcemia.
  - **Vitamin D intoxication:** It may be observed in dialysis patients overtreated with vitamin D analogs. Hypercalcemia is usually mild and improves with dose adjustment or discontinuation of the drug.
- **Decreased renal excretion:**
  - Acute renal failure
  - Volume depletion
  - Thiazide diuretics can be associated with a mild hypercalcemia likely due to increased proximal reabsorption from volume contraction.

DIAGNOSIS

Clinical Presentation

- Mild hypercalcemia is often asymptomatic and incidentally discovered on routine blood tests. Long-term manifestations include osteoporosis, nephrolithiasis, and chronic kidney disease (CKD).

- Severe hypercalcemia is often associated with neurologic and gastrointestinal (GI) symptoms.
  - **GI symptoms** include anorexia, nausea, vomiting, and constipation.
  - **Neurologic symptoms** include weakness, fatigue, confusion, stupor, and coma.
  - **Renal manifestations** include polyuria and nephrolithiasis. Polyuria combined with nausea and vomiting can cause volume depletion, resulting in impaired calcium excretion and worsening of hypercalcemia.

Diagnostic Testing

Laboratories

- **Calcium** should be interpreted in the context of the plasma albumin concentration (corrected calcium) or ionized calcium should be measured.
- **Phosphorus** may be low in settings of elevated PTH (primary hyperparathyroidism) or PTHrP (e.g., humoral hypercalcemia of malignancy). Phosphorus may be high in vitamin D toxicity or increased bone resorption without hyperparathyroidism (Paget disease).
- **Intact PTH** levels are elevated or inappropriately normal in primary hyperparathyroidism. PTH is almost always suppressed in patients with hypercalcemia because of other causes, except FHH, tertiary hyperparathyroidism, and lithium use.
- **PTHrP** can be measured to confirm the diagnosis of humoral hypercalcemia of malignancy.
- **1,25(OH)$_2$D$_3$** (calcitriol) levels are elevated in granulomatous disorders and calcitriol overdose.
- **25(OH)D** levels are elevated with noncalcitriol vitamin D intoxication (rare).
- **Urinary calcium:** Patients with FHH can be distinguished from primary hyperparathyroidism by low **urinary calcium** concentrations (<200 mg calcium per 24 hours or fractional excretion of calcium <1%).

TREATMENT

- **Volume repletion:**
  - **Correction of hypovolemia is the initial goal** and often requires at least 3 to 4 L of 0.9% saline in the first 24 hours.
  - Continuing maintenance IV fluids after restoring ECF volume promotes further calcium excretion.
  - Electrolyte concentrations should be monitored every 8 to 12 hours during induction and maintenance of diuresis.
- **Diuretics:** Although loop diuretics impair tubular reabsorption of calcium, they are generally not used for acute hypercalcemia as they may result in further volume depletion. They are useful, however, if evidence of volume overload develops. Thiazide diuretics should be avoided as they enhance calcium reabsorption by the kidney.
- **Bisphosphonates:** Intravenous bisphosphonates inhibit bone resorption and should be administered early because their effect is delayed.
  - **Pamidronate,** 60 to 90 mg, is infused over 2 to 4 hours.
    - A hypocalcemic response is seen within 2 days, peaks at 7 days, and may persist for ≥2 weeks.
    - Treatment can be repeated after 7 days if hypercalcemia recurs.

○ **Zoledronate** is a more potent bisphosphonate that is given as a 4 mg dose infused over at least 15 minutes.

○ During treatment with bisphosphonates, renal dysfunction can occur from the precipitation of calcium bisphosphonate. Hydration should precede their use, and renal insufficiency is a relative contraindication.

○ Side effects include hypocalcemia, hypomagnesemia, hypophosphatemia, and renal dysfunction.

• **Calcitonin:** Calcitonin inhibits bone resorption and increases renal calcium excretion. As a treatment for acute hypercalcemia, it can be dosed as follows:

○ Salmon calcitonin, 4 to 8 IU/kg IM or SC, q6h to q12h, lowers plasma calcium by 1 to 2 mg/dL within several hours in 60% to 70% of patients.

○ The hypocalcemic effect wanes after several days because of tachyphylaxis.

○ Calcitonin is less potent than other inhibitors of bone resorption, but has no serious toxicity, is safe in renal failure, and may have an analgesic effect in patients with skeletal metastases.[5]

○ It can be used early in the treatment of severe hypercalcemia to achieve a rapid response.

○ Side effects include flushing, nausea, and, rarely, allergic reactions.

• **Glucocorticoids** lower calcium concentrations by

○ inhibiting cytokine release

○ direct cytolytic effects on some tumor cells

○ inhibiting intestinal calcium absorption

○ increasing urinary calcium excretion

○ They are effective in hypercalcemia due to hematologic malignancies including myeloma, tumoral or granulomatous production of calcitriol, and vitamins D and A intoxication.

○ The initial dose is 20 to 60 mg/d of prednisone. Plasma calcium concentration may take 5 to 10 days to fall. After plasma calcium stabilizes, the dose should be gradually reduced to the minimum needed to control symptoms of hypercalcemia.

• **Gallium nitrate:** It inhibits bone resorption as effectively as the IV bisphosphonates and has a similar delayed onset of 2 days.

○ It is given as a 100 to 200 mg/m^2/d continuous infusion for up to 5 days, unless normocalcemia is achieved sooner.

○ There is a significant risk of nephrotoxicity and it is contraindicated if the plasma createnine is >2.5 mg/dL.

• **Dialysis:** Both **hemodialysis** and **peritoneal dialysis** using dialysate with low calcium are very effective means of treating hypercalcemia. Very low calcium dialysis baths should be used with caution as rapid development of hypocalcemia can occur.

• **Parathyrodectomy** in cases of hyperparathyroidism is indicated if the following criteria are met.[6]

(a) Corrected plasma calcium >1 mg/dL above upper limit of normal

(b) Hypercalciuria >400 mg/d

(c) Renal insufficiency

(d) Reduced bone mass (T-score <−2.5 by DEXA)

(e) Age <50 years

(f) Nephrolithiasis

(g) Lack of feasibility of long-term follow-up

HYPOCALCEMIA

GENERAL PRINCIPLES

Pathophysiology

- Hypocalcemia can result from either decreased calcium absorption from the GI tract or decreased calcium resorption from bone.
- **Decreased calcium absorption:**
  - **Vitamin D deficiency:** Vitamin D (calcidiol) deficiency is a very common problem. Limited exposure to sunlight is the leading cause.
    - Nutritional deficiency of vitamin D can lead to rickets and osteomalacia.
    - As vitamin D is fat soluble, the deficiency can be seen in malabsorption syndromes.
    - Anticonvulsants can result in vitamin D deficiency by stimulating the hepatic metabolism of calcidiol.
  - **CKD:** The loss of renal functional mass and reduced activity of 1-α hydroxylase from phosphorus retention both contribute to the decreased renal conversion of calcidiol (25(OH)D) to calcitriol (1,25(OH)$_2$D$_3$). With decreasing levels of calcitriol, patients with CKD are prone to develop hypocalcemia. However, the balance is partly maintained by increasing levels of PTH as glomerular filteration rate declines.
  - **Vitamin D-dependent rickets:** This condition is the result of either impaired hydroxylation of calcidiol to calcitriol (type I) or end-organ resistance to calcitriol (type II).
    - Type I patients respond to physiologic doses of calcitriol.
    - Patients with type II disease have mutations in the vitamin D receptor. They tend to have dramatically increased concentrations of calcitriol and respond poorly to calcitriol therapy.
- **Decreased PTH level or effect:**
  - **Hypoparathyroidism** can be associated with acquired and inherited diseases that result from either impaired synthesis or release of PTH.
    - The most common cause is polyglandular autoimmune syndrome type I, associated with chronic mucocutaneous candidiasis and primary adrenal insufficiency.
    - Occasionally, pernicious anemia, diabetes mellitus, vitiligo, and autoimmune thyroid disease are also associated with hypoparathyroidism.
    - Hypoparathyroidism may be iatrogenic after thyroidectomy.
    - It can also occur secondary to radiation, infiltrative disorders, or deposition of metals such as iron, copper, or aluminum.
  - **Hypomagnesemia:** Severe magnesium deficiency results in decreased PTH secretion from the gland.[7] Patients with hypocalcemia due to hypomagnesemia do not respond to calcium or vitamin D replacement until the magnesium deficit has been replaced.
  - **Familial hypocalcemia** results from activating mutations in the calcium-sensing receptor. Subsequent downregulation of PTH transcription leads to hypocalcemia from inappropriately low PTH levels due to receptor malfunction.

- Pseudohypoparathyroidism (Albright hereditary osteodystrophy) is a hereditary disorder in which the target cell response to PTH is decreased. Renal calcium excretion is increased and the PTH level is increased. Phenotypic characteristics include short stature, obesity, shortened metacarpals and metatarsals, and heterotopic calcification.
  - Calcimimetics have been used for the control of elevated PTH levels in patients with secondary hyperparathyroidism. In one study, 81% of patients treated with these agents experienced hypocalcemia induced by calcimimetics.[8]
- Extravascular deposition/intravascular chelation:
  - Less commonly, hypocalcemia occurs as a result of either extravascular deposition or intravascular chelation of calcium (Table 8-2).
  - Hungry bone syndrome: A profound reduction in calcium concentration can occur after surgical removal of parathyroid.
    - This "hungry bone syndrome" is due to a rapid bone mineralization in the absence of PTH.
    - Symptoms can occur soon after surgery, and patients' calcium levels should be carefully monitored (q4h to q6h).

TABLE 8-2 CAUSES OF HYPOCALCEMIA

Decreased PTH Level or Effect
Hypomagnesemia
Hypoparathyroidism (surgical or autoimmune)
Familial hypocalcemia
Pseudohypoparathyroidism
Postradiation
Infiltrative
Deposition of metals (iron, copper, or aluminum)

Disorders of Vitamin D Metabolism
Vitamin D deficiency
Drugs (anticonvulsants)
Renal disease
Vitamin D-dependent rickets

Extravascular Deposition/Intravascular Chelation
Hungry bone syndrome (after parathyrodectomy, correction of vitamin D deficiency)
Rhabdomyolysis
Tumor lysis syndrome
Acute pancreatitis
Citrate-containing blood products
Continuous dialysis with citrate
Plasma exchange with citrate
Parentral/enteral phosphate

Miscellaneous
Septic shock

PTH, parathyroid hormone.

- Hungry bone syndrome has also been described after the administration of calcimimetics for secondary hyperparathyroidism in dialysis patients.[9,10]
- Hypocalcemia also occurs after thyroid surgery (5% of cases).
  - ○ **Hyperphosphatemia:** High concentrations of phosphorus form complexes with extracellular calcium, resulting in hypocalcemia.
    - This phenomenon can occur during rapid release of intracellular phosphorus, as seen in rhabdomyolysis and tumor lysis syndrome (TLS).
    - Iatrogenic causes of this can occur during the administration of intravenous phosphorus or phosphorus-containing enemas.
  - ○ **Acute pancreatitis:** The release of pancreatic lipase digests retroperitoneal and omental fat. The fatty acids, once released, bind to the calcium. The hypocalcemia is aggravated by the hypoalbuminuria and hypomagnesemia associated with acute pancreatitis.
  - ○ **Citrate-containing blood products:** Massive transfusions of citrate-containing blood products can cause intravascular chelation of calcium, leading to hypocalcemia.[11] The use of citrate in continuous renal replacement therapy or plasma exchange can also cause this.[12]
  - ○ **Gadolinium-based contrast agents:** Gadodiamide and gadoversetamide may interfere with assays for serum calcium, and unexpected hypocalcia detected immediately after the administration of these agents should be rechecked before action is taken.[13]
- **Septic shock:** Endotoxic shock has been associated with hypocalcemia through unclear mechanisms. Hypocalcemia may be partially responsible for the hypotension, as myocardial function correlates with ionized calcium levels.

DIAGNOSIS

Clinical Presentation

- **Symptoms** depend not only on the degree of hypocalcemia but also on the rate of decline of the plasma calcium concentration.
  - ○ Precipitation of symptoms is also influenced by plasma pH and the presence or absence of concomitant hypomagnesemia, hypokalemia, or hyponatremia.
  - ○ **Neuromuscular excitability** symptoms are the most common ones.
    - The patient may experience circumoral and distal extremity paresthesias or carpopedal spasm.
    - Other manifestations include mental status changes, irritability, and seizures.

Physical Examination

- On **physical exam,** hypotension, bradycardia, laryngeal spasm, and bronchospasm may be present.
  - ○ Neurologic exam is significant for latent tetany, elicited as classical **Chvostek's** (facial twitch elicited by tapping on the facial nerve just below the zygomatic arch with the mouth slightly open) and **Trousseau's sign** (development of wrist flexion, metacarpophalangeal joint flexion, hyperextended fingers, and thumb flexion after a blood pressure cuff has been inflated to 20 mm Hg above systolic pressure for a duration of 3 minutes).

○ Cardiovascular effects include hypotension, prolonged QT interval, and impaired excitation contraction coupling, leading to congestive heart failure.

○ Long-standing hypocalcemia can also be associated with subcapsular cataracts.

Diagnostic Testing

Laboratories

- **Total calcium concentration should be corrected to the serum albumin.**
  - ○ Decreased total plasma calcium concentration is found in hypoalbuminemia without changes in the ionized calcium level. In general, for every 1.0 g/dL decrement in plasma albumin, there is a 0.8 mg/dL decline in the reported total plasma calcium level.
- **Magnesium** deficiency should be ruled out.
- **Phosphorus** will be low in conditions associated with low vitamin D activity, except for kidney failure, where there is decreased renal clearance of phosphorus. The plasma phosphorus will be increased in rhabdomyolysis or TLS.
- **PTH** that is low or inappropriately normal in the setting of hypocalcemia is indicative of hypoparathyroidism. A high PTH is often found with vitamin D deficiency states, CKD, and pseudohypoparathyroidism.
- **25(OH)D** and **1,25(OH)$_2$D$_3$** levels are useful in assessing for vitamin D deficiency and vitamin D-dependent rickets, respectively.

TREATMENT

- In symptomatic hypocalcemia or if corrected calcium concentration of <7.5 mg/dL **IV calcium gluconate** should be administered (100 to 300 mg, or 1 to 3 mL of 10% calcium gluconate solution, over 10 to 15 minutes), the first ampule can be administered over several minutes followed by a constant infusion at a rate of 0.5 to 1.0 mg/kg/h.
  - ○ Adjustments in the rate should be based on serial plasma calcium determinations.
  - ○ Treatment of hypocalcemia is ineffective without adequate treatment of hypomagnesemia.
  - ○ In the setting of metabolic acidosis, hypocalcemia should be corrected before the acidosis.
- Mild hypocalcemia can be treated with **oral calcium supplements** with or without vitamin D. Elemental calcium, 1 to 3 g/d can be given and is best absorbed when taken between meals.
- Patients with hypoparathyroidism generally need both calcium and vitamin D supplementation.
  - ○ **Calcitriol** is one of the most potent of the **vitamin D** preparations and has the fastest onset and shortest duration of action.
  - ○ A dose of 0.5 to 1.0 mcg/d is usually required in patients with hypoparathyroidism.
  - ○ Cholecalciferol and ergocalciferol are less potent but inexpensive.
- In cases of hypoparathyroidism, there is decreased distal tubular calcium reabsorption as a result of a lack of PTH. The increase in the filtered load of

calcium that results from calcium and vitamin D replacement therapy can lead to hypercalciuria, nephrolithiasis, and nephrocalcinosis.

- If urinary calcium excretion exceeds 350 mg/d, despite plasma calcium concentration in the low-to-normal range, sodium intake should be restricted; if this is not effective, a thiazide diuretic should be added.

REFERENCES

1. Friedman PA, Gesek FA. Calcium transport in renal epithelial cells. *Am J Physiol.* 1993;264:F181–F198.
2. Brown AJ, Slatopolsky E. Vitamin D analogs: therapeutic applications and mechanisms for selectivity. *Mol Aspect Med.* 2008;29:433–452.
3. Kasper DL, Braunwald E, Hauser S, et al. *Harrison's Principles of Internal Medicine.* 6th ed. New York, NY: McGraw-Hill; 2004.
4. Garvin PJ, Castaneda M, Linderer R, et al. Management of hypercalcemic hyperparathyroidism after renal transplantation. *Arch Surg.* 1985;120(5):578–583.
5. Deftos LJ, First BP. Calcitonin as a drug. *Ann Intern Med.* 1981;95(2):192–197.
6. Bilezikian JP, Silverberg SJ. Asymptomatic primary hyperparathyroidism. *N Engl J Med.* 2004;350:1746–1751.
7. Wiegmann T, Kaye M. Hypomagnesemic hypocalcemia. *Arch Intern Med.* 1977;137(7): 953–955.
8. Charytan C, Coburn JW, Chonchol M, et al. Cinacalcet hydrochloride is an effective treatment for secondary hyperparathyroidism in patients with CKD not receiving dialysis. *Am J Kidney Dis.* 2005;46:58–67.
9. Nowack R, Wachtler P. Hypophosphatemia and hungry bone syndrome in a dialysis patient with secondary hyperparathyroidism treated with cinacalcet – proposal for improved monitoring. *Clin Lab.* 2006;52:583–587.
10. Lazar ES, Stankus N. Cinacalcet-induced hungry bone syndrome. *Semin Dial.* 2007; 20(1):83–85.
11. Sihler KC, Napolitano LM. Complications of massive transfusion. *Chest.* 2010;137(1):209–220.
12. Hetzel GR, Schmitz M, Wissing H, et al. Regional citrate versus systemic heparin for anticoagulation in critically ill patients on continuous venovenous haemofiltration: a prospective randomized multicenter trial. *Nephrol Dial Transplant.* 2011;26(1):232–239.
13. Gandhi MJ, Narra VR, Brown JJ, et al. Clinical and economic impact of falsely decreased calcium values caused by gadoversetamide interference. *Am J Roentgenol.* 2008;190(3): W213–W217.

Disorders of Phosphorus Metabolism

9

Yekaterina Gincherman

GENERAL PRINCIPLES

- The average diet contains 1000 to 1400 mg of phosphorus, mainly from meat, cereals, and dairy products. Of this, up to 85% is absorbed in the small intestine.[1]
- The remainder is lost in the stool, with an additional 200 mg/d that is secreted into the colon.
- The vast majority of the body's phosphorus content is stored in the skeletal framework. Of the 700 g of phosphorus found in the average individual, 85% of it is in the skeleton and 15% in soft tissues. Extracellular fluid (ECF) contains <1% of total body phosphorus.[2]
- Even in skeletal stores, the phosphorus pool is not stagnant. There is a dynamic capture and release of phosphorus that allows regulation of the serum phosphorus levels.
- The kidney plays a central role in phosphorus balance and excretion. Between 80% and 95% of filtered phosphate is reabsorbed primarily in the proximal tubule.[3]
- Plasma phosphorus levels are regulated by a number of mechanisms that control the skeletal stores of phosphorus as well as renal handling of phosphorus. Of central importance are:
  - **Parathyroid hormone (PTH):** The major role of PTH is to preserve constant serum calcium concentration.
    - At the level of proximal tubule, PTH acts on receptors at apical and basolateral sodium-phosphorus cotransporters to promote phosphorus wasting.
    - PTH also acts directly on bone to increase phosphate entry into the ECF and indirectly on the intestine by stimulating the synthesis of calcitriol.
  - **Vitamin D** increases plasma phosphate because of enhanced intestinal phosphorus absorption by increasing sodium-phosphate cotransport across the apical bush border membrane.
  - **Fibroblast growth factor-23 (FGF-23):** This molecule belongs to a group of substances called *phosphatonins*. Their main effect is to promote renal excretion of phosphate and lower plasma phosphorus levels.
    - In contrast to PTH, FGF-23 also leads to decreased production of calcitriol and, therefore, has a net effect of reducing plasma phosphorus concentration.[4]
    - The reduction of glomerular filtration rate (GFR) in kidney disease, which leads to subsequent phosphorus retention, is a potent stimulus for FGF-23 release.[5]
  - **Insulin** stimulates an intracellular shift in plasma phosphate, thus lowering the plasma phosphorus concentrations.

HYPERPHOSPHATEMIA

GENERAL PRINCIPLES

Definition
- Hyperphosphatemia is defined by a plasma phosphorus concentration that exceeds the normal range of 2.3 to 4.3 mg/dL.
- Although the condition is defined by values outside the normal reference range, some studies suggest that higher phosphorus levels, even within the normal range, may predispose to vascular disease.[6,7]

Pathophysiology
- The **three main mechanisms** that lead to hyperphosphatemia are impaired renal excretion, transcellular shift into the ECF, and increased phosphate intake (Table 9-1).
- **Impaired renal excretion:**
  - **Renal failure:**
    - With declining GFR, the fractional excretion of phosphate begins to increase and reabsorption is suppressed. Once GFR reaches around ≤25 mL/min, it can no longer keep up with the dietary intake and the plasma phosphorus level begins to rise. Hence, hyperphosphatemia is a frequent finding in advanced chronic kidney disease (CKD).
  - **Decreased PTH effect:**
    - Because PTH decreases proximal tubular reabsorption of phosphate, deficiency of this hormone (hypoparathyroidism) or a resistance to its actions (pseudohypoparathyroidism) leads to increased tubular transport of phosphate, resulting in hyperphosphatemia.
  - **Direct stimulation of proximal tubule reabsorption:**
    - Conditions such as acromegaly, tumoral calcinosis, and the administration of bisphosphonates are known to directly stimulate renal phosphorus reabsorption. In the case of acromegaly, this is thought to be mediated by elevated levels of insulin-like growth factor 1.
- **Transcellular shift:**
  - **Acidosis** inhibits phosphate entry into the cells, leading to mild elevation in plasma phosphorus levels.
  - **Hypoinsulinemia** (same mechanism as acidosis)
- **Increased phosphate load:**
  - **Dietary indiscretion** by the patient with CKD
  - **Iatrogenic,** for example, when a patient with CKD is given **Fleet® enemas**
  - **Vitamin D intoxication** can result in increased intestinal absorption of phosphorus.
  - **Increased release of phosphorus from cellular stores**
    - **Rhabdomyolysis** can cause severe hyperphosphatemia acutely, which precipitates hypocalcaemia secondary to malignant calcium phosphate deposition in soft tissues.
    - **Tumor lysis syndrome** usually follows chemotherapy for hematologic malignancies or rapidly growing solid tumors.
    - **Massive hemolysis**

TABLE 9-1 CAUSES OF HYPERPHOSPHATEMIA

Impaired Renal Excretion
Renal failure (acute and chronic)
Hypoparathyroidism
  Developmental
  Autoimmune
  After surgery/radiation
  Activating mutation in calcium-sensing receptor
Parathyroid suppression with **hypercalcemia**
  Vitamin D or A intoxication
  Granulomatous disease
  Bone metastasis
  Immobilization
Pseudohypoparathyroidism
Acromegaly
Tumoral calcinosis
Bisphosphonates
Heparin
Magnesium abnormalities (hyper and hypo)

Transcellular Shift
Rhabdomyolysis
Tumor lysis syndrome
Massive hemolysis
Acidosis
Hypoinsulinemia
Hyperthermia
Hemolytic anemia
Fulminant hepatic failure

Increased Phosphate Intake or Absorption
High phosphate diet (in the setting of CKD)
Flee® enemas
Vitamin D intoxication
Rapid administration of IV phosphorus supplementation

CKD, chronic kidney disease; IV, intravenous.

DIAGNOSIS

Clinical Presentation

- **Symptoms** of acute hyperphosphatemia are generally **attributable to accompanying hypocalcaemia** and include **tetany, seizures, and dysrhythmias.**
- Hypocalcaemia is thought to result from tissue deposition of calcium once calcium × phosphate product reaches >55 and suppression of 1-α hydroxylase by hyperphosphatemia.
- Tissue deposition of calcium can occur in blood vessels, skin, kidneys, and other organs.

- Calciphylaxis is the term used for tissue ischemia that may result from the calcification and subsequent thrombosis of small blood vessels.
- Chronic hyperphosphatemia contributes to renal osteodystrophy.

Diagnostic Testing

Laboratories
- **Plasma creatinine** helps assess renal function.
- **Intact PTH** is elevated in CKD, but is low in the setting of hypoparathyroidism.
- **Creatine kinase** is markedly elevated in rhabdomyolysis.
- **Uric acid** levels are often markedly elevated in tumor lysis syndrome in addition to hyperphosphatemia.
- **Markers of hemolysis** (lactate dehydrogenase, haptoglobin, bilirubin, and so forth) are helpful in the appropriate setting.
- **Calcium** levels are usually low in acute hyperphosphatemia but should only be treated if symptoms occur, as treatment can precipitate, worsening malignant calcium phosphate deposition.

Treatment

- **Acute hyperphosphatemia** in patients who do not have renal insufficiency can be managed by correcting the underlying cause and by saline diuresis.
- **Chronic hyperphosphatemia** is almost always a result of CKD, and the treatment is aimed at reducing the intestinal absorption of phosphate.
  - ○ **Reduce enteric absorption of phosphorus:**
    - **Dietary restriction of phosphate.** The first step is to institute dietary restriction of phosphate to 600 to 900 mg/d.
    - **Niacinamide.** Niacinamide is the amide form of vitamin B and has been shown to reduce phosphorus levels in the dialysis population by decreasing the phosphorus uptake in the gut.[8]
  - ○ **Calcium-based phosphate binders:**
    - Binders are agents that form insoluble complexes with dietary phosphorus to prevent absorption of phosphorus in the gut.
    - Calcium-based binders are often used as first-line agents in patients with CKD who are not on dialysis, as they are widely accessible and inexpensive. However, adding a calcium load to a population at risk for vascular calcification should be done with great caution and frequent monitoring. In patients who already have hypercalcemia or evidence of vascular calcification, an alternative should be utilized.
      - □ **Calcium carbonate** (TUMS) starting at 500 mg (200 mg elemental calcium) tid with meals to a maximum of 3750 mg/d (1500 mg elemental calcium).
      - □ **Calcium acetate** (PHOSLO) starting at 667 mg (167 mg elemental calcium) tid with meals to a maximum of 6000 mg/d (1500 mg elemental calcium).
  - ○ **Non–calcium-based phosphate binders:** They are more expensive, cause GI discomfort.
    - **Sevelamer carbonate** (RENVELA) starting at 800 mg tid with meals; maximum dose 7200 mg/d.
    - **Lanthanum carbonate** (FOSRENOL) starting at 250 mg tid with meals; maximum dose 3000 mg/d.

○ **Hemodialysis:**
  ■ In the dialysis population, elevated phosphorus levels may reflect dietary indiscretions, binder noncompliance, or frequently missed dialysis treatments. Resumption of all of the above is often sufficient to improve plasma phosphorus concentrations.
  ■ Among dialysis modalities, daily nocturnal home hemodialysis is even more effective than intermittent hemodialysis in phosphorus removal.
  ■ In the acute setting, dialysis may be warranted in patients with symptomatic hypocalcemia from severe hyperphosphatemia in conjunction with renal failure.

HYPOPHOSPHATEMIA

GENERAL PRINCIPLES

Definition
• Hypophosphatemia is defined as plasma phosphorus levels below the normal range of 2.3 to 4.3 mg/dL.

Pathophysiology
• Three main mechanisms for hypophosphatemia are redistribution of extracellular phosphate into the intracellular space, decrease in intestinal absorption of phosphate, or increase in renal excretion of phosphate (Table 9-2).
• **Redistribution of extracellular phosphate** (especially important in hospital setting):
  ○ **Respiratory alkalosis** leads to a rise in intracellular pH, which in turn stimulates glycolysis, and phosphate is incorporated into adenosine triphosphate (ATP).
  ○ **Refeeding syndrome** can occur in chronically malnourished individuals, typically 2 to 5 days after they are started on enteral or parenteral feeding.[9] Caloric replacement increases insulin secretion that stimulates cell growth and enhances cellular uptake of phosphate for various molecular pathways.
  ○ **Treatment of diabetic ketoacidosis (DKA)** with intravenous (IV) insulin leads to rapid flux of phosphorus into the cells.
  ○ **Hungry bone syndrome** after partial parathyroidectomy causes movement of phosphate into the cells, leading to hypophosphatemia.
• **Decreased intestinal absorption** (uncommon):
  ○ **Malnutrition:** Poor intake alone is very rarely sufficient to cause hypophosphatemia, but if the quantity of phosphorus ingested remains less than the amount lost in colonic secretions for a prolonged period of time, hypophosphatemia may ensue. Typically, this occurs in conjunction with one of the following exacerbating conditions.
  ○ **Malabsorption syndromes:** In addition to poor intake and absorption of phosphorus and vitamin D, the accompanying diarrhea also contributes to significant gastrointestinal (GI) losses.
  ○ **Oral phosphate binders:** Indiscriminate use of phosphate binders in end-stage renal disease patients who may not be eating very well may lead to low phosphorus levels.

TABLE 9-2	CAUSES OF HYPOPHOSPHATEMIA

Cellular redistribution
Respiratory alkalosis
Refeeding syndrome
Insulin
Intravenous glucose
Hungry bone syndrome
Sepsis
Blast crisis
Growth-stimulating factor therapy
Decreased intestinal absorption
Malabsorption syndromes
Oral phosphate binders
Vitamin D deficiency
Alcoholism
Increased renal excretion
Primary hyperparathyroidism
Vitamin D deficiency (secondary hyperparathyroidism)
Decreased calcium intake
After renal transplant
Barter syndrome
Familial hypercalciuric hypercalcemia
Osmotic diuresis (DKA, recovering ATN)
Familial X-linked hypophosphatemic rickets
Autosomal-dominant hypophosphatemic rickets
Fanconi's syndrome
Wilson Disease
Oncogenic osteomalacia
Hemolytic uremic syndrome
Hyperaldosteronism
Diuretics
Glucocorticoids
Heavy metals
Cisplatin, ifosfamide, foscarnet, rapamycin
Toluene

DKA, diabetic ketoacidosis.

- ○ **Vitamin D deficiency:** Severe deficiency of this vitamin can lead to hypophosphatemia.
  - ■ The secondary hyperparathyroidism resulting from vitamin D deficiency contributes further to hypophosphatemia through increasing renal phosphate excretion.
- ○ **Alcoholism:** Alcoholics often have poor intake of both phosphate and vitamin D, resulting in total body phosphorus depletion. Use of dextrose-containing IV fluids leads to insulin secretion, which further lowers plasma phosphate by intracellular redistribution, as discussed above.
- • **Increased renal excretion:**
  - ○ **Hyperparathyroidism:** PTH causes urinary phosphate loss.[10]

- Hypophosphatemia is usually mild in primary hyperparathyroidism because PTH also stimulates calcitriol synthesis, resulting in increased intestinal absorption of phosphate.
    - However, in severe vitamin D deficiency, the resultant increase in PTH is not accompanied by the compensatory rise in calcitriol levels and hypophosphatemia can be severe.
- **After renal transplant:** Renal phosphate wasting is common after successful renal transplant due to persistently elevated PTH.
- **Osmotic diuresis:** In DKA or recovering acute tubular necrosis (ATN), excessive phosphate losses occur in urine, along with other solutes.
- **Fanconi's syndrome:** A defect in proximal tubular reabsorption will cause phosphorus wasting. Although congenital forms of Fanconi's syndrome are very rare in adults, the syndrome can be a manifestation of proximal tubule toxicity from light chains in multiple myeloma.
- **Familial X-linked hypophosphatemic rickets (XLH)** is caused by mutations in the *PHEX* gene. The condition is characterized by growth retardation, renal phosphate wasting, hypophosphatemia, and rickets. Plasma concentrations of calcitriol are low.
- **Autosomal-dominant hypophosphatemic rickets** has a similar phenotype to XLH but is inherited in an autosomal-dominant fashion. Mutations in the FGF-23 are responsible for the disease.
- **Oncogenic osteomalacia:** Paraneoplastic production of FGF-23 by mesenchymal tumors is responsible for phosphaturia in cases of oncogenic osteomalacia.

DIAGNOSIS

Clinical Presentation

- Symptoms and signs of hypophosphatemia are due to inability to make ATP and occur if total body phosphate depletion is present and the plasma phosphorus level is <1 mg/dL.
- **Neuromuscular symptoms:** weakness, rhabdomyolysis, impaired diaphragmatic function, paresthesias, dysarthria, confusion, seizures, and coma.
- **Hematologic symptoms:** hemolysis and platelet dysfunction.
- Chronic hypophosphatemia leads to rickets in children and osteomalacia in adults.

Diagnostic Testing

Laboratories

- **Fractional excretion of phosphorus and 24-hour urine phosphorus:**
    - Fractional excretion of phosphorus >5% or a urine phosphate excretion of >100 mg per 24 hours in the setting of hypophosphatemia indicates excessive renal loss.
    - Excretion rates are lower in states of impaired intestinal absorption or hypophosphatemia from transcellular shifts.
    - One exception is vitamin D deficiency, which causes phosphaturia from secondary hyperparathyroidism.
- **Plasma calcium** is typically low in secondary hyperparathyroidism from vitamin D deficiency, but high or normal in primary hyperparathyroidism.

- **25(OH) vitamin D level:** Low levels suggest vitamin D deficiency.
- **PTH** is elevated in primary or secondary hyperparathyroidism.
- **Hypomagnesemia** and **hypokalemia** accompany hypophosphatemia in the setting of refeeding syndrome.

TREATMENT

- **Moderate hypophosphatemia** (1 to 2.5 mg/dL):
  - ○ This is usually asymptomatic and can be managed primarily by treating the underlying cause. **Oral agents** can be used to help restore serum phosphorus to normal levels.
    - ▪ **Neutra-Phos** (250 mg phosphorus and 7 mEq each sodium and potassium per capsule)
    - ▪ **Neutra-Phos K** (250 mg phosphorus and 14 mEq potassium per capsule)
    - ▪ **K-Phos Neutral** (250 mg phosphorus, 13 mEq of sodium, and 1 mEq of potassium per tablet)
- **Severe hypophosphatemia** (<1 mg/dL):
  - ○ Most often requires **IV phosphate.**
    - ▪ **Potassium phosphate** (1.5 mEq potassium per mmol phosphate)
    - ▪ **Sodium phosphate** (1.3 mEq sodium per mmol phosphate)
    - ▪ IV infusion should be stopped when the plasma phosphorus level is >1.5 mg/dL or when PO therapy is possible.
    - ▪ Because of the need to replenish intracellular stores, 24 to 36 hours of phosphate infusion may be required.
    - ▪ Hyperphosphatemia must be avoided, as it can cause hypocalcaemia and ectopic calcification.
    - ▪ IV phosphate should be given cautiously in renal failure.

REFERENCES

1. Goodman WG, Quarles LD. Mineral homeostasis and bone physiology. In: Olgaard K, ed. *Clinical Guide to Bone and Mineral Metabolism in CKD.* New York, NY: National Kidney Foundation; 2006:3–25.
2. Bushinsky DA. Disorders of calcium and phosphorus homeostasis. In: Greenberg A, ed. *Primer on Kidney Diseases.* 4th ed. Philadelphia, PA: Elsevier; 2005:120–130.
3. Rose BD, Post TW. *Clinical Physiology of Acid-Base and Electrolyte Disorders.* New York, NY: McGraw-Hill; 2000:71–111.
4. Gutierrez O, Isakova T, Rhee E, et al. Fibroblast growth factor-23 mitigates hyperphosphatemia but accentuates calcitriol deficiency in chronic kidney disease. *J Am Soc Nephrol.* 2005;16(7):2205–2215.
5. Filler G, Liu D, Huang SH, et al. Impaired GFR is the most important determinant for FGF-23 increase in chronic kidney disease. *Clin Biochem.* 2011;44(5-6):435–437.
6. Ruan L, Chen W, Srinivasan SR, et al. Relation of serum phosphorus levels to carotid intima-media thickness in asymptomatic young adults (from the Bogalusa heart study). *Am J Cardiol.* 2010;106:793–797.
7. Kovesdy CP, Kuchmak O, Lu JL, et al. Outcomes associated with phosphorus binders in men with non-dialysis-dependent CKD. *Am J Kidney Dis.* 2010;56(5):842–851.

8. Cheng SC, Young D, Huang Y, et al. A randomized, double blind, placebo-controlled trial of niacinamide for reduction of phosphorus in hemodialysis patients. *Clin J Am Soc Nephrol.* 2008;3:1131–1138.

9. Kraft MD, Btaiche IF, Sacks GS. Review of the refeeding syndrome. *Nutr Clin Pract.* 2005;20(6):625–633.

10. Gardner D, Shoback D. *Greenspan's Basic and Clinical Endocrinology.* New York, NY: McGraw-Hill; 2007:282–287.

Acid–Base Disorders

Biju Marath and Steven Cheng

GENERAL PRINCIPLES

- Maintenance of acid–base status is essential for normal cellular function.
- Minute changes in the concentration of $[H^+]$ can have dramatic impact on the blood pH.
- The body maintains acid–base homeostasis through three primary mechanisms:
  - Chemical buffering by extracellular and intracellular buffers.
  - Controlling pCO_2 through modulation of alveolar ventilation.
  - Altering net acid excretion (NAE) or the reabsorption of HCO_3^-.

Definitions

- An **acid** is a substance that donates H^+ ions and a base is a substance that accepts H^+ ions.[1,2]
  - **Physiologic balance of the acid–base status** can be described by the following equation:

$$CO_2 + H_2O \leftrightarrow H_2CO_3 \leftrightarrow H^+ + HCO_3^-$$

  - Acids and bases may be "strong" or "weak"
    - Strong acids (i.e., hydrochloric acid) and strong bases (i.e., sodium hydroxide) are those that are almost completely ionized in the body.
- The **blood pH** is a mathematic expression of the $[H^+]$ of the blood.
  - $pH = -\log [H^+]$
  - pH is thus inversely related to the $[H^+]$.
    - The normal extracellular $[H^+]$ is 40 nmol/L, correlating to a pH of 7.4.
    - In general, the range of H^+ compatible with life is 16 to 160 nmol/L, or a pH between 7.8 and 6.80.
  - The **Henderson–Hasselbach equation** shows the pH as a mathematical relationship between HCO_3^- and pCO_2.

$$pH = 6.1 + \log[HCO_3^-]/(0.03 \times pCO_2)$$

- **Acidemia** is an increase in the $[H^+]$ and a decrease in the pH.
- **Alkalemia** is a decrease in the $[H^+]$ and a rise in the pH.

Classification

- Acid and base disturbances are generally classified by the genesis of the disorder.
  - Changes in the pCO_2 are referred to as "Respiratory" processes.
    - A decrease in pH due to an increase in pCO_2 is termed "Respiratory Acidosis."
    - An increase in pH due to a decrease in pCO_2 is termed "Respiratory Alkalosis."

○ Changes in the $[HCO_3^-]$ are referred to as "Metabolic" processes.
  ■ A decrease in pH due to a decrease in $[HCO_3^-]$ is termed "Metabolic Acidosis."
  ■ An increase in pH due to an increase in $[HCO_3^-]$ is termed "Metabolic Alkalosis."

Pathophysiology

- Acid–base homeostasis is under constant challenge. For example, the typical Western diet generates 1 mEq of acid/kg/d.
- Maintaining a pH compatible with life in the context of a significant acid load requires immediate buffering of the acid (primarily through HCO_3^-), a ventilatory response to blow off CO_2, and a system of excretion to rid the system of the excess acid load and regenerate HCO_3^-.[3]
  ○ **Buffering:**
    ■ Buffering is the ability of a solution to resist change in pH when a strong acid or alkali is added.
    ■ HCO_3^- is the most important physiologic buffer in the extracellular fluid (ECF) space.
    ■ As seen in the previous equation, HCO_3^- can combine with free H^+ to form H_2CO_3, which can subsequently convert to CO_2 and H_2O (see ventilatory response, below)
    ■ Intracellular buffers include proteins, phosphates, and hemoglobin.
    ■ Bone can also absorb a significant acid load and, on dissolution, release buffer compounds such as calcium carbonate and calcium bicarbonate.
  ○ **Ventilatory response:**
    ■ The ability to sense changes in pH and control pCO_2 via alveolar ventilation allows the body to further respond to the acid–base imbalance.
    ■ In response to an acid load, a reduction in pCO_2 attenuates the change in pH by shifting the equation toward the generation of CO_2 and H_2O.
      □ The normal pCO_2 is 40 mm Hg.
      □ The level falls with increased ventilation, and rises with decreased ventilation.
  ○ **Excretion:**
    ■ Ultimately, NAE and reabsorption/regeneration of HCO_3^- is required to return the system to balance.
    ■ This is accomplished through the renal elimination of titratable acids (dihydrogen phosphate) and nontitratable acids (ammonium).
    ■ Bicarbonate reabsorption must also be maximized to excrete the daily acid load.
      □ The majority of bicarbonate reabsorption occurs at the proximal tubule.
      □ Bicarbonate reabsorption is regulated by plasma HCO_3^- levels and effective circulating volume.
- Acid–base disorders arise when the capacity for resisting change in pH is exceeded or when mechanisms used to maintain physiologic pH are impaired (Figure 10-1).
- **Acidosis can occur from any of the following:**
  ○ **Metabolic insults:**
    ■ **A large acid load**
      □ Exogenous sources from toxic ingestions, such as ethylene glycol or other alcohols
      □ Endogenous sources during conditions such as lactic acidosis or ketoacidosis, during which the body continually generates acids

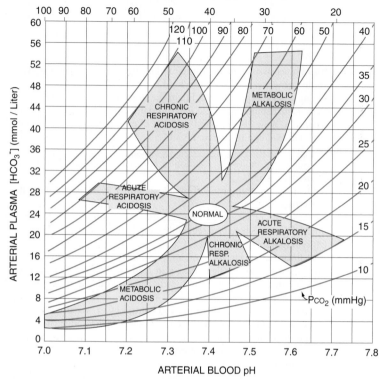

FIGURE 10-1. Acid–base map (see text). HCO_3^-, bicarbonate; pCO_2, partial pressure of CO_2; resp., respiratory. (Adapted from DuBose TD, Cogan MG, Rector FC Jr. Acid-base disorders. In: Brenner BM, ed. *Brenner and Rector's The Kidney.* 5th ed. Philadelphia: WB Saunders; 1996:949.)

- ■ A loss of bicarbonate buffer
  - □ Gastrointestinal (GI) loss (diarrhea).
  - □ Renal loss (proximal renal tubular acidosis [RTA]).
  - ■ An inability to excrete the acid load (distal RTA).
  - ○ Respiratory failure causes acidosis through the elevation of pCO_2.
- • Alkalosis can occur from any of the following:
  - ○ Metabolic insults:
    - ■ Loss of H^+-rich fluids.
      - □ Contraction alkalosis pairs loss of H^+-rich fluids (i.e., nasogastric suctioning) with increased bicarbonate reabsorption during the subsequent volume contraction.
    - ■ Excess reabsorption of bicarbonate.
      - □ Renal bicarbonate reabsorption can be stimulated by volume contraction, hypochloremia, hypokalemia.
  - ○ A decrease in pCO_2 due to hyperventilation (respiratory alkalosis).

TABLE 10-1 EXPECTED COMPENSATORY RESPONSES FOR PRIMARY ACID–BASE DISTURBANCES

Disorder	Primary Change	Compensatory Response
Metabolic acidosis	Decreased HCO_3^-	1.2-mm Hg decrease in pCO_2 for every 1-mEq/L fall in HCO_3^-
Metabolic alkalosis	Increased HCO_3^-	0.7-mm Hg increase in pCO_2 for every 1-mEq/L rise in HCO_3^-
Respiratory acidosis	Increased pCO_2	Increase in HCO_3^-
Acute	0.08 Decrease in pH for every 10-mm Hg rise in pCO_2	1-mEq/L increase in HCO_3^- for every 10-mm Hg rise in pCO_2
Chronic	0.03 Decrease in pH for every 10-mm Hg rise in pCO_2	3.5-mEq/L increase in HCO_3^- for every 10-mm Hg rise in pCO_2
Respiratory alkalosis	Decreased pCO_2	Decrease in HCO_3^-
Acute	0.08 Increase in pH for every 10-mm Hg fall in pCO_2	2-mEq/L decrease in HCO_3^- for every 10-mm Hg fall in pCO_2
Chronic	0.03 Increase in pH for every 10-mm Hg fall in pCO_2	4-mEq/L decrease in HCO_3^- for every 10-mm Hg fall in pCO_2

HCO_3^-, bicarbonate; pCO_2, partial pressure of CO_2.

- **Compensation:**
  - Compensatory responses minimize the change in pH by minimizing the alteration in the $[HCO_3^-]$ to $[pCO_2]$ ratio.
  - Metabolic disturbances are thus attenuated by a respiratory compensation.
    - In metabolic acidosis, a compensatory respiratory response decreases pCO_2 to attenuate the reduction in pH.
    - In metabolic alkalosis, a compensatory respiratory response increases pCO_2 to attenuate the rise in pH.
  - Respiratory disturbances are thus attenuated by a metabolic compensation.
    - In respiratory acidosis, a compensatory metabolic response increases $[HCO_3^-]$.
    - In respiratory alkalosis, a compensatory metabolic response decreases $[HCO_3^-]$.
    - Of note, compensatory metabolic responses require time to exert their maximal effect. As a result, the extent of metabolic compensation can sometimes be used to gauge the duration of the respiratory insult.
  - Expected values for compensatory responses are found in Table 10-1.
  - Compensations, however, are never complete. Although compensation attenuates the change in pH, it is not sufficient to restore pH to its initial value before the primary disturbance occurred.

METABOLIC ACIDOSIS

GENERAL PRINCIPLES

Definition
- Metabolic acidosis is a clinical disorder characterized by low pH and low HCO_3^-.
- The appropriate respiratory compensation is hyperventilation resulting in low pCO_2.

DIAGNOSIS

- Metabolic acidosis is further categorized into those that have an increased anion gap (AG, also known as an **AG acidosis**) and those that have a normal AG (also known as a **non-AG acidosis**).

Diagnostic Testing
- Differentiating the various forms of metabolic acidosis is critical for management.
- **Step 1: AG versus non-AG.**
  - In patients with an AG acidosis, the acid dissociates into H^+ and an "unmeasured" anion.
  - Detection of this "unmeasured anion" is possible through the AG, a simple difference between the measured cations and anions that predominate in the ECF space.
    - $AG = [Na^+] - ([Cl^-] + [HCO_3^-])$
    - Normal AG is 10 ± 3 mEq/L
      - This normal AG typically reflects the presence of unmeasured negative charges from plasma albumin.
      - Because of this, a fall in serum albumin of 1 g/dL (from normal of 4 g/dL) decreases the AG by 2.5 mEq/L.
    - An increase in the AG reflects an accumulation of other unmeasured anions, such as lactate and acetate, from the various causes of an AG acidosis.
    - The amount by which the AG increases (ΔAG) typically approximates the amount by which the serum HCO_3^- decreases (ΔHCO_3).
      - The relationship between ΔAG/ΔHCO_3 is often referred to as the **delta ratio.**
      - A significant disparity between the ΔAG and the ΔHCO_3 suggests a superimposed metabolic disorder.
- When ΔAG $\ll \Delta HCO_3$, the disproportional reduction in serum HCO_3 should raise suspicion of a superimposed nongap metabolic acidosis.
- When ΔAG $\gg \Delta HCO_3$, the decrease in serum HCO_3 has been attenuated by another process, and one should look for sources of a superimposed metabolic alkalosis or a pre-existing chronic respiratory acidosis with a compensatory increase in serum bicarbonate.
  - To further identify the nature of the unmeasured anion, additional laboratory tests can be sent, including serum lactate levels and assays for ketone bodies (as described above).
- **Step 2 (non-AG): renal versus GI defect.**
  - In a non-AG acidosis, the differential includes renal causes (RTA) and enteric bicarbonate losses. These can be differentiated by using the urine AG.

○ The urine AG is the difference between the measured cations (Na and K) and anions (Cl) in the urine. The value is calculated with the following formula:

$$\text{Urine AG} = [Na^+] + [K^+] - [Cl^-]$$

○ In physiologic states with normal acid–base handling, the urine AG has a slightly positive value (0 to ~30).
○ In states of acidosis, the kidney normally increases ammonia production to allow enhanced excretion of the acid load. Higher urine ammonium concentration is balanced by higher Cl levels. Thus, with an appropriately high ammonium in the urine, the urine AG becomes negative because the chloride concentration exceeds Na + K.
○ If urinary acidification is inadequate due to RTA, the urine ammonium levels remain low and the urine AG remains positive.

Differential Diagnosis
See Table 10-2.

Anion Gap Metabolic Acidosis
AG metabolic acidosis encompasses disorders of organic acidosis resulting from increased acid production.

- **Lactic acidosis:**
  ○ Under normal conditions, humans produce relatively small amounts of lactate, the final production of anaerobic metabolism of pyruvate.

TABLE 10-2 DIFFERENTIAL DIAGNOSIS OF METABOLIC ACIDOSIS	
Normal Anion Gap (hyperchloremic)	**Increased Anion Gap (organic)**
GI loss of HCO_3^-	Increased acid production
Diarrhea	Lactic acidosis
Intestinal fistula or drainage	Ketoacidosis
Ureterosigmoidostomy	Failure of acid excretion
Anion-exchange resins	5-Oxoprolinemia
Ingestion of calcium chloride or	Renal failure
magnesium chloride	Toxic alcohol ingestion
Renal loss of HCO_3^-	Ethanol
RTA	Methanol
Carbonic anhydrase inhibitor	Propylene glycol
Hypoaldosteronism	Ethylene glycol
Potassium-sparing diuretics	Other ingestions
Miscellaneous	Salicylate
Recovery from ketoacidosis	Paraldehyde
Dilutional acidosis	Isoniazid
Addition of hydrochloric acid	
Parenteral alimentation	

GI, gastrointestinal; HCO_3^-, bicarbonate; RTA, renal tubular acidosis.

- An **increase in production** can occur from any of the following:
  - Decrease in tissue oxygenation (e.g., hypoxemia, septic shock)
  - Excessive energy expenditures (e.g., seizures, hyperthermia)
  - Deranged oxidative metabolism (e.g., intoxications, malignancy)
  - Impaired lactate clearance (e.g., liver failure)
  - D-lactic acidosis production by D-lactic acid-producing organisms. A separate assay for D-lactate should be ordered if clinical suspicion is high (e.g., blind loop syndromes), as the standard lactate assay does not detect this isomer.
  - Treatment of lactic acidosis must be directed at the underlying cause. Therapy with HCO_3^- has not been found to be effective clinically and may even have deleterious effects.
- **Diabetic ketoacidosis (DKA):**
  - It results from a lack of sufficient insulin to metabolize glucose and short-chain fatty acids. Fatty acids are instead oxidized to the ketoacids (β-hydroxybutyric and acetoacetic acid), resulting in acid–base disturbance.
  - Ketoacids are relatively strong acids and dissociate almost completely, causing a metabolic acidosis with an elevated AG.
    - Initially, the AG may parallel the decrease in HCO_3^- level.
    - With therapy, the AG may normalize prior to the HCO_3^- due to rapid renal elimination of the ketoacid, as renal perfusion improves with volume restoration.
  - Diagnosis of DKA is made by the combination of **AG metabolic acidosis, hyperglycemia, and the presence of serum or urine ketones.**
    - The diagnostic test to detect ketones uses a nitroprusside reagent that reacts with acetoacetate only.
    - In early DKA, the ratio of β-hydroxybutyric acid to acetoacetic acid is 5:2.
    - During treatment of DKA, the formation of acetoacetate is favored, so the nitroprusside test may falsely demonstrate a rise in ketones as this ratio varies.
  - Mainstays of therapy for DKA are insulin, volume repletion, and the management of electrolyte abnormalities. Bicarbonate therapy has not been found to improve outcome in limited clinical trials.
- **Alcohol or starvation ketoacidosis:**
  - It should be suspected in patients with a history of **alcohol abuse with an unexplained high-AG metabolic acidosis.**
  - Combination of alcohol ingestion and poor dietary intake is the cause of the ketoacidosis.
  - Ratio of β-hydroxybutyric acid to acetoacetic acid is up to 20:1. Therefore, the nitroprusside test may grossly underestimate the degree of ketoacidemia in these patients.
  - Therapy consists of vigorous volume, glucose, and electrolyte repletion.
- **Toxic alcohol ingestions:**
  - The examples include **methanol** and **ethylene glycol.**
    - Methanol and ethylene glycol are low-molecular-weight alcohols that readily enter cells.
    - The metabolites are formate (with methanol) or glycolate (with ethylene glycol) and are responsible for the high AG.
  - Initial acid–base status may be normal soon after ingestion. However, an early clue is an **increased osmolar gap.**

- ○ **Osmolar gap = measured serum osmolality – calculated osmolality**
  - ■ **Calculated serum osmolality = $2[Na^+]$ + [glucose]/18 + [urea]/2.8**
  - ■ A difference of >15 to 20 mOsm/kg suggests toxic alcohol ingestion.
  - ■ An osmolar gap can also be due to other conditions that are not associated with a high-AG acidosis, including ethanol and isopropyl alcohol.
- ○ Patients with methanol poisoning present with abdominal pain, vomiting, headache, and visual disturbances (optic neuritis).
- ○ Ethylene glycol intoxication is similar to that of methanol, but does not produce optic neuritis. Calcium oxalate crystals (metabolite of ethylene glycol) in the urine also suggest ethylene glycol intoxication.
- ○ Most morbidity of methanol and ethylene glycol results from damage mediated by metabolites.
- ○ Blocking the metabolism is of prime importance in the treatment of these ingestions. This can be done by use of fomepizole (4-methylpyrazole).
  - ■ Fomepizole blocks alcohol dehydrogenase, thereby retarding metabolism of methanol and ethylene glycol.
  - ■ Hemodialysis may also be required to correct severe metabolic abnormalities and to enhance toxic metabolite elimination.
- • **Salicylate overdose:**
  - ○ Symptoms include nausea, vomiting, tinnitus, altered mental status, coma, and death.
  - ○ Symptoms correlate poorly with plasma levels, but almost always are present with very high levels (>50 mg/dL).
  - ○ Treatment:
    - ■ Alkalinizing the urine with HCO_3^- infusion may reduce symptoms and promote renal excretion.
    - ■ Hemodialysis should be considered for patients with extremely high levels, severe symptoms, significant renal failure, or refractory acidosis.
- • **Acetaminophen ingestion:**
  - ○ It results from the accumulation of 5-oxoproline (pyroglutamic acid).
  - ○ Glutathione metabolism is thought to be the mechanism.
  - ○ Cessation of the drug leads to resolution of the problem.
- • **Acute or chronic renal failure** may lead to high-AG acidosis.
  - ○ Failure to excrete the daily acid load by retention of anions (e.g., phosphates, sulfates) is the pathogenesis of metabolic acidosis.
  - ○ For both acute and chronic renal failure, the AG rises more slowly than the HCO_3^- level drops.
    - ■ In acute renal failure, the HCO_3^- level falls by ~0.5 mEq/L/d, unless hypercatabolism increases daily acid production.
    - ■ In chronic renal failure, the AG rises by ~0.5 mEq/L for each 1-mg/dL rise in serum creatinine.

Nongap (Hyperchloremic) Metabolic Acidosis

- • GI loss:
  - ○ Diarrhea and enteric fistulas account for the majority of nongap metabolic acidosis.
- • RTA:
  - ○ They are heterogeneous group of disorders defined by the presence of metabolic acidosis due to diminished NAE by the kidney, despite a normal glomerular filtration rate.[4]

TABLE 10-3	CHARACTERISTICS OF RTA		
	Type I (classic distal)	Type II (proximal)	Type IV (distal hyperkalemic)
Basic defect	Decreased distal acidification	Diminished proximal HCO_3^- reabsorption	Aldosterone resistance or deficiency
Urine pH	>5.3	Variable: >5.3 if above reabsorptive threshold; <5.3 if below	Usually <5.3
Plasma HCO_3^-	<10 mEq/L	14–20 mEq/L	>15 mEq/L
Plasma K^+	Usually reduced or normal	Usually reduced or normal	Elevated
Diagnosis	Response to $NaHCO_3$ or ammonium chloride	Response to $NaHCO_3$	Measure aldosterone
Nonelectrolyte abnormalities	Nephrocalcinosis, rickets, renal stones	Osteomalacia	Associated with diabetes mellitus

HCO_3^-, bicarbonate; $NaHCO_3$, sodium bicarbonate; RTA, renal tubular acidosis.

○ On the basis of pathophysiologic mechanisms, RTA can be classified as follows (Table 10-3):
  ■ Type I (classic distal) RTA:
    □ It is characterized by defects in secretion, permeability, or voltage gradients, resulting in the inability of the kidney to excrete hydrogen.
    □ Except for the voltage-type defects, in all other forms of type I RTA, potassium becomes the preferred cation for excretion, leading to hypokalemia.
    □ Main causes of type I RTA are hypercalcemia, nephrocalcinosis, autoimmune diseases (especially Sjögren syndrome), drugs (amphotericin B, lithium, and ifosfamide), and toxins like toluene.
    □ It can also occur as a primary disorder in children and can be hereditary.
    □ Diagnosis is based on the inability to lower the urine pH to <5.4 and the response to $NaHCO_3$ treatment.
    □ Treatment for type I RTA is indicated to correct the acidosis and minimize stone formation and nephrocalcinosis. In adults, 1 to 2 mEq/kg/d of alkali is usually necessary.
  ■ Type II (proximal) RTA:
    □ It is an uncommon disorder due to the impairment of proximal tubular reabsorption of HCO_3^-.
    □ Increased delivery of bicarbonate to the distal nephron leads to substantial potassium and sodium loss as well.
    □ It is a self-limiting disorder, because the reabsorptive capacity of HCO_3^- in the distal nephron remains intact.

- Initially, the plasma HCO_3^- concentration will drop to between 14 and 20 mEq/L, resulting in a lowered filtered load that will not exceed reabsorptive capacity.
- At this point, acidification will return to normal in the distal nephron.
- Therefore, the urine pH is variable depending on whether bicarbonate escapes proximal reabsorption.
- Infusion of bicarbonate should raise the urinary pH, and the fractional excretion of HCO_3^-, thereby establishing the diagnosis.
- Main causes include hereditary causes (e.g., Wilson disease or cystinosis), metal toxicity (lead, cadmium, or mercury), and multiple myeloma or amyloidosis.
- **Fanconi syndrome** refers to type II RTA in the setting of more global proximal tubule dysfunction, with impairment of glucose, amino acid, and phosphate reabsorption. In children, treatment may require large amounts of alkali (10 to 25 mEq/kg/d) to avoid growth retardation and osteopenia from the acidosis.

- **Type IV (distal hyperkalemic) RTA:**
  - It is metabolic acidosis secondary to aldosterone deficiency or resistance.
  - Hypoaldosteronism (e.g., primary or secondary to diabetes mellitus) impairs distal hydrogen and potassium secretion, leading to hyperkalemic metabolic acidosis.
  - Hyperkalemia also suppresses $NH4^+$ synthesis in the proximal tubule, further worsening the kidneys' ability to excrete an acid load.
  - Generalized tubular defects, like obstructive uropathy, cyclosporine, or lupus, may also result in type IV RTA by affecting H^+ secretion at the cortical collecting duct.
  - Treatment options for patients with hyperkalemia and metabolic acidosis include a low-potassium diet, sodium bicarbonate replacement, and loop diuretics. Patients with hypoaldosteronism often require mineralocorticoid replacement. Patients with general tubular defects usually do not have a significant degree of acidosis but may require treatment for hyperkalemia.

- *Other causes:*
  - **Dilutional acidosis** is due to the rapid expansion of extracellular space with non-HCO_3^- fluid. The fall in HCO_3^- level is usually small and quickly corrected by renal generation of HCO_3^-.
  - **Parenteral alimentation of amino acids** without concomitant administration of alkali may produce hyperchloremic metabolic acidosis. This can be avoided by replacing the chloride salt of amino acids with acetate salt. The acetate is then metabolized to HCO_3^- and replaces that which was consumed in amino acid metabolism.
  - **Ingestion of sulfur or other inorganic acids** can cause profound hyperchloremic metabolic acidosis.

TREATMENT

- Treatment of metabolic acidosis is usually **best accomplished by treating the underlying disease.**[5,6]
- In certain situations (e.g., lactic acidosis or DKA), alkali therapy is not beneficial and may be deleterious. However, **in patients with severe acidosis, rapid**

administration of HCO_3^- may be necessary for cardiovascular stability. With severe acidemia, the initial goal is to raise the pH to >7.20. The amount of HCO_3^- required to correct the acidemia can be estimated by the HCO_3^- deficit:

$$HCO_3^- \text{ deficit} = HCO_3^- \text{ space (L)} \times (\text{desired } HCO_3^- - \text{actual } HCO_3^-)$$

where HCO_3^- space (theoretic volume of HCO_3^- distribution) = 0.5 – 0.8 × body weight in kg.
- The HCO_3^- space is not constant, but increases with increasing severity of the acidosis.
- In normal state, this space is 50% of body weight, but increases to as high as 80% in severe acidosis (bicarbonate <10 mEq/L). This results from greater use of nonbicarbonate buffers as acidosis worsens.
- In acute settings, intravenous (IV) sodium HCO_3^- (50 mEq in 50-mL ampules) can be given as a bolus or continuous infusion (two to three ampules mixed in D_5W).
- In chronic metabolic acidosis, oral alkali can be given as sodium bicarbonate tablets or as sodium or potassium citrate solution. Typical starting doses would be sodium bicarbonate 650 mg two to three times daily (16 to 24 mEq/d), with the dose increased if necessary.

METABOLIC ALKALOSIS

GENERAL PRINCIPLES

Definition
- Metabolic alkalosis is a clinical disorder characterized by elevated pH due to an increase in HCO_3^-. Compensatory hypoventilation results in a rise of pCO_2.

DIAGNOSIS

- Disorders of metabolic alkalosis can be divided into *chloride-responsive* (chloride depletion acts as a maintenance factor), *chloride-resistant* (chloride depletion does not act as a maintenance factor), and *unclassified* categories (Table 10-4).

TABLE 10-4	TYPES OF METABOLIC ALKALOSIS	
Chloride Responsive	**Chloride Resistant**	**Unclassified**
Vomiting	Hyperaldosteronism	Alkali administration
Gastric drainage	Cushing syndrome	Milk-alkali syndrome
Villous adenoma	Bartter/Gitelman	Massive transfusion of
Chloride diarrhea	syndrome	blood products
Diuretics	Black licorice	Hypercalcemia
Posthypercapnia cystic	Profound potassium	Refeeding syndrome
fibrosis cation-	depletion	
exchange resins		
(e.g., antacids)		

Diagnostic Testing

- Chloride-responsive metabolic alkalosis occurs in volume-depleted states with low urine chloride levels (<25 mEq).
  - In metabolic alkalosis, urine chloride levels may be a more accurate determination of volume state than are urine sodium levels.
  - The urinary chloride level may be elevated if it is obtained while a diuretic is still in effect. However, more than 24 to 48 hours after the last diuretic dose, the urine chloride is appropriately low, reflecting volume depletion.
- Chloride-resistant metabolic alkalosis occurs in euvolemic states and is associated with elevated urine chloride levels (>40 mEq/L).

Differential Diagnosis

- **Chloride-responsive metabolic alkalosis:**
  - **Vomiting or gastric drainage:**
    - It is one of the most common causes of metabolic alkalosis.
    - Gastric secretions contain as much as 100 mmol/L of acid. Gastric parietal cells generate one HCO_3^- molecule for each H^+ secreted.
    - Maintenance of metabolic alkalosis occurs due to the subsequent volume contraction.
  - **Diuretics:**
    - Diuretics that exert their effect at the thick, ascending limb of the loop of Henle (loop diuretics) or at the distal tubule (thiazide diuretics) stimulate H^+ secretion through renin/aldosterone to initiate metabolic alkalosis.
    - In addition, these diuretics maintain metabolic alkalosis by volume depletion.
  - In the **posthypercapnic state,** the renal compensation to chronic hypercapnia is an elevation in HCO_3^-. When hypercapnia is corrected too quickly, the patient has an elevated level of HCO_3^- until renal readjustment can occur.
- **Chloride-resistant metabolic alkalosis:**
  - **Primary hyperaldosteronism:**
    - This leads to hypokalemic metabolic alkalosis secondary to aldosterone stimulation of distal H^+ secretion.
    - It often occurs in concert with hypertension and volume expansion.
  - **Corticosteroid excess:**
    - Many of these corticosteroids have considerable mineralocorticoid effects to produce hypokalemic metabolic alkalosis.
    - Cushing's syndrome can cause this due to the overproduction of corticosteroid.
    - Black licorice contains glycyrrhizic acid, which decreases the enzymatic conversion of cortisol to cortisone. Cortisol thus continues to activate mineralocorticoid receptors, mimicking mineralocorticoid excess.
  - Bartter syndrome is a rare condition presenting in children with increased renin levels and hyperaldosteronism without hypertension or sodium retention.
    - The disease occurs due to mutations in the $Na^+/K^+/2Cl^-$ channel in the thick ascending limb of the loop of Henle, leading to Na^+, K^+, and Cl^- wasting.
    - Bartter syndrome may be difficult to distinguish from surreptitious diuretic use and may require screening urine for presence of diuretics.

- **Unclassified metabolic alkalosis:**
  - Administration of HCO_3^- or organic anions that metabolize into HCO_3^- (citrate or acetate) can lead to metabolic alkalosis, especially in patients with renal insufficiency.
  - **Milk-alkali syndrome** is seen in patients who consume a large amount of antacids containing calcium and alkali (e.g., calcium carbonate).
    - Hypercalcemia decreases parathyroid-hormone-mediated HCO_3^- loss and also causes alkalosis through contraction.
    - This may be supported by decreased glomerular filtration rate.
    - In addition, the alkalosis acts to reduce calcium excretion and enhances the effect of hypercalcemia.
  - **Massive transfusion of blood products** (>10 U packed RBCs) can produce moderate metabolic alkalosis secondary to elevated citrate that metabolizes into HCO_3^-.
  - Similarly, metabolic alkalosis may be seen in patients undergoing **plasmapheresis,** as replacement plasma has citrate.

TREATMENT

- However, when the pH elevation becomes life threatening (>7.60), rapid reduction in pH can be achieved by hemodialysis.[5,6]
- In these acute settings, **administration of hydrochloric acid or other acids is not advocated** due to significant potential complications.
- For nonurgent cases, therapy is based on whether the case is chloride responsive or chloride resistant.
- **Chloride-responsive metabolic alkalosis:**
  - It typically **responds to the administration of oral or IV sodium chloride** in 0.9% or 0.45% solution with potassium supplements.
    - This lowers the plasma HCO_3^- level by reversing the contraction alkalosis, decreasing sodium retention, and promoting HCO_3^- excretion.
    - Optimal rate of fluid replacement is ~50 to 100 mL/h in excess of the sum of all sensible and insensible losses.
    - In edematous states (e.g., patient with heart failure), the administration of saline may not be an option.
      - In some instances, ongoing diurèsis may be necessary to prevent pulmonary edema, despite intravascular contraction.
      - Acetazolamide (250 to 375 mg PO daily or bid) is a carbonic anhydrase inhibitor that decreases proximal sodium reabsorption while increasing renal excretion of HCO_3^-. Its effect on attenuating metabolic alkalosis can be monitored with urine pH, which should increase to >7.0.
  - Concurrent hypokalemia must be corrected for metabolic alkalosis to resolve.
  - In addition, for gastric causes, the use of H_2-blockers or proton-pump inhibitors minimizes the gastric acid loss.
  - For diuretic-induced metabolic alkalosis, the use of potassium-sparing diuretics can reduce the degree of the acid–base disturbance.
- **Chloride-resistant metabolic alkalosis:**
  - It does not respond to the administration of volume.
  - For mineralocorticoid excess states, successful treatment requires restoration of normal mineralocorticoid activity, including surgical removal of an adrenal

adenoma or by the use of potassium-sparing diuretics in addition to potassium supplements.

○ Bartter syndrome may respond to nonsteroidal anti-inflammatory drugs, potassium-sparing diuretics, and potassium supplements.

RESPIRATORY ACIDOSIS

GENERAL PRINCIPLES

Pathophysiology
- Acute respiratory acidosis results from acute alveolar hypoventilation when only the buffering defense is available.
- Chronic respiratory acidosis is caused by chronic decreased effective alveolar ventilation. Over time, the renal compensatory mechanisms operate at maximal capacity.

DIAGNOSIS

- Respiratory acidosis is a disorder caused by processes that increase pCO_2, resulting in a decrease in pH and a compensatory increase in HCO_3^-.
- The increase in pCO_2 is due to decreased alveolar ventilation. The physiologic buffer systems generate the immediate response to the low pH during the acute phase.
- Over the next several days, renal compensation is initiated through an increase in NAE termed the *chronic phase.*
- The third response to respiratory acidosis is the restoration of effective ventilation.

Differential Diagnosis
- **The causes of acute respiratory acidosis** include neuromuscular abnormalities, airway obstruction, thoracic-pulmonary disorders, vascular disease, respiratory muscle fatigue, and mechanical ventilation.
- **The causes of chronic respiratory acidosis** include thoracic-pulmonary disorders (e.g., chronic obstructive pulmonary disease) and neuromuscular abnormalities.
- When a patient in a steady state of chronic hypercapnia suffers a new insult, the pCO_2 acutely rises. This is termed acute respiratory acidosis superimposed on chronic respiratory acidosis.

TREATMENT

- Treatment is restoration of effective ventilation.
- In chronic respiratory acidosis, treatment is difficult, but maximizing pulmonary function may lead to significant improvement.

RESPIRATORY ALKALOSI

GENERAL PRINCIPLES

Pathophysiology
- **Acute respiratory alkalosis** results from acute alveolar hyperventilation when only the buffering defense is available.

○ Patients may present with paresthesias, muscle cramps, tinnitus, and even seizures.
- **Chronic respiratory alkalosis** is caused by chronic increased effective alveolar ventilation. During this period, the renal compensatory mechanisms are fully exerted.

DIAGNOSIS

- Respiratory alkalosis is **the most common acid–base disorder in seriously ill patients.**
- Respiratory alkalosis is a disorder caused by processes that decrease pCO_2, resulting in an increase in pH and a compensatory decrease in HCO_3^-. The decrease in pCO_2 is due to increased alveolar ventilation.
- The buffering response constitutes the acute phase, and the renal response defines the chronic stage of respiratory alkalosis.
- The third response to respiratory alkalosis is the restoration of appropriate ventilation.

Differential Diagnosis
- Causes of respiratory alkalosis include central stimulation of respiration (e.g., fever, anxiety, and head trauma), peripheral stimulation of respiration (e.g., pulmonary embolism and pneumonia), liver insufficiency, sepsis, and mechanical ventilation.

TREATMENT

- The key to therapy is treating the underlying cause. **Correcting significant hypoxemia may be more important than the acid–base disturbance.**

SOME EXAMPLES OF MIXED ACID–BASE DISTURBANCES AND THEIR EVALUATION

A SIMPLE CHANGE IN MEDICINES

A patient with chronic lung disease with edema received diuretics. An arterial blood gas (ABG) test done a week earlier showed pH, 7.38; pCO_2, 50 mm Hg; and HCO_3^-, 29 mmol/L. He presents now with weakness, dizziness, and a low blood pressure. His ABG test values are pH, 7.46; pCO_2, 56 mm Hg; and HCO_3^-, 39 mmol/L. A review of his baseline laboratory values reveals a mild respiratory acidosis with adequate metabolic compensation. The change was the introduction of diuretics.

- **Step 1:** pH is elevated, indicating alkalemia.
- **Step 2:** HCO_3^- is elevated, indicating metabolic alkalosis. The pCO_2 is elevated as well, but this signifies an acidosis of respiratory origin. As the pH is alkalemic, the primary change in this acid–base disorder is a metabolic alkalosis, and the elevated pCO_2 (above baseline) is an attempt at compensation.
- **Step 3:** Information for calculation of AG is not given; hence, it is assumed to be within normal limits.
- **Step 4:** The next step is to gauge the appropriateness of the compensatory response. Acutely, if the HCO_3^- is changed by 10 mmol/L, the expected change in the pCO_2 would be to 57 mm Hg (Table 10-1), which is quite close to this patient's value.

- **Step 5:** It appears that this patient with chronic compensated respiratory acidosis developed an acute metabolic alkalosis. Given the clinical circumstances, it is clear that the diuretic therapy caused hypovolemia and contraction alkalosis, making the pH alkalemic.
- **Step 6:** Appropriate therapy is withdrawal of diuretics and volume repletion.

Mind the Gaps

A 25-year-old female with acute respiratory distress syndrome in the medical intensive care unit (ICU) requires inverse ratio ventilation to maintain adequate oxygenation. At 2 days after initiation of this therapy, her morning ABG reads pH, 7.12; pCO_2, 38 mm Hg; and HCO_3^-, 12 mmol/L. Other laboratory data are as follows: Na, 130 mmol/L; Cl, 93 mmol/L; K, 5.0 mmol/L; blood urea nitrogen, 40 mg/dL; and glucose, 100 mg/dL.

- **Step 1:** pH is very low, indicating severe acidemia.
- **Step 2:** HCO_3^- is quite low, suggesting metabolic acidosis.
- **Step 3:** The patient has a significant AG (25). The HCO_3^- level is appropriate for the gap.
- **Step 4:** pCO_2 is slightly decreased; however, no evident compensation has occurred.
- **Step 5:** Thus, a formulation is made for severe AG metabolic acidosis without compensation.

Her renal function is normal, as are lactic acid levels; serum ketones are not detectable. Serum osmolality is noted to be 330 mOsm/L. As her calculated osmolality is 280 mOsm/L, she has an osmolal gap of 50, which is abnormal. However, most of the usual offenders that can cause an elevated osmolal gap (ethanol, methanol, ethylene glycol, and so forth) are unlikely here, as the patient is in an ICU. The offending agent is identified after a careful review of medicines: the patient was started on high-dose infusions of lorazepam to enhance sedation during inverse ratio ventilation. Lorazepam infusions contain propylene glycol, which can cause metabolic acidosis with AGs and osmolal gaps, should sufficiently high doses be used. Such high doses are sometimes required in the ICU, exposing the patient to the risk of propylene glycol toxicity. Propylene glycol levels can be measured and correlate quite strongly with osmolality and osmolal gap.

A Gap in the Gap

A 25-year-old diabetic was admitted to the ICU with profound ketoacidosis, pH of 7.1, and AG of 25. Treatment was started with IV saline and insulin infusion. A few hours later, the following ABG results were received: pH, 7.28; pCO_2, 28 mm Hg; HCO_3^-, 13 mEq/L; and AG, 18.

- **Step 1:** pH is decreased, suggesting acidemia.
- **Step 2:** HCO_3^- is low, suggesting metabolic acidosis. The pCO_2 is low, reflecting respiratory compensation for the acidemia.
- **Step 3:** The AG is 18. Expected HCO_3^- for this AG is 19 (taking 12 as normal AG and 25 as normal HCO_3^- value). However, the observed HCO_3^- is 13. This suggests the presence of a non-AG metabolic acidosis in addition to an AG metabolic acidosis and respiratory compensation.
- **Step 4:** Expected pCO_2 is 28 mm Hg. As observed, pCO_2 is 28 mm Hg as well, the compensatory response is appropriate.

- **Step 5:** It is clear that the patient who presented with an AG metabolic acidosis now has a non-AG acidosis in addition, with persistent (although improved) acidemia and appropriate respiratory compensation. Two fundamentally important factors in addressing a metabolic acidosis are to look for an AG and to decide if the acidosis is entirely due to the gap process or to a combination of a gap acidosis along with a nongap acidosis. Matching the observed HCO_3^- to the expected HCO_3^- for the gap observed helps in detecting a hidden nongap acidosis.

The development of nongap acidosis is common in ketoacidosis due to ketoacid metabolism of and excretion in the urine. Administration of insulin helps metabolize the ketone bodies to HCO_3^-. The HCO_3^- generated is used to buffer intracellular acidosis. Thus, although the AG closes (due to the removal of ketones), the HCO_3^- level and acidemia lag behind, accounting for the nongap acidosis.

When All Is Not What It Seems

- At times, mixed acid–base disorders can be difficult to detect if not carefully and systematically scrutinized. A patient in the ICU developed pancreatitis, and nasogastric suction was instituted for 2 to 3 days. The course was complicated by sepsis and shock. The following laboratory values were received: pH, 7.41; pCO_2, 40 mm Hg; HCO_3^-, 25 mEq/L; Na, 140 mmol/L; and Cl, 90 mmol/L. The pH, pCO_2, and HCO_3^- values are in the normal range. Thus, if the casual observer decided to stop here, the fact that there is an AG of 25 would be completely missed.
- The presence of an AG is strong evidence of a metabolic acidosis. Expected HCO_3^- for an AG of 25 is 12 mEq/L. The HCO_3^- level in this patient is 25, suggesting a coexisting metabolic alkalosis.
- A review of the clinical scenario explains the acid–base abnormalities. The metabolic alkalosis was generated by nasogastric suction. At this point, septic shock developed. The resulting metabolic acidosis counterbalanced the pH and HCO_3^- concentration. This is a good example of a mixed disorder with a metabolic alkalosis and abnormal AG.
- Triple acid–base disorders are combinations of metabolic acidosis and alkalosis with either respiratory acidosis or respiratory alkalosis. (The two respiratory disorders cannot coexist; one cannot breathe fast and slow simultaneously.)

REFERENCES

1. Halperin M, Goldstein M. *Fluid, Electrolyte, and Acid-Base Physiology: A Problem-Based Approach,* 3rd ed. Philadelphia, PA: WB Saunders; 1999.
2. Rose B, Narins R, Post, T. *Clinical Physiology of Acid-Base and Electrolyte Disorders.* New York, NY: McGraw-Hill, Medical Publishing Division; 2001.
3. Schrier R. *Renal and Electrolyte Disorders,* 6th ed. Philadelphia, PA: Lippincott Williams & Wilkins; 2003.
4. DuBose T, Hamm L. *Acid-Base and Electrolyte Disorders: A Companion to Brenner and Rector's The Kidney.* Philadelphia, PA: WB Saunders; 2002.
5. Adrogué HJ, Madias NE. Medical progress: management of life-threatening acid–base disorders—first of two parts. *N Engl J Med.* 1998;338:26–34.
6. Adrogué HJ, Madias NE. Medical progress: management of life-threatening acid–base disorders—second of two parts. *N Engl J Med.* 1998;338:107–111.

Overview and Management of Acute Kidney Injury

11

Andrew Siedlecki and Anitha Vijayan

GENERAL PRINCIPLES

- Acute kidney injury (AKI) is among the most commonly encountered diseases in the hospital setting, with national prevalence of 13%.
- AKI is synonymous with the historical term acute renal failure.
- In the acute setting, a small elevation in serum creatinine (SCr; 0.3 mg/dL) is independently associated with increased mortality and substantial financial cost to the healthcare system.
- Awareness of AKI is limited by the sensitivity of SCr, the standard biomarker of kidney damage, and therefore requires clinical context to either anticipate or mitigate the disease course.
- Early recognition of AKI by the physician is essential to the care of the hospitalized patient.

Definition

- Criterion for AKI is met when one of the following conditions is true: **an abrupt (within 48 hours) reduction in kidney function due to a rise in SCr by ≥0.3 mg/dL or documented oliguria of <0.5 mL/kg/h for more than 6 hours.**[1]
- A 50% increase in SCr also warrants alarm, but such nonfixed changes in SCr have been difficult to verify in large epidemiologic studies.
- This definition of AKI has gained the support of the Kidney Disease: Improving Global Outcomes (KDIGO) foundation, which generates guidelines for the international field of nephrology.[2]

Classification

- Criteria for AKI are standardized to facilitate communication between practitioners and to clarify the results of outcomes-based analyses.
- A simplified staging system compiled by the Acute Kidney Injury Network (AKIN) group that categorizes the severity of AKI is shown in Table 11-1. This criteria evolved from the staging system that was previously outlined in the RIFLE (Risk, Injury, Failure, Loss, End-Stage Renal Disease) criteria.[3]
- Staging has yet to be confirmed as a significant predictor of patient morbidity or mortality, and continues to be evaluated with covariates that represent high-risk populations.
- Although the terminology has changed from ARF to AKI, the disease remains subclassified into **prerenal, postrenal, and intrinsic renal injury.**
- Prerenal azotemia refers to problems with renal perfusion, either from decreased intravascular volume, decreased blood pressure, or decrease in effective circulating

TABLE 11-1	CLASSIFICATION/STAGING SYSTEM FOR AKI[4]	
Stage	Serum Creatinine Criteria	Urine Output Criteria
1	Rise in SCr ≥0.3 mg/dL or ≥150%–200% from baseline	<0.5 mL/kg/h for >6 h <0.5 mL/kg/h for >12 h
2	Rise in SCr >200%–300% from baseline	<0.3 mL/kg/h for >24 h or anuria >12 h
3	Rise in SCr >300% from baseline, or SCr >4 mg/dL with an acute increase of at least 0.5 mg/dL	

AKI, acute kidney injury; SCr, serum creatinine.

volume. Postrenal azotemia is caused by obstruction to urine flow and accounts for ~5% to 15% of all cases of AKI.

- **Intrinsic renal injury** can be from **glomerular, microvascular, interstitial, or tubular** causes. **Acute tubular necrosis (ATN)** is a disease of the sick hospitalized patient and will be discussed in detail in this chapter. Other intrinsic causes of AKI are discussed elsewhere in the book.

Epidemiology

- Generally AKI is a disease of the hospitalized patient, with ~13.5% of all hospitalized patients meeting the diagnostic criteria for AKI. As can be expected, the number is much higher in patients with multiorgan failure and in the intensive care unit (ICU).[5] In contrast, only ~1% of all patients presenting to the emergency room have the diagnosis of AKI.
- AKI is associated with high mortality, which has not changed significantly in the last 55 years. The average mortality in an ICU patient with AKI is quoted anywhere from 45% to 60%. Studies have demonstrated that AKI is an independent factor contributing to the mortality and not just an innocent bystander, as previously believed. In a study of hospitalized patients who received intravenous (IV) radiocontrast procedures, the risk of mortality was increased by 5.5-fold in those who developed AKI (compared to patients who did not develop renal injury), after accounting for comorbid conditions.[1,6]
- Some of the possible **reasons for the persistent poor survival in AKI** include:
  ○ **Delay in diagnosis of AKI:** By the time a patient's SCr increases 0.3 mg/dL, renal function would have declined by at least 25%.[7] Creatinine remains a late marker of AKI and is being challenged by more sensitive and biologically significant markers such as Neutrophil gelatinase associated lipocalin (NGAL) and cystatin C.[8]
  ○ **Inability of dialysis to provide actual renal replacement:** The endocrine, cytokine, and immunologic functions of the kidney are not being replaced with dialysis.
  ○ **Delay in initiation of dialysis:** The optimal timing of renal replacement therapy (RRT) remains a question, with limited studies suggesting that early initiation of dialysis might improve the outcome.

○ **Inadequate dialysis prescription:** Studies have shown that prescribed dialysis efficiency is rarely achieved in AKI. However, two recent trials in AKI suggested that increasing the dose of RRT may not necessarily improve outcome. These studies are discussed in the chapter on renal replacement therapy.

DIAGNOSIS

- The initial diagnostic evaluation of a patient suspected of AKI is triggered by either an **increase in SCr** or **decrease in urine output over several hours.**
- A stepwise approach should always focus on delineating whether AKI is the result of prerenal or postrenal processes, with the understanding that intrinsic renal injury will likely take a more thorough battery of testing and may not be forthcoming by evaluation of the patient's volume status and urinary outlet alone.
- By definition, **prerenal and postrenal lesions** impose functional restraints on renal performance and anticipate dramatic improvement in solute clearance after removal of such lesions, if achieved in a timely fashion. Prerenal and postrenal AKI are discussed in detail in the following chapter.
- In contrast, **intrinsic AKI** is *not* expected to reverse swiftly and the clinical course and prognosis depend on the underlying cause.
- In the ICU, the most common cause is ATN, usually due to both ischemic and toxic insults (multifactorial ATN).

Clinical Presentation

- The following questions should be answered by the end of the history and physical exam in a patient with AKI.
- Is the patient volume depleted?
- Does the patient have a urinary tract obstruction?
- Has this patient been exposed to a major nephrotoxin (medications, IV contrast, over-the-counter agents, herbal products, and so forth)?
- Could this patient have intrinsic renal disease?
- Does the patient have a preexisting condition (e.g., decompensated congestive heart failure, liver cirrhosis, diabetes, peripheral vascular disease) increasing vulnerability to renal injury?
- Is there a need for further serologic testing and/or renal biopsy?

History

- **Urine patterns and frequency:**
  ○ Estimate daily urine volumes and recent trends (1 "Dixie" cup = 75 mL, 1 coffee cup = 225 mL, 1 cola can = 350 mL, 24-hour urine container = 2.5 L).
  ○ Elicit any history of hematuria, dysuria, or pyuria.
  ○ Urgency, frequency, dribbling, and incontinence, especially in elderly men, may point toward prostatic disease.
  ○ Onset of urinary symptoms may also provide a temporal clue to the duration of illness.
  ○ For hospitalized patients, a careful review of the intake, output, and daily weights is essential.

- **Volume status:**
  - History of dizziness, orthostatic instability, dependent lifestyle, prolonged nursing home stay, and unmonitored chronic diuretic use, may point toward intravascular depletion, whereas weight gain, edema, or periorbital swelling (especially in the mornings) may signify fluid retention.
  - Consider the possible mechanisms of fluid loss—hemorrhage, diarrhea, polyuria, and situations leading to excessive insensitive losses (e.g., fever or diminished intake due to dysphagia, surgical wounds closing by secondary intention)—as they all predispose to volume depletion.
  - Review the patient's records or hospital chart in detail for episodes of blood pressure swings.
  - For postoperative patients with AKI, it is essential to review the intra- and postoperative hemodynamic records.
- **Medications:**
  - A thorough review of the patient's medications is essential in pinpointing the correct diagnosis.
  - This **includes over-the-counter medicines** (nonsteroidal anti-inflammatory drugs [NSAIDs], high dose acetaminophen), herbal products, and other health and food supplements.
  - Scout for **nephrotoxins** in the hospital chart (e.g., NSAIDs, renin–angiotensin–aldosterone system inhibitors, aminoglycosides, polymyxins).
  - In hospitalized patients, exclude covert nephrotoxic exposure, such as iodine-based IV contrast media with radiologic studies and angiograms.
  - Some drugs may precipitate or exacerbate urinary retention and should be considered as possible causes of postrenal AKI (e.g., tricyclic antidepressants, carbidopa, disopyramide and certain antihypertensive agents).
  - Several herbal products, such as herbal appetite suppressants (*Hoodia Gordonii*[9]) and herbal diuretics (*Radix Tripterygii*[10]), have been implicated in AKI because of volume depletion.
  - Herbals containing aristolochic acid may cause interstitial nephritis and tubular necrosis.[11]
- **Infections:**
  - The source and severity of infection, as well as the treatment strategies for the infection, in a patient with AKI must be carefully reviewed.
  - **Sepsis** initiates an innate immune response and can lead to renal vasoconstriction and ATN.
  - Some infectious organisms **directly** lead to renal involvement: For example, *Legionella* infection can cause an interstitial nephritis.
  - **Indirect causes** include bacterial endocarditis or hepatitis C with cryoglobulinemia, both of which can cause an immune complex deposition glomerulonephritis.
  - Finally, the many different **antibiotics** in use today can cause nephrotoxicity, either directly or by causing acute allergic interstitial nephritis.
- **Other potential etiologies:**
  - Patients should be carefully questioned for other symptoms of systemic diseases.
  - Severe myalgias, dark urine (with or without decreased urine output), and appropriate clinical scenarios (exercise, crush injury, recent surgery, drug or alcohol use, medications, immobilization, and so forth) may point toward **rhabdomyolysis.**

- ○ Arthralgias, arthritis, skin rash, oral ulcers, hair loss, and significant cytopenias in the past may suggest the possibility of a **connective tissue disorder** (e.g., systemic lupus erythematosus).
- ○ Sinusitis, cough, and hemoptysis may suggest diseases such as **Wegener's granulomatosis** or **Goodpasture syndrome.**
- ○ A history of recent sore throats or significant skin infections may suggest acute **poststreptococcal glomerulonephritis.**
- ○ Bone pain and anemia may suggest underlying **multiple myeloma.**
- ○ Also important is a history of chronic liver disease. If cirrhosis is present, assess the severity and degree of compensation of cirrhosis of the liver.
  - ■ **Hepatorenal syndrome** is a devastating complication usually seen with advanced, decompensated liver disease.
  - ■ Patients with ascites are prone to develop **spontaneous bacterial peritonitis** that can lead to sepsis and ATN.
  - ■ Any history suggestive of purpura must alert the clinician to the possibility of **cryoglobulinemia** (especially in a patient with hepatitis C), or Henoch–Shonlein purpura or other vasculitis.
- • **Risk factors:**
  - ○ Appraisal of a patient's **comorbidities** may identify a handicapped autoregulatory system.
  - ○ For example, in decompensated heart failure, a patient's increased sympathetic tone may cause an increased susceptibility to nephrotoxic radiocontrast.
  - ○ Similarly, the presence of hypertension, diabetes, or significant peripheral vascular disease should also raise the possibility of dysfunctional microvasculature due to increased atherosclerotic burden, intimal hyperplasia, and decreased arterial capacitance.

Physical Examination
- • **Volume status:**
  - ○ Determination of the patient's **volume status** by a thorough examination is an absolute prerequisite in the examination of the renal patient.
  - ○ Check the patient's pulse and blood pressure. If blood pressure is normal or high, evaluate for orthostatic hypotension in the sitting and standing positions, paying careful attention to the pulse as well.
  - ○ Assess for jugular venous distention and edema.
  - ○ Mucous membranes and skin turgor need to be checked for assessment of hydration.
- • **Cardiac exam:**
  - ○ This should focus on the location and character of apical impulse, presence of S_3 (volume overload) or S_4 (pressure overload), and functional regurgitant murmurs suggesting valve ring dilatation because of volume overload.
  - ○ The presence of dyspnea and tachypnea suggest fluid overload. Acidosis may induce Kussmaul respiration, but this deep-sighing character is not to be confused with the dyspnea of pulmonary edema.
  - ○ Inspiratory crackles at the lung bases occur in pulmonary edema.
- • **Abdominal examination:**
  - ○ Hepatomegaly, splenomegaly, and ascites can occur due to passive congestion in fluid-overload states.

○ The liver may be pulsatile if volume overload has resulted in severe functional tricuspid regurgitation.

○ Exclude obstruction by assessing bladder distention, performing a prostate exam, and placing a Foley catheter if indicated.

• **Other systemic signs:**

○ Rash (e.g., vasculitis, atheroemboli, interstitial nephritis, lupus), arthritis (e.g., vasculitis, connective tissue disorders), pulmonary hemorrhage (vasculitis, lupus) can also provide diagnostic clues.

○ Large lower extremity muscle groups tender to palpation may alert the physician to a developing compartment syndrome and rhabdomyolysis.

○ A complete and thorough examination is required in addition to the above to elicit possible causes of the AKI, to assess the degree of compensation, and to detect features suggestive of uremic syndrome.

Diagnostic Testing

Laboratories

• **Examination of urine:**

○ Urinalysis and microscopic examination of the urine sediment **by a trained physician** is probably the most important test in the evaluation of AKI.

○ The urinalysis should be bland, not reveal protein, blood, cells, or casts in prerenal azotemia and in uncomplicated postrenal failure, unless there is underlying chronic kidney disease.

○ The urinalysis and sediment may help to not only separate renal causes from pre- and postrenal etiologies but also to differentiate between a tubular, glomerular, or interstitial process (Table 11-2).

○ If the urine dipstick tests strongly positive for blood but no red blood cells are seen, **myoglobinuria or hemoglobinuria** should be suspected, suggesting rhabdomyolysis or severe intravascular hemolysis leading to AKI.

TABLE 11-2	URINALYSIS (UA) IN AKI			
	UA Protein	UA Blood	FeNa (%)	Sediment
Prerenal	No	No	<1	Bland; hyaline casts
Acute tubular necrosis	+	+	>1	Muddy brown granular casts; epithelial cells and epithelial cell casts
Glomerulonephritis	++	++	<1	Dysmorphic RBCs; RBC casts
Acute interstitial nephritis	+	+	>1	Eosinophils; WBCs and WBC casts; rarely, RBC casts
Postrenal	+/−	+/−	>1	Monomorphic RBCs and WBCs or crystals may be seen

AKI, acute kidney injury; RBC, red blood cells; WBC, white blood cells.

- It must be kept in mind that in certain diseases that affect the preglomerular blood vessels, such as thrombotic microangiopathies (e.g., thrombotic thrombocytopenic purpura or hemolytic-uremic syndrome), the urine sediment may be bland despite a bona fide renal etiology.
- The overall clinical presentation must therefore always be kept in mind. Indeed, the urine can be bland despite the diagnosis of ischemic ATN. This is typical in the elderly patients with underlying dilated cardiomyopathy. Details of various types of casts and interpretations can be found in Chapter 1.

- **Urinary indices:**
  - In oliguric AKI, the differentiation of prerenal failure from ATN is critical in guiding the decision to restrict or resuscitate the fluid.
  - Various parameters in the urine have been evaluated to make such a differentiation. The basic principle of these parameters is fairly uniform: **In the face of diminished perfusion, the intact renal parenchyma tries to conserve as much sodium as possible** to restore extracellular fluid volume and, hence, renal perfusion. Thus, the **urine is very concentrated and allows excretion of very little sodium.**
  - However, once the renal parenchyma is damaged, the tubules lose their ability to concentrate the urine and to conserve sodium. It must be kept in mind that these indices are usually not useful in nonoliguric states. Some of these indices are presented in Table 11-3.
  - **FENa = [(urine Na/plasma Na)/(urine creatinine/plasma creatinine)] × 100**
    - Although fractional excretion of sodium (FENa) is useful in distinguishing prerenal AKI from ATN, its sensitivity diminishes in the setting of diuretic use.
  - **FEUrea = [(urine urea nitrogen/blood urea nitrogen)/(urine creatinine/plasma creatinine)] × 100**
    - FEUrea calculation takes advantage of urea transporters that are not altered by loop diuretic action, with a sensitivity near 85%, specificity of 92%, and positive predictive value of 98%. FEUrea >50 is consistent with ATN; <35 is consistent with prerenal injury.

- **Blood counts and coagulation screen:**
  - Review of the blood counts and screening tests for coagulation abnormalities may provide extremely valuable information about underlying disease processes leading to AKI.

TABLE 11-3 URINE DIAGNOSTIC INDICES IN THE DIFFERENTIATION OF PRERENAL AZOTEMIA FROM RENAL AZOTEMIA

	Typical Findings	
Diagnostic Index	Prerenal Azotemia	Acute Tubular Necrosis
Fractional excretion of sodium (%)	<1	>1
U_{Na}	<20	>20
Urine osmolality	>500	Variable
Plasma BUN to SCr ratio	>20	<10–15

BUN, bold urea nitrogen; SCr, serum creatinine; U_{Na}, urine sodium.

○ A peripheral smear must be examined where indicated. The presence of schistocytes in cases of AKI suggests thrombotic thrombocytopenic purpura, hemolytic-uremic syndrome, and disseminated intravascular coagulation as possible etiologies. Rarely, schistocytes can also be seen in conditions with severe renal vasculitis, such as diffuse lupus nephritis.

• **Chemistry panel:**
  ○ Review of laboratory values, including blood urea nitrogen, creatinine, electrolytes, and acid-base balance, is essential to establishing the previous baseline and trend leading to the current abnormality.
  ○ If severe metabolic acidosis is present, **anion and osmolar gaps should** be evaluated so as to not miss a severe metabolic derangement or toxic ingestion causing the AKI.
  ○ Elevated plasma **blood urea nitrogen out of proportion to sCr (>20:1)** should prompt an investigation of gastrointestinal bleeding, recent use of high-dose corticosteroids, leading to protein breakdown, or parenteral or enteral high-protein feeding.
  ○ In rhabdomyolysis, profound hyperkalemia and hyperphosphatemia (due to release from damaged myocytes), hypocalcemia (due to calcium-phosphorus binding), and a disproportionate elevation of the creatinine in relation to blood urea nitrogen may develop. **Creatinine kinase (CK) elevation** happens within 12 hours after the injury, and the rise is in proportion to the severity and extent of the muscle injury. Kidney injury has been reported with CK levels >5000 IU/L, but is typically seen with values >25,000 IU/L.

Imaging
• Assessment of obstruction should be given high priority in the patient presenting to emergency room with AKI.
• **Renal ultrasound** is readily available and extremely accurate in excluding urinary tract obstruction as a cause of AKI.
  ○ Ultrasonography is useful in **delineating renal sizes and echo texture** and should be obtained early in the workup of AKI in patients presenting to the emergency room or hospital with hyperkalemia after a foley catheter has been placed.
  ○ However, in the intensive care setting, where obstruction is an unlikely cause of AKI, the yield from ultrasound is very low and it should not be ordered routinely.
  ○ An ultrasound can provide false-negative results in the setting of profound volume depletion as well as in cases of retroperitoneal fibrosis, in which dilatation of calyces and ureters may not occur.
• Computerized tomography and magnetic resonance imaging are alternative modalities to rule out obstruction due to microcalculi or a fibrotic process, in cases where dilatation of calyces may not be seen on ultrasound.

Diagnostic Procedures
• **Serologic profile and special tests:**
  ○ In situations suggestive of intrinsic renal disease, various serologic tests (Table 11-4) are indicated to delineate the etiology. These tests are discussed in detail in other chapters covering vasculitis, lupus nephritis, and intrinsic causes of AKI.

TABLE 11-4	EXAMPLES OF SEROLOGIC OR SPECIAL TESTS ASSOCIATED WITH CAUSES OF AKI

Test	Associated Condition
• ANA, double-stranded DNA	• Lupus nephritis
• C-ANCA (often + proteinase 3 ab)	• Wegener granulomatosis
• P-ANCA (often + myeloperoxidase ab)	• Microscopic polyangiitis, Churg–Strauss syndrome
• Rheumatoid arthritis factor	• Vasculitis, cryoglobulinemia
• Cryoglobulins	• Cryoglobulinemia-associated MPGN
• Anti-GBM antibodies	• Goodpasture syndrome
• Antistreptolysin-O titer	• PSCGN
• Complement levels (low)	• PSCGN, cryoglobulinemic MPGN I, LN, shunt nephritis, GN with SBE, atheroemboli
• Hepatitis B and C antibodies	• Membranous GN or MPGN
• HIV	• Collapsing focal segmental glomerulosclerosis, interstitial nephritis
• Urine and serum protein electrophoresis and immune fixation and serum-free light chains	• Myeloma kidney (cast nephropathy), monoclonal deposition disease, amyloidosis

ANA, antinuclear antibody; AKI, acute kidney injury; C-ANCA, cytoplasmic anti-neutrophil cytoplasmic antibody; GBM, glomerular basement membrane; GN, glomerulonephritis; HIV, human immunodeficiency virus; LN, lupus nephritis; MPGN, membranoproliferative glomerulonephritis; P-ANCA, peri-nuclear anti-neutrophil cytoplasmic antibody; PSCGN, poststreptococcal glomerulonephritis; SBE, subacute bacterial endocarditis.

- **Tissue diagnosis:**
  - ○ **Renal biopsy is usually not required** to establish the diagnosis of ATN.
  - ○ However, if the cause of AKI is not apparent, or if there is a suspicion of **rapidly progressive glomerulonephritis,** then renal histology is required to make a diagnosis and aid in management.
  - ○ This must be done in a timely fashion, as certain disease processes irreversibly destroy renal parenchyma if they are not treated expeditiously.
  - ○ In cases of suspected acute interstitial nephritis with a clear inciting agent, discontinuation of the agent and observation of the renal function can be chosen over a kidney biopsy, especially in high-risk patients.
  - ○ In cases of suspected glomerulonephritis (based on historical features, urine abnormalities, and blood and serologic tests), a renal biopsy is necessary before immunosuppressive therapy is instituted. For instance, even when diagnosis of lupus nephritis is obvious, most nephrologists obtain a tissue diagnosis to correctly define and classify the disease, and to outline progression and future therapy options.
- **Newer biomarkers:**
  - ○ There is great interest in the development of newer serum and urine markers for early diagnosis of AKI, as SCr is neither a true biomarker nor an early marker of disease.

○ SCr slowly identifies renal injury and does so indirectly, because it is derived from muscle filaments and not kidney structure.

○ An ideal biomarker would instead reflect actual cellular injury derived from the kidney (like troponin for myocardial infarction), and detect such injury within hours of the event.

○ If therapy can be started in the early stages of AKI (initiation phase), then this can potentially prevent the continued deterioration of renal function.

○ Promising biomarkers include serum and urine neutrophil gelatinase-associated lipocalin, which increases as early as 1 hour after coronary artery bypass grafting in patients who later develop AKI.[12]

○ Interleukin-18 has also shown similar results, including in the setting of delayed graft function after kidney transplantation.[13]

○ Other molecules of interest include cystatin C and kidney injury molecule-1. Further studies are underway to determine if any of these markers will enhance the diagnostic utility of creatinine in AKI.

TREATMENT

- Management of AKI **depends on the underlying etiology** and will be discussed under each category.
- However, some uniform guidelines that are noted below cover all diagnoses.
- **Avoidance of additional nephrotoxic agents** and further hypotension can hasten renal recovery.
- **Acid-base and electrolyte disturbances:**
  ○ **Hyperkalemia** and **metabolic acidosis** are frequently encountered in AKI. The individual management of these conditions is discussed elsewhere. In the setting of AKI, these two conditions are the foremost reasons to initiate RRT.
- **Nutritional support:**
  ○ Nutrition is one of the important facets of supportive care.
  ○ AKI is a stressful, catabolic state, and adequate nutrition is essential with enteral or parenteral support and should be initiated in a timely manner.
  ○ Unlike CKD, where protein restriction is recommended, protein requirements in AKI vary from 1.0 g/kg (prior to dialysis initiation or during hemodialysis) to 2.5 g/kg (in continuous RRT).
- **Dose adjustment of medications:**
  ○ **Adjusting doses of concurrent medications** to the renal function is **essential in preventing further renal injury** as well as **avoiding systemic toxicity.**
  ○ Even seemingly innocuous medications such as magnesium-containing antacids and phosphorus-containing enemas (Fleets®) can be damaging in the setting of renal dysfunction.
  ○ Various guidelines are available to make recommended dose adjustments for the level of renal function. The pharmacist is also a valuable resource in making medication adjustments in renal failure.
  ○ If the patient requires initiation of hemodialysis or continuous RRT, then dose adjustments are again necessary in some cases to ensure adequate drug levels.
- The criteria for **initiation of** RRT are noted in Chapter 15, Renal Replacement Therapy in Acute Kidney Injury.

REVIEW OF ACUTE TUBULAR NECROSIS

- ATN refers to the AKI resulting from **ischemic or toxic injury to the tubules**. The common etiologies of ATN are detailed in Table 11-5.
- Several disease processes contribute to the overall prevalence of AKI in the tertiary care setting.
- The most commonly studied scenarios include sepsis, cardiothoracic surgery, iodine-based radiocontrast, and nephrotoxic medications.[14]
- Three major components that comprise the diverse pathophysiology of AKI include ischemia, inflammation, and direct tubular damage.[15,16]
- The **natural history of ATN** progresses through **four phases**:
  - ○ **Initiation** refers to an early phase in which ischemia leads to cell injury.
  - ○ **Extension** refers to the phase in which tubular cell polarity is disrupted with a loss of viable and damaged cells into the urinary space, causing tubular casts with obstruction and backleak. Electrolyte transport across the tubular brush border is deranged.
  - ○ During the **maintenance** phase, the cells undergo dedifferentiation, fibroblast migration, and proliferation, and result in fully established renal failure.
  - ○ In the **recovery** phase, stem cells repopulate the tubular epithelium and cell polarity is slowly restored, allowing for an incremental capacity to shuttle solute across the brush border in a physiologic manner.
- All of these phases may not be clinically obvious and one may progress to the next rapidly.
- In oliguric patients, an osmotic diuresis may be seen in the recovery phase (post-ATN diuresis), and meticulous attention should be paid to fluid balance and electrolyte replacement.
- ATN can last from days to several weeks in patients with baseline normal renal function, with the potential for renal recovery even after weeks of oliguria.

TABLE 11-5	CAUSES OF AKI		
Ischemia	**Toxins**	**Drugs**	
• Prolonged diuresis	• Radiocontrast	• Aminoglycosides	
• Large vessel surgical cross-clamp	• Myoglobin (rhabdomyolysis)	• Cisplatin	
• Sepsis	• Unbound heme fragments (intravascular hemolysis)	• Amphotericin B	
	• Ethylene glycol/methanol	• Intravenous bisphosphonates	
	• Tumor lysis (uric acid, phosphate)	• Crystalline nephropathies (indinavir, acyclovir)	
	• Miscellaneous (snake venom, paraquat)		

AKI, acute kidney injury.

- Of the patients with ATN, ~90% can regain sufficient renal function to discontinue dialysis, if they had baseline normal renal function.
- However, these patients are at a higher risk of developing CKD and end-stage renal disease and need to be followed closely.[17]

Pathophysiology of Ischemic Kidney Injury

- Ischemic ATN in many circumstances is a **progression or persistence of the prerenal condition that leads to structural damage of the tubular epithelium.**
- Although 25% of the cardiac output flows into the renal circulation, most of the blood flow is relegated to the cortex, and the medulla is maintained in a relative hypoxic state.
- The S_3 segment of the proximal tubule is especially vulnerable in ischemic states and most of the damage occurs in this segment.
- Overwhelming levels of angiotensin II, endothelin-1, and circulating catecholamines cause intense intrarenal vasoconstriction, overcoming the protective effects of prostaglandins and nitric oxide.[18,19]
- Other factors also come into play: The ischemic response stimulates release of inflammatory cytokines, which in turn leads to increased expression of adhesion molecules on the leukocytes and their ligands on the endothelium. This environment results in increased leukocyte-endothelium adhesion and endothelial injury.
- Congestion and obstruction of capillaries in the outer medulla causes persistent medullary ischemia.
- Tubular cell damage begins with a aberrant trafficking of integrin proteins and ion-transport channels, which leads to loss of cellular voltage gradients, detachment of the epithelial brush border, and disengagement of the epithelial basement membrane.[15]
- Disruption of membrane transport proteins with continued perturbation of cellular metabolism causes tubular backleak and further loss of glomerular filtration rate (GFR).
- The cumulative effect of these insults is apoptosis or, in some cases, frank necrosis.

Nephrotoxic Injury

- Various endogenous and exogenous toxins can lead to tubular damage and AKI. A list of some of the important toxins is presented in Table 11-5.
- Contrast-induced nephropathy is discussed in detail in Chapter 14.
- Rhabdomyolysis, a frequently encountered nephrotoxic injury, is described below.

Rhabdomyolysis

- Destruction of skeletal myocytes releases cytosolic contents (potassium, phosphorus, myoglobin, CK) into extracellular space and systemic circulation.
- The incidence of AKI in rhabdomyolysis is reported to be between 10% and 50%. In cases of traumatic rhabdomyolysis, the incidence of AKI is as high as 85%.
- The **common causes** include immobilization (e.g., alcoholic patient or patient with seizures or stroke; patient found at home after a fall; or postsurgery patients with large muscle mass or obesity, or undergoing urological or bariatric surgeries), trauma (gunshot wound with vascular compromise, motor vehicle

accidents, crush injury following earthquakes or building collapse), or extreme exertion (exercise in severe heat, new recruits at army camps, and so forth). Other causes include cocaine use, medications like statins, and hypophosphatemia.

- Vasoconstriction plays a major role in nephrotoxicity associated with unbound myoglobin.[20] Dimeric heme proteins can have direct cytotoxic effect on tubular epithelial cells; the mechanism remains ill defined.
- Renal ischemia is believed to result from activation of endothelin receptors as well as scavenging of nitric oxide. Myoglobin is also believed to generate free radicals that can induce oxidative injury to the tubules. This may be inhibited in an alkaline pH.

Management of ATN

- Ischemia-induced AKI occurs in many different clinical scenarios. Recommendations for therapy in any given case have to be tailored according to the clinical circumstances.
- Here, we present a broad and basic framework of therapy. The management of other individual causes is presented in relevant chapters elsewhere.

Restoration of Effective Circulatory Volume

- **Restoration of effective circulatory volume** is one of the crucial aspects of management in patients with ischemic renal injury.
  - The initial fluid of choice is a **crystalloid solution,** such as normal saline in most situations, administered until euvolemia is restored.
  - Theoretical benefit of colloid such as albumin, gelatin, and dextrans outside the operating room are often outweighed by complications such as coagulopathy, anaphylactoid reactions, heart failure, and renal failure.[21]
  - Fluids must be administered with caution in oliguric AKI in order to avoid volume overload and subsequent heart failure or respiratory failure.
  - If fluid resuscitation is not successful in improving blood pressure, inotropic or pressor agents may be needed.
- In the special circumstance of rhabdomyolysis, **early volume repletion** is essential in preventing AKI.[22]
  - Initially normal saline should be infused at a rate of 1 to 2 L in the first hour and then continued at 150 to 300 mL/h, depending on the urine output and the patient's volume status.
  - **Sodium bicarbonate infusions are not recommended** and can have deleterious effects if acid-base status is not monitored closely—especially in the setting of hypocalcemia—given the risk of increased calcium binding in the setting of alkalosis.[23,24]
  - Anuric or oliguric AKI signals extensive tubular injury and requires a downward titration of IV fluids.
  - Early initiation of RRT should be considered in anuric or oliguric patients, given the risk of life-threatening hyperkalemia with ongoing muscle damage.

Withdrawal and Avoidance of Nephrotoxins

- It is extremely important to **avoid further injury** to the suffering kidney.
  - Contrast media should be avoided wherever possible.
  - NSAIDs, angiotensin-converting enzyme inhibitors, and angiotensin 2 receptor blockers should be held.

○ Nonnephrotoxic antibiotics should be prescribed whenever possible.
○ If a potentially toxic antibiotic usage is unavoidable, the dose should be carefully adjusted, and drug levels should be closely monitored; if possible, pharmacokinetic principles should be applied (e.g., aminoglycosides).

Diuretics
- **The diuretic challenge** is often used in patients with oliguric AKI, in an attempt to convert them to a nonoliguric state. This may be helpful in the management of the patient with regard to hyperkalemia and hypervolemia.
  ○ **Diuretics do not improve survival or hasten renal function recovery in AKI.**
  ○ Theoretically, diuretics discourage cellular debris from obstructing the tubular lumen because of enhanced urinary volume. However, little evidence exists that forced diuresis can mitigate the intraparenchymal obstructive process.
  ○ The use of diuretics to convert from an oliguric to nonoliguric state should not sway the physician away from early nephrology consultation or institution of RRT in a timely fashion.
  ○ If diuretics are used, then **doses utilized must be high enough to reach the loop of Henle** in order to be effective in the setting of reduced GFR. For example, with a GFR of <30 mL/min, a 160 to 200 mg IV bolus of furosemide might be needed.
  ○ If there is a diuretic response, then it can be continued as intermittent doses or as a continuous infusion. Studies have not shown a difference in outcome with either method.
  ○ Volume status should be ascertained carefully prior to and during diuretic administration, to avoid intravascular volume depletion.

Renal Replacement Therapy
- RRT is the mainstay of care for unremitting AKI. Details regarding the different modes of dialysis for treatment of AKI are discussed in Chapter 15.

Experimental Agents for the Treatment of AKI
- Several medications have been **investigated in clinical trials, but none are approved** for use in the prevention or treatment of AKI.
  ○ **Dopamine** has vasodilatory and diuretic properties; however, it offers no clinical response at low dose and causes severe hypotension at high doses.[25]
  ○ **Fenoldopam** is a dopamine-1 receptor agonist that has selective activity in the kidney vasculature, but also causes systemic hypotension, negating its renal benefit. In high-risk patients, fenoldopam may have benefit if it can be administered in a directed fashion to the renal vasculature,[26] but this is not practiced routinely.
  ○ **Anaritide** initially failed to show efficacy in the setting of heart failure; however, by tailoring administration to the high-risk patient population in the cardiothoracic ICU, the drug has demonstrated selective benefit.[27]
- The difficulty of treating established AKI has generated interest in the study of prophylactic agents. The **following medications** were **evaluated in phase III clinical trials** for AKI in select settings but **are not recommended as standard therapy.**
  ○ **Iloprost,** a prostacyclin analog, has vasodilatory effect on the renal medulla and has been shown to reduce the incidence of AKI in high-risk patients undergoing radiologic studies enhanced with iodinated radiocontrast.[28] This drug's benefit is yet to be confirmed in patients who participated in the US healthcare system.

○ Rolofylline, an adenosine-1 receptor antagonist, was not effective in the treatment of patients with cardiorenal physiology. However, the selected clinical trial design has been criticized for not administering the drug as a continuous infusion and assessment of benefit before the drug was metabolized.[29]

• Most of clinical trials evaluating therapeutic agents in the setting of ATN have been hampered by the lack of an early biomarker. Several studies are underway to find an ideal renal biomarker, which hopefully will pave the way to find therapeutic strategies for ATN.

REFERENCES

1. Chertow GM, Burdick E, Honour M, et al. Acute kidney injury, mortality, length of stay, and costs in hospitalized patients. *J Am Soc Nephrol.* 2005;16:3365–3370.
2. Lameire N. KDIGO Clinical Guidelines. http://www.kdigo.org/clinical_practice_guidelines_3. Last accessed 12/27/10 <www.kdigo.org.>
3. Hoste EA, Clermont G, Kersten A, et al. RIFLE criteria for acute kidney injury are associated with hospital mortality in critically ill patients: a cohort analysis. *Crit Care.* 2006; 10:R73.
4. Mehta RL, Kellum JA, Shah SV, et al. The Acute Kidney Injury Network. Acute Kidney Injury Network: report of an initiative to improve outcomes in acute kidney injury. *Crit Care.* 2007;11(2):R31.
5. Lafrance JP, Miller DR. Defining acute kidney injury in database studies: the effects of varying the baseline kidney function assessment period and considering CKD status. *Am J Kidney Dis.* 2010;56:651–660.
6. Coca SG, Yusuf B, Shlipak MG, et al. Long-term risk of mortality and other adverse outcomes after acute kidney injury: a systematic review and meta-analysis. *Am J Kidney Dis.* 2009;53:961–973.
7. Brenner B, Lazarus M, eds. *Acute Renal Failure.* New York, NY: Churchill Livingstone; 1993.
8. Koyner JL, Vaidya V, Bennett MR, et al. Urinary biomarkers in the clinical prognosis and early detection of acute kidney injury. *Clin J Am Soc Nephrol.* 2010;5:2154–2165.
9. van Heerden F. Hoodia gordonii: a natural appetite suppressant. *J Ethnopharmacol.* 2008;119:434–437.
10. Xi Z, Ningning X. Effects of long-term use of the heat-clearing, diuresis-promoting and collateral-mediating Chinese drugs on changes of proteinuria in patients with chronic nephritis. *J Tradit Chin Med.* 2006;26:213–217.
11. Liu Q, Wang Q, Yang X, et al. Differential cytotoxic effects of denitroaristolochic acid II and aristolochic acids on renal epithelial cells. *Toxicol Lett.* 2009;1841:5–12.
12. McIlroy DR, Wagener G, Lee HT. Neutrophil gelatinase-associated lipocalin and acute kidney injury after cardiac surgery: the effect of baseline renal function on diagnostic performance. *Clin J Am Soc Nephrol.* 2010;5:211–219.
13. Hall IE, Yarlagadda S, Coca SG, et al. IL-18 and urinary NGAL predict dialysis and graft recovery after kidney transplantation. *J Am Soc Nephrol.* 2010;21:189–197.
14. Waikar SS, Liu K, Chertow GM. Diagnosis, epidemiology and outcomes of acute kidney injury. *Clin J Am Soc Nephrol.* 2008;3:844–861.
15. Schrier RW, Wang W, Poole B, et al. Acute renal failure: definitions, diagnosis, pathogenesis, and therapy. *J Clin Invest.* 2004;114:5–14.
16. Jang HR, Ko G, Wasowska BA, et al. The interaction between ischemia-reperfusion and immune responses in the kidney. *J Mol Med.* 2009;87:859–864.
17. Goldberg R, Dennen P. Long-term outcomes of acute kidney injury. *Adv Chronic Kidney Dis.* 2008;15:297–307.
18. Abels BC, Branch RA, Sabra R. Interaction between thromboxane A2 and angiotensin II in postischemic renal vasoconstriction in dogs. *J Pharmacol Exp Ther.* 1993;264:1285–1292.

19. Arendshorst WJ, Brannstrom K, Ruan X. Actions of angiotensin II on the renal microvasculature. *J Am Soc Nephrol.* 1999;10:S149–S161.
20. Poole B, Wang W, Chen YC, et al. Role of heme oxygenase-1 in endotoxemic acute renal failure. *Am J Physiol Renal Physiol.* 2005;289:F1382–F1385.
21. Ragaller MJ, Theilen H, Koch T. Volume replacement in critically ill patients with acute renal failure. *J Am Soc Nephrol.* 2001;12:S33–S39.
22. Bosch X, Poch E, Grau JM. Rhabdomyolysis and acute kidney injury. *N Engl J Med.* 2009;361:62–72.
23. Bagley WH, Yang H, Shah KH. Rhabdomyolysis. *Intern Emerg Med.* 2007;2:210–218.
24. Brown CV, Rhee P, Chan L, et al. Preventing renal failure in patients with rhabdomyolysis: do bicarbonate and mannitol make a difference? *J Trauma.* 2004;56:1191–1196.
25. Karthik S, Lisbon A. Low-dose dopamine in the intensive care unit. *Semin Dial.* 2006;19:465–471.
26. Weisz G, Filby SJ, Cohen MG, et al. Safety and performance of targeted renal therapy: the Be-RITe! Registry. *J Endovasc Ther.* 2009;16:1–12.
27. Swärd K, Valsson F, Odencrants P, et al. Recombinant human atrial natriuretic peptide in ischemic acute renal failure: a randomized placebo-controlled trial. *Crit Care Med.* 2004;32:1310–1315.
28. Spargias K, Adreanides E, Demerouti E, et al. Iloprost prevents contrast-induced nephropathy in patients with renal dysfunction undergoing coronary angiography or intervention. *Circulation.* 2009;120:1793–1799.
29. Massie BM, O'Connor CM, Metra M, et al. Rolofylline, an adenosine A1-receptor antagonist, in acute heart failure. *N Engl J Med.* 2010;363:1419–1428.

Prerenal and Postrenal Acute Kidney Injury

12

Judy L. Jang and Anitha Vijayan

PRERENAL KIDNEY DISEASE

GENERAL PRINCIPLES

- Prerenal azotemia is the most common cause of acute kidney injury (AKI). Rapid restoration of effective circulatory volume usually leads to prompt and complete resolution of AKI.
- A complete examination of the urine, including the sediment, in addition to a thorough history and physical examination exam is essential in ascertaining the accurate diagnosis.
- Fractional excretion of sodium (FE_{Na}) is useful in the *oliguric state only*.
- Fractional excretion of urea (FE_{Urea}) may be a useful marker to distinguish prerenal AKI from acute tubular necrosis (ATN) in the setting of diuretic use.

Definition

- Prerenal kidney injury is characterized by a state in which renal parenchymal function is preserved and is responding appropriately to diminished perfusion. Because the integrity of the renal parenchymal tissue is preserved, timely restoration of perfusion and glomerular ultrafiltration pressure should correct glomerular filtration rate (GFR).
- There is a continuum from compensated renal hypoperfusion, without a change in GFR, to prerenal injury with reduced GFR to ischemic ATN.[1,2]

Epidemiology

- Prerenal azotemia has been described as the cause of AKI in 30% to 70% of community-associated kidney injury and up to 30% of hospital-associated kidney injury, depending on various patient populations.[3]

Etiology

- The important causes of prerenal AKI are summarized in Table 12-1. These include:
  - Intravascular volume depletion
  - Decreased effective circulating volume
  - Renal vasoconstriction (e.g., sepsis, hypercalcemia, liver disease, and nonsteroidal anti-inflammatory drugs [NSAIDs], cyclooxygenase 2 [COX-2] inhibitors)
  - Pharmacologic agents that impair autoregulation and GFR (e.g., efferent arteriolar vasodilatation due to **angiotensin-converting enzyme inhibitors** [ACEIs] or **angiotensin-2 receptor blockers** [ARBs]).[1]

TABLE 12-1	MAJOR CAUSES OF PRERENAL AZOTEMIA

Decrease in effective circulating volume
Hemorrhage: traumatic, surgical, gastrointestinal, postpartum
Gastrointestinal losses: vomiting, nasogastric suction, diarrhea
Renal losses: drug-induced or osmotic diuresis, diabetes insipidus, adrenal insufficiency
Skin and mucous membrane losses: burns, hyperthermia, other causes of increased insensible losses
"Third-space" losses: pancreatitis, intestinal obstruction, severe crush injury, hypoalbuminemia

Decreased cardiac output
Diseases of myocardium, valves, pericardium, or conducting system
Pulmonary hypertension, pulmonary embolism, positive-pressure mechanical ventilation
Drugs: antihypertensive medications, afterload reduction, anesthetics, drug overdoses

Afferent arteriolar vasoconstriction
Drugs: norepinephrine, ergotamine, NSAIDs, calcineurin inhibitors
Electrolyte disturbances: hypercalcemia
Systemic illnesses: end-stage liver disease, sepsis, anaphylaxis

Efferent arteriolar vasodilatation
AECIs
ARBs

Common clinical scenarios that acutely impair autoregulation and glomerular filtration rate
ACEIs or ARBs in the setting of bilateral renal artery stenosis
Underlying CKD on ACEI or ARB and sudden volume depletion (e.g., vomiting or diarrhea)
Use of ACEIs or ARBs in conjunction with NSAIDs or COX-2 inhibitors. (e.g., elderly patient on ACEI started on NSAIDs for gout)
Use of NSAIDs in the setting of volume depletion

ACEI, angiotensin-converting enzyme inhibitor; ARB angiotensin-2 receptor blocker; CKD, chronic kidney disease; COX-2, cyclooxygenase 2; NSAID, nonsteroidal anti-inflammatory drug.

Adapted from Brenner, BM, ed. *Brenner & Rector's The Kidney.* 7th ed. Philadelphia: WB Saunders; 2004.

- There are factors that limit the ability of renal autoregulation to maintain homeostasis.
  ○ Under normal circumstances, the kidney may be able to preserve function despite significantly low perfusion pressures.
  ○ Renal function may decompensate at relatively higher mean arterial pressures in patients with limited ability to maintain afferent arteriolar dilatation due to preexisting large or small vessel disease (e.g., atherosclerosis, diabetic nephropathy). Thus, an elderly patient being treated with ACEIs

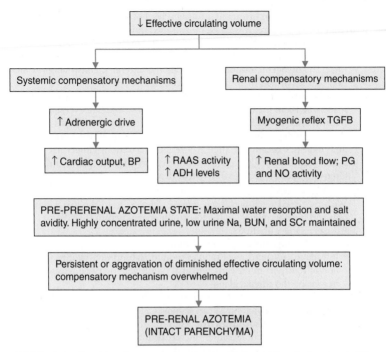

FIGURE 12-1. Algorithm for prerenal azotemia. ADH, antidiuretic hormone; BP, blood pressure; BUN, blood urea nitrogen; NO, nitric oxide; PG, prostaglandin; RAAS, renin–angiotensin–aldosterone system; SCr, serum creatinine; TGFB, tubuloglomerular feedback.

could suffer from prerenal azotemia, even with relatively modest decreases in blood pressure.

Pathophysiology

- The hallmark of the prerenal state is **decreased perfusion of the kidney.** There are immediate systemic and renal compensatory responses, recruiting multiple neurohumoral systems, directed at maintaining blood flow and GFR. The cascade of events discussed below is depicted in Figure 12-1.
- The adrenergic system functions to maintain blood pressure.
  - A decrease in blood pressure leads to increased sympathetic activity, resulting in increased peripheral vascular resistance. Thereby, cardiac output increases, leading to restoration of perfusion pressure.
  - Negative repercussions to the kidneys may result, as renal vasoconstriction due to sympathetic drive may cause decreased renal blood flow (RBF).
  - Sympathetic activity also stimulates release of renin through beta-adrenergic receptors.

- Renal **autoregulation** maintains a constant level of RBF despite fluctuations in arterial blood pressure. It is based on two mechanisms, the myogenic response and tubuloglomerular feedback.
  - A function of smooth muscle contraction in response to external stretching force, the **myogenic response**, causes afferent arteriolar constriction or dilation on rises or falls in arterial pressure.
  - **Tubuloglomerular feedback** leads to afferent arteriolar dilatation when the macula densa in the early distal tubule senses low solute delivery.[4]
  - Maintenance of GFR through falling perfusion pressures stems from the ability to **independently maneuver the afferent and efferent arterioles.** As flow increases because of afferent arteriolar relaxation, glomerular pressure is maintained through efferent arteriolar constriction, mediated through the renin–angiotensin–aldosterone system (RAAS).
- The **RAAS** is critical in renal self-defense.
  - With decreased renal perfusion, renin is released from the juxtaglomerular cells and leads ultimately to the formation of angiotensin II (AII).
  - AII has a variety of effects:
    - It produces arteriolar vasoconstriction.
    - It leads to enhanced renal tubular sodium reabsorption by direct stimulation of transport in the early proximal tubule and increased release of aldosterone by the adrenal gland.
    - It exerts complex effects on glomerular hemodynamics. With modest hypotension or congestive heart failure (CHF), AII can preserve GFR by its **preferential vasoconstrictive** action on the **efferent** arteriole. Efferent arteriolar constriction causes increased intraglomerular pressure, thus maintaining the filtration fraction. With increasing AII activity, the afferent arteriole also starts to constrict, leading to decreased filtration.[5] Blocking this effect of AII with ACEIs or ARBs leads to an earlier and more marked fall in GFR.
    - It generates nitric oxide release and stimulates production of vasodilator prostaglandins, particularly prostacyclin, which protect the afferent arteriole from vasoconstrictive influences.[6,7] This interaction leads to early decompensation of renal function in patients using NSAIDs due to loss of prostacyclin production.
    - It increases release of antidiuretic hormone (ADH) from the posterior pituitary. Mainly stimulated by volume depletion and hyperosmolality, ADH acts to exert maximal water conservation and excretion of concentrated urine. Acting through the V_1-receptors, it also causes vasoconstriction and increased peripheral resistance and blood pressure.
- Because of these autoregulatory mechanisms, renal function is able to be maintained even under conditions of diminished effective volume.
- If, however, the effective circulatory volume continues to decrease, the renal compensatory mechanisms may be overwhelmed, as the afferent arteriolar vasodilatation is no longer adequate to maintain flow.
  - Should the levels of AII become overwhelming, vasoconstriction will occur in the renal vasculature. RBF will subsequently decrease, as will urine output, resulting in a state of prerenal azotemia.[5]
  - The blood urea nitrogen and plasma creatinine levels will start to rise as the kidney strives to hold onto water and salt through persistent tubular action. If this sequence is not reversed quickly, the parenchyma will no longer remain intact and the patient may suffer ischemic ATN.

DIAGNOSIS

Clinical Presentation

- Signs and symptoms of prerenal kidney injury are usually very subtle and patients are frequently asymptomatic.
- Careful monitoring of urine output for oliguria (<400 to 500 mL/d) is critical in identifying and reversing oliguric prerenal kidney injury.
- The diagnosis of prerenal AKI ultimately rests on a combination of clinical findings and laboratory testing.

History

- A detailed history of events causing alterations in volume status should be sought.
  - A history of lightheadedness or orthostatic instability may point toward intra-vascular depletion.
  - Hemorrhage, diarrhea, polyuria, and situations leading to excessive insensi-tive losses (e.g., fever or diminished intake due to dysphagia) all predispose to volume depletion.
  - Weight gain, edema, or periorbital swelling may signify fluid retention in the extravascular space.
  - A review of the patient's records should be conducted for episodes of blood pressure swings. For postoperative patients, it is essential to review intra- and postoperative hemodynamic records for hypotension.
- Obtain history of urinary symptoms and trends. Intake and output charts, as well as weight records, of a hospitalized patient should be carefully reviewed.
- Elicit preexisting underlying factors (e.g., CHF, hypertension, or diabetes mellitus) that may adversely affect ability to exercise maximum autoregulation.
- A thorough review of medications should be conducted, with specific focus on nephrotoxic medications that can induce glomerular hypoperfusion (e.g., NSAIDs, COX-2 inhibitors, ACEIs, ARBs, calcineurin inhibitors, and so forth).

Physical Examination

- Pulse rate and blood pressure should be measured in supine and standing posi-tions in patients with suspected volume depletion.
- Mucous membranes and skin turgor need to be checked for assessment of degree of hydration.
- The presence of jugular venous distention and edema suggest volume overload. The location and character of the apical impulse, presence of S3 (volume over-load) or S4 (pressure overload), and presence of functional regurgitant mur-murs should be carefully discerned. Dyspnea, tachypnea, and crackles can occur with pulmonary edema.
- Splenomegaly, hepatomegaly, and ascites can occur because of passive conges-tion in fluid overload states.

Diagnostic Testing

- Additional procedures such as central venous pressure or pulmonary capillary wedge pressure measurement might be required if volume status is not apparent from a thorough history and physical examination.[8]

- **Urinalysis** in prenatal kidney injury is often characterized as "**bland**," with no protein or blood seen. Typically, hyaline casts can be seen under magnification.[2]
- Urine indices in the oliguric state, such as the FE_{Na} and the FE_{Urea}, are useful but imperfect tools to help differentiate the prerenal state from ATN. In oliguric AKI, the differentiation of prerenal failure from ATN is critical to guide appropriate management.
  - In prerenal AKI, the FE_{Na} **is <1%, in the absence of diuretic** use. In one study, the FE_{Na} was low in only 48% of diuretic-treated patients with prerenal azotemia.[9]
  - Urea absorption by the proximal tubule is increased in prerenal states,[10] leading to a FE_{Urea} **of <35%.** Given that most diuretics used clinically work at distal sites, FE_{Urea} should not be affected by their use and is therefore a valuable clinical measure in the setting of diuretic use. Though the positive predictive value of FE_{Urea} is 98%, FE_{Urea} values in chronic kidney disease (CKD) have not been standardized, so caution must be used.
- Interpretations of urine indices must be made in conjunction with other assessments of the patient, because there are clinically important **exceptions** to these generalizations. For instance, patients with certain types of ATN, such as contrast-induced renal injury, rhabdomyolysis, sepsis, wherein vasoconstriction plays a key role, may present FE_{Na} rates <1%, despite having tubular injury. **Acute glomerulonephritis** can also present with low FE_{Na}, but urinalysis will reveal hematuria, proteinuria and presence of red blood cells, and sometimes, casts.

TREATMENT

- The treatment of prerenal AKI should be **expeditious** to avoid ischemia to the renal tubules and ATN.

Restoration of Effective Circulatory Volume

- The fundamental problem in most cases of prerenal azotemia is diminished effective circulatory volume. Prompt and effective restoration improves RBF, leading to increased GFR and improvement or normalization of renal function.
  - In most cases of prerenal injury, administration of intravenous fluids is the mainstay of therapy.
  - The initial fluid of choice is administration of a crystalloid solution to restore the euvolemic state. **Normal saline** is usually the most effective choice.
  - Alternatives include colloid solutions such as albumin, gelatin, and dextrans. However, anaphylactoid reactions, coagulopathy, and precipitation of oliguria and AKI may sometimes be seen with these agents.[11]

Treatment of Underlying Causes

- In patients with hepatorenal syndrome (HRS), the underlying hepatic dysfunction needs to be reversed either with recovery of the injured liver (e.g., acetaminophen overdose) or with liver transplantation.
- Correction of compromised cardiac output may involve preload and afterload reduction and diuresis or appropriate use of inotropic agents, vasodilators, or other means to maintain blood pressure and perfusion.

- The HRS and cardiorenal syndrome (CRS) are discussed below.
- In patients with sepsis, immediate intervention with broad-spectrum intravenous antibiotics and pressor support will help stabilize blood pressure and improve renal perfusion.
- Medications such as diuretics or those interfering with the RAAS pathway should be discontinued without delay. Other medications that should be discontinued include NSAIDs and COX-2 inhibitors. Calcineurin inhibitors should be handled with caution, as sudden discontinuation in a patient with organ transplant can precipitate rejection. However, levels should be closely monitored and should be maintained in the recommended therapeutic range.

SPECIAL CONSIDERATIONS

Hepatorenal Syndrome

- HRS is the most frequent cause of renal dysfunction in patients with cirrhosis.
- Two types of HRS were originally defined by the International Ascites Club.[12,13]
  - **Type 1 HRS** presents as rapid and progressive impairment of renal function defined by a doubling of the initial serum creatinine to a level >2.5 mg/dL (220 μmol/L) or a 50% reduction of the initial 24-hour creatinine clearance to a level <20 mL/min in <2 weeks. This is associated with a dismal prognosis.
  - **Type 2 HRS** presents as impairment in renal function with serum creatinine levels >1.5 mg/dL (132 μmol/L) that does not meet criteria for type 1 HRS. Type 2 HRS develops gradually over weeks and is associated with a better survival.
- Renal vasoconstriction is the main hemodynamic derangement that defines HRS.
  - The main variable responsible for these hemodynamic changes is portal in the setting of cirrhosis, causing a splanchnic arterial vasodilation. This vasodilation occurs mainly because of the production of nitric oxide as a consequence of endothelial stretching and possibly bacterial translocation.[12]
  - The accumulation of plasma volume in the splanchnic bed causes a compensatory response because of decreased central blood volume with activation of systemic vasoconstrictor and antinatriuretic systems (RAAS, sympathetic system, ADH). This accounts for the sodium and water retention, as well as renal vasoconstriction, as the kidney senses a relative hypovolemic state.
  - Recent studies suggest that the development of HRS may also be due, in part, to reduction in cardiac output.
- HRS occurs in ~10% of hospitalized patients who have cirrhosis and ascites. In addition, the probability of developing HRS in patients who had cirrhosis and ascites was 18% at 1 year and increased to 39% at 5 years.[14]
- Individuals who develop HRS most often exhibit clinical features of advanced cirrhosis along with low arterial blood pressure, low urine volume, and severe urinary sodium retention (urine sodium <10 mEq/L). Dilutional hyponatremia is almost universally found.
- **Elevated serum creatinine levels define HRS.** However, these levels usually are lower than those seen in noncirrhotic patients who have AKI because of reduced muscle mass and low endogenous production of creatinine in cirrhosis.

- **Suggested diagnostic criteria for HRS** include[13,15]:
  - Acute or chronic hepatic disease with advanced hepatic failure and portal hypertension.
  - Low GFR, as indicated by plasma creatinine levels >1.5 mg/dL or 132 μmol/L.
  - Exclusion of other apparent causes for renal failure, such as shock (sepsis or hypovolemia), volume depletion, use of nephrotoxic drugs (e.g., NSAIDs), and obstruction.
  - No improvement in renal function despite withdrawal of diuretics and volume challenge with intravenous albumin.
- The only **definitive cure** for HRS is recovery of hepatic function either with **liver transplantation** or **spontaneous recovery** of the diseased liver.
- **Temporizing measures** can provide a bridge to liver transplantation or recovery.
  - The combination of drugs to induce splanchnic vasoconstriction (octreotide) and renal vasodilation (midodrine) has been beneficial in improving renal function in HRS.[16]
  - Even though intravenous albumin appears to augment the response to these agents, its use remains controversial. However, in the setting of large-volume paracentesis, intravenous albumin should be administered to prevent renal dysfunction, especially in the setting of spontaneous bacterial peritonitis.
  - Alternatively, vasopressin analogs (e.g., terlipressin), which can also cause splanchnic vasoconstriction along with renal vasodilation, can be used instead of the combination.[17] The limitation of terlipressin is its unavailability in many countries, including the United States.
  - The **transjugular intrahepatic portosystemic shunt** is another potential modality of therapy for HRS. A self-expandable metal stent is inserted between the hepatic vein and the intrahepatic portion of the portal vein using a transjugular approach, with a resulting decrease in portal pressure. It is primarily reserved for treatment of variceal bleeding and refractory ascites, although small studies have suggested some improvement in renal function.[18]
  - Molecular adsorbent recirculating system (MARS) is a modified form of dialysis using albumin-containing dialysate that is recirculated and perfused online through charcoal and anion exchanger columns, and enables the removal of water-soluble and albumin-bound substances. It is believed that this system removes some of the vasoactive substances that mediate the hemodynamic changes that lead to HRS, thereby improving systemic hemodynamics and renal perfusion. Short-term studies suggest survival benefit with MARS in HRS, but larger studies are required before this expensive therapy can be widely recommended.[19] It is not approved for use in the United States.
  - Hemodialysis is extremely controversial in HRS. Generally, hemodialysis is usually offered only if the patient is awaiting liver transplantation or there is a chance of liver recovery. In the absence of these possibilities, dialysis adds little to overall survival in this condition.

Cardiorenal Syndrome

- The coexistence of renal and cardiac dysfunction, in which acute or chronic dysfunction in one organ may induce acute or chronic dysfunction in the other organ, has been termed CRS.

- A classification of CRS with five subtypes has been proposed that reflects the bidirectional nature of the heart and kidney interaction, the timeframe, and the pathophysiology[20]:
  - CRS Type 1: **rapid worsening of cardiac function results in AKI**
  - CRS Type 2: chronic worsening of cardiac function causes progressive CKD
  - CRS Type 3: abrupt and primary worsening of renal function (e.g., AKI, ischemia, glomerulonephritis) leads to acute cardiac dysfunction (e.g., CHF, arrhythmia, ischemia)
  - CRS Type 4: primary CKD contributes to cardiac dysfunction (e.g., ventricular hypertrophy, diastolic dysfunction, increased risk of adverse cardiovascular events)
  - CRS Type 5: acute or chronic systemic disorders cause both cardiac and renal dysfunction
- The classical CRS seen in the hospital setting is Type 1 CRS and the discussion below will focus only on this condition.
- Renal insufficiency is found in 30% to 40% of patients admitted to the hospital for heart failure.[21]
- The pathophysiology of CRS Type 1 involves interconnected hemodynamic and neurohormonal mechanisms.
  - Impaired cardiac output in heart failure causes renal arterial underfilling and increased venous pressure. In response, neurohormonal sympathetic activation occurs and increases systemic vasoconstriction, leading to a reduction in GFR. This, in turn, activates the RAAS, which generates more AII, aldosterone, endothelin-1, and ADH, in an attempt to maintain euvolemia through fluid retention, vasoconstriction, or both.[22]
  - The activity of these systems remains elevated over the long term in patients with heart failure, resulting in systemic and pulmonary congestion, a hallmark of CRS.
- **Features of CRS Type 1** include low systolic blood pressure, tendency for hyperkalemia, diuretic resistance, and anemia. Preexisting renal dysfunction as well as other risk factors such as hypertension and diabetes mellitus may contribute to worsening renal failure and poor outcome associated with decompensated cardiac disease.[23,24]
- The **management of the CRS** remains a challenge in spite of advances in medical therapy.
  - In the setting of overt volume overload, **large doses of loop diuretics** (e.g., furosemide 120 to 200 mg) may need to be administered intravenously to achieve a desirable diuresis.
  - For synergy, **thiazide diuretics** or analogs (e.g. metolazone) should be added, to block sodium absorption in the distal convoluted tubule and increase natriuresis.
  - Small studies have shown that nitrates allow for decreased doses of diuretics.
  - Inotropic agents have been used successfully in the cardiogenic shock stage but need further evaluation with lesser degrees of cardiac failure.
  - Nesiritide, a potent vasodilator, has been used to rapidly reduce cardiac filling pressures and improve dyspnea in patients with heart failure. However, nesiritide should be used with caution, as deterioration of renal function has been seen in some cases.[25]
  - Hemofiltration, though shown to be beneficial in achieving faster fluid removal in small trials, is invasive and expensive. Larger, multicenter evaluations are needed before its use can be widely recommended.
  - **Anemia** should be treated with judicious use of intravenous iron, erythropoietic-stimulating agents and blood transfusion, as correction of anemia has been shown to decrease rehospitalizations and improve quality of life in heart failure patients.

POSTRENAL KIDNEY DISEASE

GENERAL PRINCIPLES

- Obstructive uropathy should be considered in patients with decreased or absent urine output, change in voiding pattern, unexplained renal insufficiency, or pain suggesting urinary tract distension.
- Ultrasound is a cost-effective and efficient way to evaluate for urinary tract obstruction (UTO).
- The degree of obstruction may be underestimated in severely dehydrated patients. In such cases, repeating the ultrasound after adequate volume replacement may highlight the hydronephrosis.
- Rarely, in cases of retroperitoneal fibrosis or lymphomas, the ureters are encased and hydronephrosis is not seen despite severe UTO.
- UTO may present with polyuria if the obstruction is incomplete.
- Prompt relief of obstruction is essential to avoid parenchymal destruction.
- Fluid replacement during a postobstructive diuresis (due to retained volume and solutes) should be judicious. Overzealous fluid replacement may lead to replacement of the postobstructive diuresis by a diuresis secondary to intravenous fluids.

Definition

- **Obstructive uropathy** describes an impediment to urine flow due to structural or functional change anywhere from the renal pelvis to the tip of the urethra. This resistance to flow increases pressure proximal to the point of obstruction. Renal parenchymal damage may or may not be associated.
- **Obstructive nephropathy** describes any functional or pathologic changes in the kidney that result from UTO.

Classification

- Obstructive uropathy is classified based on the duration, level, and degree of obstruction.[26]
  - The duration is characterized as either acute or chronic (hours to weeks vs. months to years).
  - Obstruction is considered upper tract if it is located above the ureterovesical junction and lower tract if located below it.
  - The degree of obstruction is either complete or partial.
  - The common causes of obstruction are noted in Tables 12-2, 12-3 and 12-4.

Epidemiology

- UTO accounts for <5% of cases of AKI in the hospitalized patients.
- However, in patients presenting to the emergency room with AKI, it can be seen in ~20% of the patients.
- The condition has a bimodal distribution:
  - In childhood, obstructive uropathy is primarily due to congenital abnormalities of the urinary tract.
  - Incidence rises after age 60 because of the increased presentation of benign prostatic hyperplasia (BPH) and prostate cancer in older men.
- Early identification is critical as the extent to which the renal function recovers with treatment is inversely proportional to the duration and degree of obstruction. Hydronephrosis is found at postmortem examination in 2% to 4% of patients.[27]

TABLE 12-2	CONGENITAL CAUSES OF OBSTRUCTIVE UROPATHY

Ureter

Ureteropelvic junction obstruction
Ureteroceles
Ectopic ureter
Ureteral valves

Bladder

Myelodysplasias (e.g., meningomyelocele)
Bladder diverticula

Urethra

Prune-belly syndrome
Urethral diverticula
Posterior urethral valves

Etiology

- Obstructive uropathy may be the result of anatomic or functional abnormalities anywhere in the urinary tract. These abnormalities are either congenital (Table 12-2) or acquired (Tables 12-3 and 12-4). The etiology varies depending on the age and sex of the patient.
  - In children, obstruction is due mainly to anatomic abnormalities, including urethral valves or stricture and stenosis at the ureterovesical or ureteropelvic junction.
  - Nephrolithiasis is the most common cause of obstructive uropathy in young adults.
  - In females, pregnancy (due to the effects of progesterone and mechanical pressure by the gravid uterus) and gynecologic tumors account for most of the cases.
  - In the older adults, the most common causes are BPH or prostate cancer, retroperitoneal or pelvic tumors, and stones.

TABLE 12-3	ACQUIRED INTRINSIC CAUSES OF OBSTRUCTIVE UROPATHY

Intraluminal	Intramural
Intrarenal	**Anatomic**
Tubular precipitation of proteins: Bence-Jones proteins	Tumors (renal pelvis, ureter, bladder, urethra)
Tubular precipitation of crystals: uric acid, medications (e.g., acyclovir, indinavir, sulfonamides)	Strictures (ureteral or urethral)
	Infections
	Granulomatous disease
	Instrumentation or trauma
	Radiation therapy
Extrarenal	**Functional Disorders of the Bladder**
Nephrolithiasis	Diabetes mellitus with autonomic bladder
Blood clots	Multiple sclerosis
Papillary necrosis	Spinal cord injury
Fungus balls	Anticholinergic agents

TABLE 12-4	ACQUIRED EXTRINSIC CAUSES OF OBSTRUCTIVE UROPATHY

Reproductive and Urologic

Uterus (pregnancy, prolapse, tumors)
Ovary (abscess, cysts, tumors)
Fallopian tubes (pelvic inflammatory disease)
Prostate (benign hyperplasia, adenocarcinoma)

Gastrointestinal

Crohn's disease
Appendicitis
Diverticulitis
Colorectal carcinoma

Vascular Disorders

Aneurysms (abdominal aortic, iliac)
Venous (ovarian vein thrombophlebitis, retrocaval ureter)

Retroperitoneal Disorders

Fibrosis (idiopathic, drug related, inflammatory, malignancy)
Infection/abscess
Radiation therapy
Tumor and/or lymphadenopathy (primary or metastatic)
Iatrogenic complication of surgery

Pathophysiology

- Obstruction to the urinary flow affects the kidney through a variety of factors with complex interactions that alter both glomerular hemodynamics and tubular function.[28]
  - The GFR drops after the onset of UTO because of a decrease in net hydrostatic pressure across the glomerular capillary wall. Initially, this is due to an increase in intratubular pressure, but in the latter stages of obstruction, it is secondary to a fall in intraglomerular pressure. This reduction in intraglomerular pressure is a manifestation of decreased RBF, caused by AII- and thromboxane A_2-mediated vasoconstriction.
- Obstructive nephropathy is also associated with several abnormalities of tubular function believed to be caused by increased pressure within the tubules, leading to altered transport of sodium, water, and several other ions and solutes.
- In long-standing obstruction, the parenchyma atrophies, and fibrosis and scarring of the tubulointerstitium follow.[29]

DIAGNOSIS

Clinical Presentation

- Clinical manifestations vary with the site, degree, and rapidity of onset of obstructive uropathy.[29,30] The diagnosis should be considered in patients with any of the following:
  - **Pain:**
    - Kidney and ureteral pain is usually along the T11 to T12 distribution.

- Upper ureteral or renal pelvic lesions cause **flank pain or tenderness,** whereas lower ureteral obstruction may present with **colicky pain** radiating to the ipsilateral testicle or labia.
- Severe pain accompanied by **nausea and vomiting** may result from acute complete ureteral obstruction (e.g., obstructing ureteral calculus).
- In patients with partial or slowly developing obstruction (e.g., pelvic tumor), pain may be minimal or absent.

○ **Palpable mass:**
  - Hydronephrosis may rarely present as a palpable flank mass, particularly in long-standing cases.
  - A **palpable mass in the suprapubic** area may represent a distended bladder.

○ **Change in voiding pattern and symptoms:**
  - Unilateral obstruction does not cause decreased urine volume unless it occurs in the only functioning kidney.
  - Complete obstruction at the level of the bladder or urethra results in **anuria.**
  - Partial or intermittent obstruction can result in **polyuria** or polyuria alternating with oligoanuria. **Difficulty in voiding** or abnormalities in the urine stream may be present.
  - Urinary **urgency and frequency,** as well as dysuria, may be seen in infection, complicating obstruction.

○ **Unexplained renal failure:**
  - Obstruction should be considered in all patients with renal failure without a history of kidney disease and relatively benign urinary sediment.
  - Obstructive uropathy by itself can lead to renal failure due to pressure atrophy, intrarenal reflux, and ischemia, or it can be superimposed on another renal parenchymal disease and accelerate the rate of its progression.

○ **Other complications:**
  - Recurrent **urinary tract infections** without any explanation (and failure of adequate antibiotics to clear them) should always raise the suspicion of stasis and obstruction.
  - **Hypertension** may be seen with both unilateral and bilateral obstruction of any duration. Unilateral obstruction causes elevated renin levels with activation of the RAAS axis, leading to hypertension. In cases of bilateral obstruction, hypertension is due to increased extracellular fluid volume secondary to impaired sodium excretion.
  - **Nephrolithiasis,** in addition to being a cause, can be a result of UTO. Chronic obstruction promotes infection. Infection with urease-producing organisms leads to increased urine pH, precipitating struvite stone formation. Infection in this setting is extremely difficult to eradicate unless the stone is removed.
  - **Hyperkalemic hyperchloremic metabolic acidosis** may sometimes complicate partial obstruction. In this "pseudohypoaldosterone" state, tubules damaged by obstruction cannot respond fully to aldosterone, leading to difficulty in excreting potassium and hydrogen ions. Any elderly, nondiabetic patient who has a chemical picture suggestive of hyperkalemic hyperchloremic acidosis should be carefully evaluated for obstruction.
  - Impaired concentrating ability of the kidney (nephrogenic diabetes insipidus) caused by renal tubular defects results in **polyuria** and polydipsia. Elderly patients with impaired thirst mechanisms may present with dehydration and hypernatremia.
  - **Polycythemia** has been associated with hydronephrosis and is likely related to increased production of erythropoietin by the obstructed kidney.

History

- Obstructive (hesitancy, weak stream, intermittency) and irritative (frequency, nocturia, urgency) symptoms are important to obtain, given that prostatic disease is the most common cause of lower tract obstruction. Hematuria may also relate to many other potential pathologic conditions causing UTO.
- Pain in the flank or suprapubic region, with specific radiation patterns, is suggestive.
- A history of urinary tract infections, stones, diabetes, or neurologic disease that could make bladder evacuation difficult is also important to determine.
- Recent surgery or history of tumors or radiation to the pelvis may provide clues to the etiology.
- Medication history must be carefully explored to assess functional causes of obstruction, such as anticholinergic medications.

Physical Examination

- A complete physical exam should be performed to help determine the volume status of the patient.
- Special emphasis should be placed on ensuring that the abdomen and flanks are carefully examined for the presence of any palpable masses. A distended bladder may be felt in the suprapubic region. Costovertebral tenderness should be elicited.
- A digital rectal examination should be performed. Females should receive a pelvic examination.

Diagnostic Testing

- Urinalysis, serum chemistries, and blood cell counts should be obtained. Imaging studies and diagnostic procedures are done depending on symptoms and suspected level of obstruction.

Laboratories

- Urinalysis is expected to be **bland** in uncomplicated UTO.
- Clues to underlying etiologies may be provided by abnormalities in the urine.
  - **Hematuria** may suggest the presence of stones, infection, or tumor.
  - Crystals on urine microscopy may be seen with metabolic abnormalities, leading to production of stones. Thus, the type of crystal seen provides information on not only the presence of a stone but possibly also the type of stone causing obstruction.
- Serum chemistries may detect renal insufficiency, suggesting that obstruction may be bilateral and severe or complete. Other metabolic abnormalities, such as hyperkalemia and acidosis, may be present.

Imaging

- Plain radiography can provide a gross estimate of kidney size. It may reveal renal pelvic, ureteral, or bladder calculi, the majority (90%) of which are radiopaque. However, ultrasonography (US) provides better information and is readily available; hence, plain films are rarely obtained if one suspects AKI from urinary obstruction.
- US is the **initial imaging test** of choice in most patients. It is readily available, noninvasive, inexpensive, and avoids contrast exposure. US can determine renal size and may reveal dilation of the collecting system (hydronephrosis), which is suggestive of postrenal AKI. Figure 12-2 shows an US image of obstruction with preserved renal cortex.

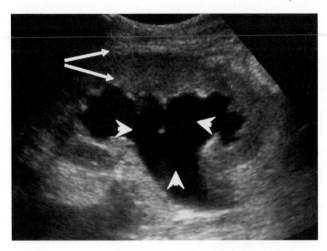

FIGURE 12-2. Ultrasound image of the kidney demonstrating the dilated calyces (*arrowheads*) with preserved renal cortex (*between arrows*). (Courtesy of William D. Middleton, MD, Washington University School of Medicine, St. Louis, MO.)

○ It is important to review the ultrasound with the radiologist, especially with regard to the extent of the damage to the renal cortex. If the renal cortex is extremely thinned out, then chances are that the obstruction was long standing and relieving it will not improve renal function.

○ False-positive results can be seen in cases of extrarenal pelvis, congenital megacalyces, renal cysts, calyceal diverticula, and diuresis. A dilated collecting system without obstruction can be seen in cases of ileal conduits, vesicoureteral reflux, primary megaureter, and acute pyelonephritis.

○ Absence of hydronephrosis (and **false-negative results**) can occur with severe dehydration, early or mild obstruction, staghorn calculi, or if retroperitoneal fibrosis or tumor encases the collecting system, preventing dilation of the ureter.

○ If obstruction is strongly suspected as the cause of AKI and ultrasound is inconclusive, the physician must strongly consider seeking a urology consultation for cystoscopy.

- **Computed tomography (CT)** has become a very useful tool to assess UTO. It may be performed rapidly and does not require the use of intravenous contrast. The ability to evaluate the cause of obstruction affords CT an invaluable advantage. Unenhanced helical CT is the modality of choice and is particularly accurate for obstruction due to ureteral calculi.

- Magnetic resonance imaging can be used, but it is not superior in accuracy to US or CT. In addition, it is time-consuming and expensive.

- **Intravenous urography** can be useful to define anatomy and to identify the level of obstructive uropathy. However, it is rarely used, given the potential for **exacerbation of renal failure with intravenous contrast.**

- **Antegrade or retrograde pyelography** is preferred to studies that require intravenous administration of contrast agents in patients with renal insufficiency.

Antegrade pyelography entails percutaneous placement of a catheter into the renal pelvis, whereas retrograde studies are done through a cystosope. These procedures help to delineate the obstruction further.

- **Radionuclide scans** can detect obstruction without use of contrast agents but require some renal function. Performed by injection of radionuclide tracer, images are then obtained with a gamma-scintillation camera and reveal delayed excretion of the tracer. Sensitivity of the test is enhanced when used in conjunction with **diuresis renography.** Administration of a loop diuretic (e.g., furosemide) causes a rapid washout of the tracer in cases of functional obstruction, but cannot do so if there is mechanical obstruction to urine flow. This can help to differentiate between intrinsic renal injury versus obstruction.
- **Voiding cystourethrography** is helpful for bladder neck and urethral obstructions, as well as vesicoureteral reflux.

TREATMENT

- Therapy is aimed at achieving three main goals[31]:
  - **Elimination of any life-threatening complication of obstruction.** This involves rapid restoration of intravascular volume, treatment of severe metabolic complications (e.g., hyperkalemia, acidosis), and initiation of aggressive management of infection.
  - **Preservation of renal function.** If the problem is bilateral obstruction, immediate steps to relieve the obstruction are mandated. The longer the obstruction, the higher the risk for irreversible renal parenchymal damage. The location of the obstruction dictates the procedure of choice.
    - Lower obstructive uropathy may require a catheter or more proximal drainage. If a transurethral catheter cannot be placed, a urology consultation may be needed to place a suprapubic catheter.
    - For an upper tract obstruction, the placement of percutaneous nephrostomy tubes or ureteral catheters or stents should be requested, and performed immediately by interventional radiology or urology.
  - **Determination of the cause of obstruction and definitive treatment.** Definitive diagnosis and therapy can be planned and pursued once the patient has been stabilized and the urinary system decompressed.

COMPLICATIONS

Postobstructive Diuresis

- **Polyuria,** associated with substantial losses of water and solutes, is commonly seen after relief of severe, bilateral obstruction.
  - The factors causing this phenomenon are osmotic diuresis caused by retained urea and other osmoles, volume overload, tubular concentration defects, and accumulation of natriuretic factors (e.g., atrial natriuretic peptide).
  - Osmotic diuresis and volume overload are predominant early and cease with excretion of the excess solute and water. However, tubular insensitivity to ADH at times may persist longer.

- Volume depletion will develop once the obstruction is relieved if urine losses are not replaced.
  - As the diuresis can be substantial, volume status, urine output, and chemistry values in blood and urine need to be **closely monitored** to gauge **fluid and electrolyte support** (e.g., hypotonic vs. isotonic fluids, requirement for potassium, magnesium, and phosphorus).
  - It is reasonable to start with 0.45% saline and replace approximately two-thirds of the urine losses. If signs of hypo- or hypervolemia develop, the replacement rate can be adjusted accordingly. The replacement fluid rate can be gradually decreased over the course of the next few days.
  - Hypokalemia, hypophosphatemia, and hypomagnesemia are frequently seen during postobstructive diuresis.
- Fluid replacement during postobstructive diuresis should be performed cautiously. Overzealous fluid replacement will lead to persistent high urine flow rates despite the resolution of the osmotic diuresis.

PROGNOSIS

- Recovery of renal function clearly correlates with the degree and duration of obstruction.
  - Recovery from complete obstruction can be seen within 1 week if no irreversible renal injury has occurred, but may take up to 12 weeks to achieve a new lower baseline if some damage has occurred.
  - Recovery from partial obstruction will typically be seen within 7 to 10 days.
- Correction of the obstruction may not be necessary in UNILATERAL obstruction, if the patient is largely asymptomatic, the plasma creatinine concentration is normal, and there is little or no parenchymal atrophy on US.
  - In a prospective study in patients with unilateral obstructive uropathy with a **normal-functioning contralateral kidney,** the preoperative renographic clearance and perfusion of the corresponding kidney were the only predictors of recoverability of unilateral renal obstruction. Kidneys with a renographic GFR <10 mL/min/1.73 m^2 were irreversibly damaged. Improvement or stabilization of function was expected after relief of obstruction of kidneys with a renographic GFR ≥10 mL/min/1.73 m^2.[2,32]

REFERENCES

1. Brenner BM, ed. *Brenner and Rector's the Kidney.* 8th ed. Philadelphia, PA: Saunders Elsevier; 2008.
2. Thadhani R, Pascual M, Bonventre JV. Acute renal failure. *N Engl J Med.* 1996;334:1448–1460.
3. Nolan CR, Anderson RJ. Hospital-acquired acute renal failure. *J Am Soc Nephrol.* 1998;9:710–718.
4. Blantz RC, Konnen KS. Relation of distal tubular delivery and reabsorptive rate to nephron filtration. *Am J Physiol.* 1977;233:F315–F324.
5. Badr KF, Ichikawa I. Prerenal failure: a deleterious shift from renal compensation to decompensation. *N Engl J Med.* 1988;319:623–629.
6. Gabbai FB, Thomson SC, Peterson O, et al. Glomerular and tubular interactions between renal adrenergic activity and nitric oxide. *Am J Physiol.* 1995;268:F1004–F1008.

7. De Nicola L, Blantz RC, Gabbai FB. Nitric oxide and angiotensin II. Glomerular and tubular interaction in the rat. *J Clin Invest.* 1992;89:1248–1256.

8. Klahr S, Miller SB. Current concepts: acute oliguria. *N Engl J Med.* 1998;338:671–675.

9. Carvounis CP, Nisar S, Guro-Razuman S. Significance of the fractional excretion of urea in the differential diagnosis of acute renal failure. *Kidney Int.* 2002;62:2223–2229.

10. Goldstein MH, Lenz PR, Levitt MF. Effect of urine flow rate on urea reabsorption in man: urea as a "tubular marker". *J Appl Physiol.* 1969;26:594–599.

11. Ragaller MJ, Theilen H, Koch T. Volume replacement in critically ill patients with acute renal failure. *J Am Soc Nephrol.* 2001;12:S33–S39.

12. Ginés P, Schrier RW. Renal failure in cirrhosis. *N Engl J Med.* 2009;361:1279–1290.

13. Arroyo V, Ginés P, Gerbes AL, et al. Definition and diagnostic criteria of refractory ascites and hepatorenal syndrome in cirrhosis. International ascites club. *Hepatology.* 1996;23:164–176.

14. Ginés A, Escorsell A, Ginés P, et al. Incidence, predictive factors, and prognosis of the hepatorenal syndrome in cirrhosis with ascites. *Gastroenterology.* 1993;105:229–236.

15. Salerno F, Gerbes A, Ginés P, et al. Diagnosis, prevention and treatment of hepatorenal syndrome in cirrhosis. *Gut.* 2007;56:1310–1318.

16. Kalambokis G, Economou M, Fotopoulos A, et al. The effects of chronic treatment with octreotide versus octreotide plus midodrine on systemic hemodynamics and renal hemodynamics and function in nonazotemic cirrhotic patients with ascites. *Am J Gastroenterol.* 2005;100:879–885.

17. Sanyal AJ, Boyer T, Garcia-Tsao G, et al. A randomized, prospective, double-blind, placebo-controlled trial of terlipressin for type 1 hepatorenal syndrome. *Gastroenterology.* 2008;134:1360–1368.

18. Guevara M, Ginés P, Bandi JC, et al. Transjugular intrahepatic portosystemic shunt in hepatorenal syndrome: effects on renal function and vasoactive systems. *Hepatology.* 1998; 28:416–422.

19. Cárdenas A, Ginés P. Hepatorenal syndrome. *Clin Liver Dis.* 2006;10:371–385.

20. Ronco C, Haapio M, House AA, et al. Cardiorenal syndrome. *J Am Coll Cardiol.* 2008; 52:1527–1539.

21. Smith GL, Lichtman JH, Bracken MR, et al. Renal impairment and outcomes in heart failure: systematic review and meta-analysis. *J Am Coll Cardiol.* 2006;47:1987–1996.

22. Cadnapaphornchai MA, Gurevich AK, Weinberger HD, et al. Pathophysiology of sodium and water retention in heart failure. *Cardiology.* 2001;96:122–131.

23. Obialo CI. Cardiorenal consideration as a risk factor for heart failure. *Am J Cardiol.* 2007;99:21D–24D.

24. Fonarow GC, Heywood JT. The confounding issue of comorbid renal insufficiency. *Am J Med.* 2006;119:S17–S25.

25. Sackner-Bernstein JD, Skopicki HA, Aaronson KD. Risk of worsening renal function with nesiritide in patients with acutely decompensated heart failure. *Circulation.* 2005;111:1487–1491.

26. Korbet SM. Obstructive uropathy. In: Greenberg A, ed. *Primer on Kidney Diseases.* 3rd ed. San Diego, CA: Academic Press; 2001.

27. Beers MH, Porter RS, Jones TV, et al. *The Merck Manual of Diagnosis and Therapy.* 18th ed. Whitehouse Station NJ: Merck Research Laboratories; 2006.

28. Klahr S. New insights into the consequences and mechanisms of renal impairment in obstructive nephropathy. *Am J Kidney Dis.* 1991;18:689–699.

29. Klahr S. Obstructive nephropathy: pathophysiology and management. In: Schrier RW, ed. *Renal and Electrolyte Disorders.* 6th ed. Philadelphia, PA: Lippincott Williams & Wilkins; 2003.

30. Klahr S. Obstructive nephropathy. In: Massry SG, Glassock RJ, eds. *Massry & Glassock's Textbook of Nephrology.* 4th ed. Philadelphia, PA: Lippincott Williams & Wilkins; 2001.

31. Klahr S. Urinary tract obstruction. In: Schrier RW, ed. *Diseases of the Kidney & Urinary Tract.* 7th ed. Philadelphia, PA: Lippincott Williams & Wilkins; 2001.

32. Khalaf IM, Shokeir AA, El-Gyoushi FI, et al. Recoverability of renal function after treatment of adult patients with unilateral obstructive uropathy and normal contralateral kidney: a prospective study. *Urology.* 2004;64:664–668.

Intrinsic Causes of Acute Kidney Injury

13

Judy L. Jang

- Once hemodynamic and postrenal causes of acute kidney injury (AKI) have been excluded, acute renal dysfunction that is intrinsic to the kidneys must be considered.
- In the approach to intrinsic AKI, it is helpful to group the etiologies by the site of initial nephron pathology: the supplying microvasculature, the glomerulus, the tubule, or the interstitium (Table 13-1). Although significant clinical overlap exists, a few readily attainable clinical findings might suggest the category to which a particular case of intrinsic AKI belongs:
  - **Microvascular:** new or accelerating hypertension with evidence of microangiopathic hemolytic anemia.
  - **Glomerular:** new or accelerating hypertension and volume overload, heavy proteinuria, and/or significant hematuria, especially if red blood cell casts are present.
  - **Tubular:** urinary sediment containing characteristic tubular cell casts or crystals.
  - **Interstitial:** the presence of pyuria or white blood cell casts.
- This chapter will focus on the causes of intrinsic AKI that involve the nonglomerular segments of the nephron. Glomerular causes of renal insufficiency found in Table 13-1 are discussed elsewhere.

MICROVASCULAR AKI

- Atheroembolic renal disease, malignant hypertension, and scleroderma renal crisis may manifest as an acute decline in renal function due to injury to the small arteries and arterioles supplying the glomeruli as the primary pathologic event.
- In antiphospholipid syndrome (APS), hemolytic-uremic syndrome (HUS), thrombotic-thrombocytopenic purpura (TTP), preeclampsia, and HELLP (hemolysis, elevated liver enzymes, and low platelets) syndrome, the initial site of injury may be the supplying microvasculature and/or the glomerular capillaries themselves as a result of generalized endothelial dysfunction.
- Special emphasis is given to atheroembolic renal disease because of its increased incidence compared with others in this category. Malignant hypertension, HUS, TTP, preeclampsia, and HELLP are discussed in detail elsewhere in this manual and will only be briefly mentioned in this chapter.

TABLE 13-1	CAUSES OF INTRINSIC ACUTE KIDNEY INJURY ACCORDING TO SITE OF PRIMARY INJURY		
Microvasculature	**Glomerulus**	**Tubule**	**Interstitium**
Atheroembolic renal disease	Rapidly progressive glomerulonephritis	Crystalline nephropathy	Acute interstitial nephritis
Malignant hypertension		Myeloma kidney	Infiltrative malignancies
Scleroderma renal crisis		Acute tubular necrosis (toxic or ischemic)	Acute pyelonephritis
Antiphospholipid syndrome Preeclampsia/HELLP syndrome HUS/TTP			

HELLP, hemolysis, elevated liver enzymes, and low platelets; HUS/TTP, hemolytic-uremic syndrome/ thrombotic-thrombocytopenic purpura.

ATHEROEMBOLIC RENAL DISEASE

GENERAL PRINCIPLES

Definition
- Atheroembolic renal disease refers to AKI that arises from the occlusion of the renal microvasculature from inflammation caused by deposition of lipid debris.

Classification
- **Three patterns** of disease evolution may be apparent in atheroembolic renal disease:
  - **Acute** (35% of cases): An abrupt deterioration in renal function occurs 3 to 7 days after the inciting event, usually with multisystem organ involvement from a massive embolic shower.
  - **Subacute** (56% of cases): Repeated smaller embolic showers or progressive **obliterative arteritis** in previously involved vessels leads to a stepwise deterioration in renal function, with stabilization by 3 to 8 weeks. This is the most common pattern of the disease.
  - **Chronic** (9% of cases): Renal insufficiency is slowly progressive and is hard to distinguish from worsening hypertensive nephrosclerosis or ischemic renovascular disease.[1]

Epidemiology
- Atheroembolic renal disease is most commonly a disease of the elderly white male.
- The mean age of presentation is 66 to 70 years and men are affected four times as commonly as women, paralleling the prevalence bias of atherosclerotic vascular disease.[2,3]
- The incidence of clinically significant renal atheroemboli is not well defined. It occurs much more commonly with aortography and aortic surgeries.[4]

Pathophysiology
- Setting the stage for the occurrence of atheroembolic renal disease is the presence of aortic atherosclerosis upstream of the kidneys.

- Although spontaneous atheroemboli may occur, more often there is an inciting event leading to plaque destabilization and distal showering of lipid.
  - In the majority of provoked cases, plaque destabilization occurs from vascular wall trauma during either vascular surgeries or percutaneous endovascular procedures.
  - It has also been suggested that anticoagulation and thrombolytic administration may be causative.[2,3] However, despite widespread use of anticoagulants and thrombolytic agents, the incidence of renal atheroemboli in the absence of preceding vascular procedures is low.
- The **lipid lodges in the small arterioles and incites thrombus formation,** causing distal ischemia and infarction. Within days there may be recanalization of the thrombus and restoration of blood flow, but an inflammatory foreign body arteritis then ensues, leading to progressive fibrosis and eventual obliteration of the vessel lumen. Continued nephron ischemia thus occurs.[5]

Prevention

- Preventive measures include **secondary prevention of atherosclerotic risk factors.**
- The possibility of using a brachial or axillary approach for endovascular procedures needs to be considered, as most atherosclerotic plaques are in the abdominal aorta.

DIAGNOSIS

Clinical Presentation

- The main manifestations of atheroembolic disease are listed in Table 13-2.
- Patients usually have multiple cardiac disease risk factors, a history of cerebrovascular accidents, or an abdominal aortic aneurysm.
- The typical patient is noted to **have blue or dark red discoloration of the toes** associated with increasing creatinine several days after a vascular procedure. Lipid embolism can occur from 3 days to 3 months after the inciting event.
  - The skin is the most commonly affected organ, but the reliance on characteristic skin findings (e.g., livedo reticularis, cyanotic changes) for diagnosis may contribute to the underrepresentation of this disease among dark-skinned races.
  - Other organ systems such as the gastrointestinal tract and central nervous system may be simultaneously involved.[1]
  - The **multisystem disease involvement,** together with the variable occurrence of **eosinophilia** and **depressed complement levels,** may mimic a vasculitis.[6]
- Renal histology reveals **empty clefts** in arcuate and interlobular arteries from the dissolution of lipid from these sites by the fixation process.
  - Early lesions display an inflammatory arteritis composed of eosinophils, neutrophils, and macrophages, which is later replaced by a giant cell foreign body reaction with proliferation and fibrosis of the vascular intima. Acutely, the tubules may show signs of acute tubular necrosis (ATN).
  - Late in evolution, patchy glomerular sclerosis and tubular atrophy may be visualized in areas supplied by affected vessels. Similar arteriolar inflammation or fibrosis can be found in other tissues, especially the muscle, gastrointestinal tract, and skin.[5,6]
- **Biopsy of skin lesions** may have an especially high diagnostic yield.

TABLE 13-2	CLINICAL AND LABORATORY FINDINGS IN PATIENTS WITH RENAL ATHEROEMBOLIC DISEASE

Very Common

New onset, accelerated, or labile hypertension
Skin findings: cyanotic or ulcerated digits or scrotum, livedo reticularis on back or lower extremities, nodules, and/or purpura
Eosinophiluria by Hansel stain
Peripheral blood eosinophilia
Elevated erythrocyte sedimentation rate or C-reactive protein

Common

Gastrointestinal symptoms: nausea, abdominal pain, and/or gastrointestinal bleeding
Microscopic hematuria
Mild proteinuria (rarely in the nephrotic range)
Renal artery stenosis on imaging study
Various markers of ischemic organ injury: elevated creatine kinase, amylase/lipase, and/or transaminases

Uncommon

Fevers
Central nervous system symptoms: focal neurologic deficits and/or progressive dementia
Retinal emboli with Hollenhorst plaque visible on fundoscopy
Hypocomplementemia

TREATMENT

- As no means of reversing the tissue injury exists, therapy consists of **aggressive supportive care** addressing the most common mechanisms of death in the acute multivisceral forms of the disease.
  - These include ongoing cardiac ischemia, decompensated heart failure, stroke, and malnutrition in the setting of gastrointestinal ischemia.
  - With multivisceral involvement, **further anticoagulation or intravascular manipulations should be strictly avoided,** perhaps even in the setting of recurrent cardiac ischemia.
  - Particular attention should be given to the **management of hypertension** (preferably with use of renin–angiotensin blockade) and volume overload.
  - If **renal replacement therapy (RRT)** is required, hemodialysis should be performed without anticoagulation. If this is not possible, peritoneal dialysis can be employed.
  - **Nutritional support** should be aggressive, even administered parenterally if needed, in those with significant gut ischemia.
- In addition to these basic management principles, various other strategies have been pursued.
  - Corticosteroids have not been proven to affect renal outcome.
  - Association data suggest a benefit from statin use, perhaps through atherosclerotic plaque stabilization and reductions in inflammation.[3,5]

OUTCOME/PROGNOSIS

- Patients with renal atheroemboli have poor overall prognosis.
- Progression to dialysis dependence occurs in approximately one-third of the patients who survive the initial insult, though a mild improvement in glomerular filtration rate can occur.
- In a large study of 354 patients, atheroembolic renal disease resulted in end-stage renal disease and death in 33% and 28% of patients, respectively, after an average follow-up of 2 years.[2]

OTHER MICROVASCULAR CAUSES OF INTRINSIC AKI

GENERAL PRINCIPLES

- **Scleroderma renal crisis** refers to a clinical entity of acute and progressive renal dysfunction with worsening hypertension occurring in scleroderma patients. An incompletely understood endothelial cell dysfunction with vascular hyperresponsiveness underlies its pathogenesis, as in the other tissues that scleroderma affects.
- **In APS,** antibodies with specificity for anionic phospholipids or the plasma proteins that bind to them induce activation of platelets and endothelial cells, leading to a procoagulant state. If thrombosis occurs primarily in the microvasculature, this can result in an acute or chronic thrombotic microangiopathy in multiple organs, including the kidney. Macroscopic thrombosis may involve the renal arteries in APS and may mimic the microvascular forms of the disease with acute renal failure and accelerating hypertension.[7]
  - ○ **Catastrophic APS** is said to be present if an additional procoagulant stimulus (e.g., infection, surgery, or withdrawal of anticoagulation) initiates fulminant, predominantly microvascular thrombosis that clinically involves at least three different organ systems in a span of <1 week.
- **HUS and TTP** are syndromes of systemic thrombotic microangiopathy and prominent consumptive thrombocytopenia.
  - ○ In HUS, drugs, infections, or toxins initiate endothelial and neutrophil activation or a deficiency in complement regulatory molecules leads to microvascular thrombosis.
  - ○ TTP appears to result from the accumulation of large von Willebrand multimers from reduced ADAMTS13 protease activity. The large multimers then initiate platelet aggregation and activation in the small vessels.
- **Preeclampsia** is a syndrome of new or worsening hypertension with proteinuria, occurring in the late stages of pregnancy. Endothelial dysfunction seems to occur from an imbalance of placenta-derived angiogenic and antiangiogenic factors.
- **HELLP** is a more severe variant of preeclampsia in which microangiopathic anemia is more prominent and there is also evidence of liver dysfunction.

DIAGNOSIS

Clinical Presentation

- Some of the clinical features that distinguish the diseases in this category of intrinsic AKI are discussed in Table 13-3.

TABLE 13-3 THE MICROVASCULAR CAUSES OF INTRINSIC ACUTE KIDNEY INJURY

	Malignant Hypertension	Scleroderma Renal Crisis	Microvascular APS[b]	HUS/TTP	Preeclampsia/HELLP
Incidence	Most common microvascular cause of AKI at 2.6 per 100,000 patients per year	10% of patients with scleroderma, almost always within first 5 years after diagnosis	25% of patients with primary APS	Eleven cases per million people per year	5% of pregnancies[9]
Risk factors	Longstanding hypertension, black race, abrupt interruption of BP medications, secondary causes of HTN	More extensive and rapidly progressive scleroderma skin involvement, cooler temperature environments, black race, initiation of corticosteroids at high dose, use of cyclosporine	Procoagulant states including a recent thrombotic event, withdrawal of anticoagulation, pregnancy, infection, surgery, and so forth	• Infection: enteritis with shiga-toxin–producing bacteria, HIV, pneumococcal infection • Drugs: quinine, contraceptives, calcineurin inhibitors, chemotherapeutic medications, thienopyridines • Peripartum	Previous preeclampsia or positive family history, primigravid, age >40 or <18, multifetal gestation, previous hypertension or renal disease, diabetes, obesity
Distinguishing clinical features[a]		Signs of scleroderma (sclerodactyly, interstitial lung disease, and so forth) are present and usually obvious. Autoantibodies (e.g., anti-Scl-70 or anti-ribonucleic acid polymerase) may be present. A total of 10% of patients may be normotensive at diagnosis	Signs of APS (previous thrombosis in an atypical vessel, infarcts in other vascular beds, livedo reticularis, and so forth) or SLE are present. Lupus anticoagulant or antiphospholipid antibody is present. Thrombocytopenia may be significant. Focal renal cortical atrophy may be evident. Course may be chronic, acute, or fulminant (i.e., catastrophic APS)	Hemolytic anemia and thrombocytopenia is prominent. Fever may be present. ADAMS13 activity may be low in idiopathic TTP but is variable. Presence of accelerated hypertension is less consistently seen	Elevation in BP can be relatively mild. Usually occurs after 20th week of pregnancy. Evidence of fetal compromise may be evident. Reduction in GFR is usually mild. Proteinuria often becomes nephrotic in later stages. Glomerular endotheliosis is prominent early on

Principles of management				
Treatment: Reduce BP by 25% within 2–6 hours and toward 160/100 mm Hg by 24–48 hours. Renal function may initially worsen slightly	*Prevention:* Avoidance of renal ischemia from drugs or volume depletion. At-risk patients should monitor BP closely and if a sustained rise occurs, renal function should be assessed *Treatment:* Initiate ACEI promptly. Renal function may initially worsen, but continued therapy will allow eventual improvement, with >50% of patients able to stop dialysis[8]	*Prevention:* Avoidance of precipitants (see Risk Factors) +/– aspirin or hydroxychloroquine *Treatment:* Address underlying precipitant, anticoagulation, +/– antiplatelet therapy, +/– glucocorticoids. If catastrophic APS present, initiate plasma exchange or intravenous immune globulin in addition to above	*Treatment:* ○ Typical HUS (postenteritis)—supportive care alone ○ Atypical HUS or TTP—supportive care plus plasma exchange (less desirably, high-dose plasma infusion) +/– corticosteroids	*Prevention:* Low-dose aspirin in high-risk patients[10] *Treatment:* Antihypertensive therapy and close mother and fetal monitoring until fetal maturity. Deliver fetus if maturity is reached or severe preeclampsia occurs

---

[a] As all may present with accelerating hypertension and worsening renal function, the clinical features that distinguish the diseases are emphasized.

[b] Antiphospholipid antibody syndrome may also present with large-artery thrombosis that may manifest similarly to the microvascular form of the disease.

ACEI, angiotensin-converting enzyme inhibitor; AKI, acute kidney injury; APS, antiphospholipid syndrome; BP, blood pressure; GFR, glomerular filtration rate; HELLP, hemolysis elevated liver enzymes, low platelets syndrome; HIV, human immunodeficiency virus; HTN, hypertension; HUS, hemolytic-uremic syndrome; SLE, systemic lupus erythematosus; TTP, thrombotic-thrombocytopenic purpura.

- The vasculopathy in these disorders leads to glomerular ischemia, which prompts a vicious cycle of high renin- and angiotensin-induced vasoconstriction, rises in blood pressure, and further glomerular ischemia.
  - This is most apparent in scleroderma renal crisis, in which there is fairly prompt reversal of the disease with the initiation of angiotensin-converting enzyme inhibition.[11]
- The appearance of **accelerating hypertension** and worsening renal function is common to all of the diseases in this category of AKI secondary to the shared pathophysiologic mechanism of ischemia, leading to increased renin production.
  - Marked hypertension may lead to signs of decompensated heart failure or angina.
  - Headaches, altered mental status, seizures, or focal neurologic deficits can be evident from hypertensive encephalopathy or cerebral microvascular occlusions.
  - Retinal hemorrhages, exudates, or papilledema may be observed on fundoscopic exam.
- Laboratory data may reveal findings consistent with a **microangiopathic hemolytic anemia** (schistocytosis, elevated lactate dehydrogenase, and reduced haptoglobin).
- On urinalysis, hematuria, granular casts, and worsening proteinuria may be present in varying degrees.
- Renal histology findings are remarkably similar amongst the diseases in this category, except that malignant hypertension and scleroderma renal crisis may involve the preglomerular vessels more prominently.
  - Early on, **fibrinoid necrosis** with a paucity of inflammatory infiltrate is seen in the small arteries and arterioles. **Thrombi** may be visualized in glomerular capillary loops. Glomerular endotheliosis, or swelling of endothelial cells with subendothelial deposition of hyaline material, may be seen in any of these diseases, but is more prominent in preeclampsia.
  - Later, the intima displays myxoid thickening and finally undergoes fibrous proliferation, resulting in the typical **concentric onion skin lesions** that may obliterate the lumen of smaller vessels. There is secondary ischemic sclerosis and dropout of supplied glomeruli and tubules.

TREATMENT

- Basic principles of management are presented in Table 13-3.

TUBULAR AKI

- The causes of intrinsic AKI in which the primary site of injury is the renal tubule include ATN, the crystalline nephropathies, and myeloma cast nephropathy (see Table 13-1).
- Though not helpful for diagnosing cast nephropathy, clues to the presence of the remaining causes of AKI in this category may be obtained from analysis of the urine sediment: muddy brown casts may be visualized in ATN and characteristic crystals might be seen in the crystalline nephropathies. ATN will not be discussed any further here as it is presented elsewhere in this manual.

CRYSTALLINE NEPHROPATHIES

GENERAL PRINCIPLES

Definition
- The crystalline nephropathies describe the AKI that results from the intratubular precipitation of various compounds.
  - The most common cause of crystalline nephropathy is tumor lysis syndrome (TLS), which includes the entities acute uric acid nephropathy and acute phosphate nephropathy.
  - Less commonly, crystalline nephropathy may result from the precipitation of **calcium oxalate, acyclovir, sulfonamide, methotrexate, indinavir,** or **triamterene.**
  - There are rare case reports of occurrence of crystalline nephropathy with the use of ciprofloxacin, foscarnet, and ampicillin, and with plasma cell dyscrasias.

Pathophysiology and Risk Factors
- Intratubular crystal formation and deposition is promoted by **three mechanisms:** high tubular fluid concentration of a substance, prolonged intratubular transit time, and decreased solubility.
  - The first two mechanisms occur in the setting of decreased effective circulating volume, leading to an increase in proximal tubular fluid reabsorption. This results in both high concentrations of the offending compound in the distal tubule and decreased distal flow rates.
  - Underlying chronic kidney disease is also a major risk factor for the crystalline nephropathies, because a larger amount of the compound is excreted per functioning nephron and because drugs are frequently overdosed in renal insufficiency.
  - The third mechanism, decreased solubility, is often dependent on the distal tubular fluid pH.
    - Compounds with a pKa <7, such as uric acid, calcium oxalate, sulfonamides, methotrexate, and triamterene, tend to precipitate in acidic urine, whereas compounds with a pKa >7, such as indinavir and calcium phosphate, tend to precipitate in alkaline urine.[12]

Prevention
- The mainstay of prevention is **avoidance of the two most frequent predisposing factors: volume depletion** and **drug overdosing** (usually from failure to adjust the dose for renal impairment).
- Establishing a brisk urine output (e.g., ≥100 to 150 mL/h) in high-risk patients is extremely important.
- For substances with pKa <7, urinary alkalinization by administering intravenous isotonic bicarbonate solutions or oral citrate can be considered.[12] Urine pH should be periodically followed to ensure an appropriate level of alkalinization. Acetazolamide may be added if a metabolic alkalosis ensues.
- Attempting to acidify the urine to increase the solubility of weakly basic compounds is dangerous and not recommended.
- These preventive strategies are based on underlying pathophysiologic mechanisms and evidence for reductions in crystalline nephropathy occurrence is lacking, except perhaps in the case of high-dose methotrexate administration.

DIAGNOSIS

Clinical Presentation

- The clinical contexts in which the more common crystalline nephropathies occur are summarized in Table 13-4. The clinical manifestations of ethylene glycol intoxication are discussed later.
- Extensive crystal deposition in any of the forms of crystalline nephropathy may result in pain from distention of the renal capsule, which is similar to ureteral colic.
- **Nephrolithiasis** may coexist with intratubular crystal deposition in some cases (especially with indinavir and sulfonamides).[18,19]
- Hypocalcemia due to the coprecipitation of calcium in acute phosphate nephropathy and oxalate nephropathy may result in paresthesias, lethargy, or tetany.
- High levels of acyclovir accumulating with the onset of renal failure can lead to hallucinations, delirium, and myoclonus. Similarly, toxic levels of methotrexate can also cause neurologic disturbances, as well as nausea, rash, and mucositis.

Diagnostic Testing

- A summary of the laboratory findings characteristic for the more common etiologies of crystalline nephropathy is found in Table 13-4.
- **Urine sediment findings** will often reveal **hematuria, pyuria, and mild proteinuria.** Although the offending substances have unique crystal morphologies on urine microscopy, examining the sediment is not independently diagnostic.
  - As the obstructed tubules may not empty urine into the collecting system, the absence of crystals does not exclude crystalline nephropathy.
  - The presence of crystals does not prove their pathogenic role, because calcium oxalate, calcium phosphate, and uric acid crystalluria can be seen in normal individuals. In addition, patients receiving typical offending medications can sometimes display crystalluria without AKI.
- **Renal ultrasound** may reveal **bilaterally enlarged and echogenic kidneys** and can identify concomitant macroscopic lithiasis.
- **Renal biopsy** is required to make a definitive diagnosis.
  - Light microscopy reveals **crystalline** deposits, usually in the distal tubules, with a surrounding **interstitial infiltrate** that may contain giant cells as part of a foreign body reaction. Evidence of ATN can also be present as many of the inciting agents display direct tubular cell toxicity.
  - Polarized microscopy may demonstrate birefringence depending on the offending agent.

TREATMENT

- Treatment of established AKI consists of **discontinuing the offending agent** and, if nonoliguric and not volume overloaded, applying the same principles used in prevention: **establishing brisk urine flow** with volume expansion and the judicious use of diuretics and, for weak acids, urinary alkalinization.
- Moderate-to-large doses of diuretics may be required to establish adequate urine flow, and care must be taken with bicarbonate loading to avoid severe alkalosis.

TABLE 13-4 CAUSES OF CRYSTALLINE NEPHROPATHY, THEIR DISTINCTIVE CLINICAL STRATEGIES FOR TREATMENT

Inciting Agent	Context of Occurrence	Laboratory Findings	Prevention and Treatment
Phosphate nephropathy	TLS—especially posttreatment form; very rarely in rhabdomyolysis and severe hemolysis; phosphosoda bowel prep[13]	• Crystalluria with weakly birefringent, long prisms often in rosettes • Hyperphosphatemia out of proportion to renal insufficiency and hypocalcemia; in TLS, rhabdomyolysis, and hemolysis, hyperkalemia out of proportion to renal insufficiency, and high LDH • Renal biopsy: von Kossa stain positive crystals	• *Prevention:*[a] Non-calcium-based phosphate binders; avoid treatment of hypocalcemia unless symptomatic or ECG changes present • *Treatment:*[a] Non–calcium-based phosphate binders; consider early initiation of renal replacement therapy, especially continuous modalities
Uric acid nephropathy	TLS—especially spontaneous form; very rarely in rhabdomyolysis or HGPRT deficiency	• Crystalluria with brownish, strongly birefringent, rhomboid plates, rosettes, or needles • Uric acid >15 mg/dL in absence of prerenal state, urine uric acid: urine creatinine often >1 and almost always >0.75; in TLS and rhabdomyolysis, hyperkalemia out of proportion to renal insufficiency and high LDH	• *Prevention:*[a] In those at high risk of TLS,[b] start hypouricemic therapy, usually allopurinol but may consider rasburicase in patients with multiple high-risk features, especially children • *Treatment:*[a] Rasburicase

(continued)

TABLE 13-4	CAUSES OF CRYSTALLINE NEPHROPATHY, THEIR DISTINCTIVE CLINICAL STRATEGIES FOR TREATMENT (Continued)		
Inciting Agent	Context of Occurrence	Laboratory Findings	Prevention and Treatment
Oxalate nephropathy	EG poisoning; primary hyperoxaluria; very rarely with high-dose IV ascorbic acid, xylitol, or sorbitol infusions	• Crystalluria with birefringent monohydrate needles or dihydrate envelope shapes • Hypocalcemia; in EG poisoning osmolal gap >10 mOsm/L and detectable serum and urine EG early, with later disappearance of both and development of severe anion gap acidosis • Renal biopsy: silver nitrate/rubeanic acid stain positive crystals	• *Prevention:*[a] Consider urine alkalinization; for high-risk EG ingestion,[b] prompt fomepizole or, less desirably, ethanol therapy; consider thiamine, magnesium, and pyridoxine in alcoholics; avoid treatment of hypocalcemia unless symptomatic or ECG changes present • *Treatment:*[a] Consider urine alkalinization; begin fomepizole or, less desirably, ethanol if EG level >20 mg/dL; consider early dialysis support, especially if EG >50 mg/dL and renal insufficiency or acidosis is present
Acyclovir	High-dose IV acyclovir bolus; very rarely with oral acyclovir or with oral valacyclovir	• Crystalluria with birefringent needles, occasionally engulfed by white cells	• *Prevention:*[a] Increase time of IV acyclovir infusion to ≥1 hour. • *Treatment:*[a] Lowering dose without stopping the drug may be sufficient in many[14]
Indinavir	20% on chronic therapy develop AKI, especially with longer treatment and smaller body size[15]	• Crystalluria with birefringent plates, fans, or starbursts • Isosthenuria common • Contrast computed tomography with wedge-shaped perfusion defects in up to 50%	• *Treatment:*[a] May require urologic consultation for concomitant indinavir stone if present

Drug	Clinical setting / notes	Findings	Prevention / Treatment
Methotrexate	High-dose IV therapy given for some malignancies[16]	• Crystalluria with amorphous yellow casts • High serum methotrexate level, cytopenias	• *Prevention:*[a] Urinary alkalinization to pH ≥8 • *Treatment:*[a] Urinary alkalinization to pH ≥8; leucovorin rescue ± thymidine for extrarenal toxicity until methotrexate level <0.05 μmol/L; for very high methotrexate levels, consider carboxypeptidase G2 versus daily hemodialysis with high-flux membrane
Sulfonamides	High-dose IV therapy, especially with sulfadiazine[17]	• Crystalluria with variable shapes from shocks of wheat to spheres • Positive lignin test (orange urine on mixing with 10% hydrochloric acid) • Densities in renal parenchyma and in collection system on imaging are common	• *Treatment:*[a] Dose reduction and urine alkalinization to pH >7.1 usually sufficient; may require urologic consultation for concomitant sulfonamide stone if present
Triamterene	Must distinguish from AIN, which is much more common	• Crystalluria with birefringent orange casts and spheres • Hyperkalemia out of proportion to renal insufficiency	• *Treatment:*[a] Urine alkalinization to pH >7.5; may require urologic consultation for the more common triamterene stone if obstructed

[a]Saline loading with concomitant diuretic use when urine output is inadequate is recommended for prevention and treatment of all of the crystalline nephropathies when possible.

[b]See text for definition of high-risk features.

AIN, acute interstitial nephritis; AKI, acute kidney injury; ECG, electrocardiogram; EG, ethylene glycol; HGPRT, hypoxanthine-guanine phosphoribosyl transferase; IV, intravenous; LDH, lactate; TLS, tumor lysis syndrome.

- Additionally, **early initiation of RRT** can rapidly decrease the concentration of some inciting agents (e.g., phosphate, oxalate, and acyclovir).
- Evidence for improved renal outcome with the abovementioned maneuvers is lacking.
- See Table 13-4 for details on specific management strategies for the various causes of crystalline nephropathy.

SPECIAL CONSIDERATIONS

- The pathogenesis and management of crystalline AKI from TLS and ethylene glycol intoxication are discussed further below.

Tumor Lysis Syndrome

- TLS results from the sudden release of normally intracellular compounds to the extracellular space from massive tumor cell death.
- The **main risk factor** is the presence of a **large tumor burden** with a **rapid doubling time** and thus **exquisite response to cytolytic therapy.**
  - Most cancers associated with TLS are high-grade lymphoproliferative malignancies, with up to 6% of these patients developing this complication. It has also been reported with several aggressive solid tumors, including lung and breast carcinoma.
  - Though the disease usually arises in the setting of traditional potent chemotherapy directed against nucleic acid processing, it has also been observed with interferon, endocrine therapies such as corticosteroids or tamoxifen, and radiation treatment.
  - Spontaneous TLS can also occur when aggressive cancers rapidly outstrip their nutrient supply.
- The AKI due to TLS has historically been thought of as an acute uric acid nephropathy.
  - Purine nucleosides are released by dying cells and are metabolized to hypoxanthine and xanthine. Xanthine oxidase converts both intermediates to uric acid. At normal plasma pH, 98% of uric acid exists as the more-soluble ionized salt, urate. In the normally acidic tubular fluid, it exists primarily as the less-soluble uric acid and may precipitate in the kidney.
  - As hypouricemic therapy is commonly employed for prophylaxis in at-risk patients, acute phosphate nephropathy has become an important cause of AKI in TLS. Significant amounts of phosphate complexed with adenosine exist in the intracellular compartment, especially in metabolically active cancer cells. Once released by cell death, phosphate precipitates in the renal tubules and other tissues as calcium phosphate.[20]
- **High-risk patients for TLS** include those with biological evidence of laboratory TLS (hyperkalemia, hyperphosphatemia, hypocalcemia, hyperuricemia), high-grade lymphoproliferative malignancies, large tumor burdens, and renal impairment and/or involvement at the time of TLS diagnosis.[21,22]
- **Preventive strategies** should be initiated promptly in high- and intermediate-risk patients, given the potential severity of complications from TLS.
  - **Volume expansion** to achieve brisk urine flow and hypouricemic therapy should be initiated 2 days prior to the start of chemotherapy.

- Urine alkalinization is *not* universally recommended, given the potential risk of calcium phosphate precipitation in alkaline urine.
  - Alkalemia can also worsen hypocalcemia by increasing protein binding of free calcium.
  - Data from animal studies revealed no reduction in the occurrence of uric acid nephropathy with urine alkalinization.
- Two options for hypouricemic therapy exist: allopurinol and rasburicase.
  - Allopurinol (400 to 800 mg total daily dose) competitively inhibits xanthine oxidase, thus preventing the *further* production of uric acid. Uric acid levels decrease over the next 48 hours.
  - Rasburicase is a recombinant uricase enzyme that converts *existing* uric acid to allantoin, which is 5 to 10 times more soluble in urine than uric acid. After intravenous rasburicase administration (0.05 to 0.20 mg/kg over 30 minutes), uric acid levels decrease by 86% at 4 hours compared with a 12% reduction with allopurinol.[23]
  - Comparative data between allopurinol and rasburicase regarding meaningful clinical end points, such as reductions in AKI, dialysis requirement, or death, do not exist. Therefore, the extremely high cost of rasburicase deters its use in prevention unless an allopurinol allergy is present.
- Patients with evidence of organ system dysfunction have "clinical TLS" and require therapeutic rather than preventive interventions.
  - Similar to preventive methods, maintaining adequate urine flow and suppressing further rises in the serum concentration of uric acid and phosphate is essential.
  - Rasburicase may be used to promptly reduce the uric acid level, eliminating this indication for RRT.
  - When significant hyperphosphatemia is present, early RRT may still be required along with non–calcium-based phosphate binders to prevent further phosphate precipitation and/or hypocalcemia.
    - Hypocalcemia should not be treated with intravenous calcium without first lowering the phosphorus, unless the patient is symptomatic or there are changes in the electrocardiogram.
    - With intermittent hemodialysis, phosphorus clearance is fairly inefficient and daily or twice-daily treatments may be needed to achieve negative phosphorus balance. Continuous RRT may be more effective at reducing phosphorus levels in this situation.
- Most patients with AKI will not require dialysis and will recover to their previous renal function, though patient and renal prognosis may be worse with spontaneous TLS.

Ethylene Glycol Intoxication

- Ethylene glycol is metabolized by hepatic alcohol dehydrogenase to four toxic organic compounds: glycoaldehyde, glycolic acid, glyoxylic acid, and oxalic acid.
  - Accumulation of the organic anions glycolate, glyoxylate, and oxalate leads to a severe anion gap metabolic acidosis.
  - These compounds, especially glycolic acid, are direct cell toxins and cause multiorgan dysfunction with heart failure, ATN, and nervous system depression.
  - Oxalate precipitates with calcium in several tissues, including the renal tubules, causing crystalline nephropathy.

- The clinical manifestations of ethylene glycol intoxication evolve over time as the alcohol is metabolized. This time course is prolonged in cases of ethanol coingestion due to competitive inhibition of alcohol dehydrogenase.[24]
  - During the first 30 minutes to 12 hours, ethylene glycol causes inebriation, with progression to **seizures or coma.**
  - At 12 to 36 hours postingestion, peak concentrations of organic acid intermediates lead to profound acidosis with Kussmaul respirations and **cardiopulmonary failure.**
  - At 24 to 72 hours postingestion, the oxalate end product accumulates in the tissues, resulting in AKI.
- If patients are at high risk, then treatment is initiated to prevent end-organ damage. The **criteria for initiation of treatment** are: serum ethylene glycol levels >20 mg/dL; OR a known recent ethylene glycol ingestion with an osmolal gap >10 mOsm/L; OR strong suspicion of recent ingestion plus three of the following: pH <7.3, serum bicarbonate <20 mEq/L, osmolal gap >10 mOsm/L, and/or urinary oxalate crystals.
- **Management** of ethylene glycol intoxication (see Table 13-4) should be focused on decreasing the concentration of toxic metabolites in high-risk ingestions. Reductions in the levels of toxic metabolites can be achieved by:
  - Limiting further organic acid formation through the use of competitive alcohol dehydrogenase inhibitors such as fomepizole or ethanol.[25]
  - Increasing metabolite clearance through early initiation of RRT.
  - Conversion to less-toxic metabolites by cofactor supplementation.

OUTCOME/PROGNOSIS

- In most cases of crystalline nephropathy, the **prognosis for full renal recovery is excellent.**
- In the drug-related crystalline nephropathies, recovery of renal function is expected to occur within days to weeks after cessation or even just dose reduction of the drug.
- Phosphate nephropathy due to phosphate-containing laxatives prior to colonoscopy may have a worse prognosis, because the population affected by this entity is older and has a higher prevalence of underlying chronic kidney disease.

MYELOMA CAST NEPHROPATHY

GENERAL PRINCIPLES

Definition

- Multiple myeloma is a malignancy of plasma cells, most often leading to overproduction of monoclonal immunoglobulin, the so-called M-protein.
- Myeloma cast nephropathy (myeloma kidney) refers to the intrinsic AKI that results as the **filtered light chain component of the M-protein (the Bence-Jones protein) exerts toxic and obstructive injury to the tubules.**

Epidemiology

- Renal dysfunction is seen in ~30% of patients with multiple myeloma at initial diagnosis.[26]

- The likelihood of underlying cast nephropathy is increased in cases of more profound AKI.

Etiology

- Potential etiologies of AKI in patients with myeloma include hypercalcemia-induced volume depletion, hypotension from infection, glomerular diseases such as light-chain deposition disease or amyloidosis, and cast nephropathy.[27] AKI can also be associated with bisphosphonate used in multiple myeloma, especially in a patient with underlying vitamin D deficiency.
- However, in those patients with persistent renal dysfunction, despite treatment of hypovolemia and infection, cast nephropathy is the most common cause of AKI.[28]

Pathophysiology

- The propensity of a particular myeloma light chain to produce cast nephropathy depends somewhat on the amount of Bence-Jones proteinuria and also on its tendency to aggregate together with Tamm–Horsfall protein.[26,29]
- Proximal tubular injury from additional insults and decreased effective circulating volume further increase the risk of cast formation, as both may increase the concentration of light chains in the distal tubule.
- Given these mechanisms at play, **many cases of myeloma kidney have an identifiable inciting event:**
  ○ **Volume depletion,** perhaps from hypercalcemia-induced diabetes insipidus.[26]
  ○ **Infection** resulting in ATN or decreased effective circulating volume.
  ○ **Nonsteroidal anti-inflammatory drug (NSAID)** use, through adverse effects on glomerular filtration.
  ○ **Iodinated contrast** exposure, through its ability to induce afferent arteriolar vasoconstriction.[30]

DIAGNOSIS

Clinical Presentation

- Patients with cast nephropathy generally have more advanced myeloma; hence, other features of the disease are usually present. They may have complaints of fatigue, bone pain with pathologic fractures, and recurrent infections.
- Anemia is often present. Hypercalcemia from myeloma-induced bone resorption is common and may lead to polyuria with signs of volume depletion.[30,31] The anion gap may be low from both hypercalcemia and the presence of circulating cationic paraprotein.

Diagnostic Testing

- The **urine sediment is usually bland,** with little or no proteinuria noted on urine dipstick because this only measures albuminuria.
- Urine protein electrophoresis and/or immunofixation will reveal the **presence of a monoclonal light chain** in almost all cases.
- Serum protein electrophoresis with immunofixation will also reveal the paraprotein, though this is less consistent, especially in cases of light-chain myeloma where the malignant clone produces only light chains instead of the full immunoglobulin.

- The **serum free light chain assay** is a recently introduced test, with greater sensitivity for the detection of paraprotein than protein electrophoresis or immunofixation, and it may further assist in the diagnosis.
- A skeletal survey will usually reveal osteopenia and typical punched-out lesions in bone.
- The diagnosis of multiple myeloma is typically confirmed by bone marrow biopsy, revealing clonal expansion of plasma cells.
- Definitive diagnosis of myeloma kidney requires **kidney biopsy**, although kidney-specific therapy may be ineffective.
  - Renal biopsy may only be necessary when considering plasma exchange or other diagnoses.
  - **Characteristic eosinophilic casts with a "brittle" or "fractured" appearance** may be visualized in the lumens of distal tubules on light microscopy. There may be tubular cell toxicity and surrounding **interstitial inflammation**, occasionally taking the form of a giant cell reaction.[32] Cast nephropathy can be misinterpreted as interstitial nephritis; hence, it is vital for the nephrologist to review the histology with the pathologist, to avoid misdiagnosis.

TREATMENT

- Treatment of cast nephropathy primarily consists of supportive care and **treatment of the underlying malignancy.**
  - Hypovolemia and hypercalcemia should be corrected, infections should be treated aggressively, and other nephrotoxic insults should be removed.
  - There is no evidence that forced diuresis with loop diuretics improves recovery by washing out obstructing casts. In fact, animal data suggest that there may even be an increase in the tendency to form casts with this strategy.[33]
  - **Treatment of the underlying myeloma** should be initiated promptly in consultation with an oncologist in order to reduce levels of the paraprotein as rapidly as possible.
    - High-dose corticosteroids are a part of all the available treatment regimens and are the primary noninvasive means to rapidly reduce paraprotein levels.
    - Allopurinol should be started prior to institution of therapy for myeloma to reduce the risk of subsequent TLS.
- **Plasma exchange** has been used for acute treatment of cast nephropathy as a means to more rapidly reduce paraprotein levels. Data regarding its use come from small, usually retrospective studies with conflicting results.
  - The most often quoted study supporting the use of plasma exchange in myeloma kidney prospectively enrolled 29 patients to either plasma exchange or hemodialysis as needed, or to daily continuous peritoneal dialysis only, regardless of need. All patients received concomitant corticosteroids and cytotoxic therapy. Renal recovery and survival was better in the hemodialysis and the plasma exchange group.[34]
  - A recent retrospective study of 40 patients analyzed the efficacy of plasma exchange in patients whose serum levels of free light chains were used to guide therapy and in patients with biopsy-proven cast nephropathy. A total of 14 patients with cast nephropathy had serum free light chains measured before and after plasma exchange. In seven of the nine patients whose free light chains were reduced by 50% or more, a renal response, defined as 50%

reduction in serum creatinine and dialysis interdependence at 180 days, was seen.[35]
- ○ A larger prospective study randomized 97 patients with a clinical diagnosis of myeloma kidney to either plasma exchange or no adjunctive pheresis treatment. All patients received similar chemotherapy, and hemodialysis was provided to patients in both groups when indicated. There was no statistically significant difference in outcomes between the two groups.[36] Limitations to the study included uncertainty regarding the diagnosis of cast nephropathy, as few patients had biopsy-proven disease.
- ○ On the basis of this data, **plasma exchange is not recommended for most cases of cast nephropathy,** though it **may be considered in those with a rapid decline in renal function, high paraprotein levels, and less chronicity seen on renal biopsy.**

OUTCOME/PROGNOSIS

- The median survival of patients with multiple myeloma is ~3 to 4 years.
- The occurrence of renal insufficiency shortens the median survival to 1.5 to 2 years.
- There is some potential for renal recovery in cast nephropathy with even severe renal dysfunction, with up to 40% of patients who survive the short-term period being able to regain dialysis independence.[37]

INTERSTITIAL AKI

- The causes of intrinsic AKI in which the primary site of pathology is the kidney interstitium include **acute interstitial nephritis (AIN), infiltrative malignant processes,** and **acute pyelonephritis** (see Table 13-1).
- The presence of pyuria and white blood cell casts on urine sediment analysis may allow one to tentatively narrow the differential diagnosis to these interstitial causes of intrinsic renal dysfunction.

ACUTE INTERSTITIAL NEPHRITIS

GENERAL PRINCIPLES

Definition
- AIN is a hypersensitivity reaction characterized by inflammation in the renal interstitium, sparing the glomeruli.

Epidemiology
- AIN is the predominant finding in 10% of biopsies performed in cases of AKI.[38]
- The incidence seems to be increasing, perhaps as a result of more liberal prescribing practices and the availability of new medications.

Etiology

- The **major causes of AIN are drugs** (70% of cases), **infections** (15%), and **systemic diseases** (Table 13-5). Among drug-induced AIN, antibiotics and NSAIDs, including salicylates and COX-2 inhibitors, may be responsible for 30% and 40% of cases, respectively.
- Other less-common etiologies include idiopathic causes (10%), tubulointerstitial nephritis with uveitis syndrome (5%), and sarcoidosis (1%).[39]

Pathophysiology

- AKI results from **immune-mediated tubular injury.** The localization of inflammation to the interstitium may occur through several mechanisms, including molecular mimicry with tubular epitopes or deposition of immunogenic portions of the inciting agent at a specific location in the kidney.
- Similar to other hypersensitivity reactions, AIN is not dose dependent, there is recrudescence in disease activity on reexposure to compounds with similar biochemical structure, and there is often multiorgan involvement.[40]
- Both cell-mediated and humoral immunity seem to play a role, though the former seems play a more significant role in pathogenesis.[41]

DIAGNOSIS

Clinical Presentation

- The presenting features of AIN can be quite variable, due in part to the multiplicity of agents that can initiate the syndrome. A summary of clinical and laboratory features associated with some of the more common causes of AIN is given in Table 13-6.
- The **combination of AKI, urinary symptoms** (e.g., flank pain, macroscopic hematuria, or oliguria), and **symptoms of hypersensitivity** (e.g., rash, fever, or arthralgias) should alert the clinician to the possibility of AIN.[39,48]
  - ○ Signs of hypersensitivity may be absent in up to half of AIN cases, especially in those attributable to NSAIDs.[49]
- The temporal relationship between the initiation of a new drug and the development of renal dysfunction may also aid in the diagnosis.
  - ○ Disease manifestations develop within 3 weeks of initiation of the inciting drug in ~80% of patients, with an average latency of onset of 10 days (range 1 day to >1 year).[50]
  - ○ The duration of onset may be longer with NSAIDs, with a mean latent period of 2 to 3 months.[49]
- In AIN related to infection or systemic diseases, the clinical features of the inciting disease often predominate.

Diagnostic Testing

- **Urinalysis** may reveal nonspecific findings such as hematuria and/or sterile pyuria.
  - ○ The presence of white blood cell casts is more specific, although they can also be seen in pyelonephritis and certain proliferative glomerulonephritides.
  - ○ **Eosinophiluria** (urine eosinophils numbering >1% of the urine white blood cell count) can be seen (usually detected) more reliably with Hansel stain

TABLE 13-5 CAUSES OF ACUTE INTERSTITIAL NEPHRITIS

Drugs[a]	Infections	Systemic Diseases	Other
Antimicrobial agents	**Bacteria**	Light-chain gammopathy	Wasp sting
Penicillins (especially ampicillin and methicillin)	*Brucella* species	Sarcoidosis	Chinese herbs
	C. jejuni	Sjögren's syndrome	Idiopathic
	C. diphtheriae	Systemic lupus erythematosus	
	Chlamydia species	Tubulointerstitial nephritis and uveitis syndrome	
Cephalosporins	*E. coli*		
Ciprofloxacin	*Legionella* species		
Indinavir	*L. interrogans*	Wegner's and other vasculitides	
Rifampin	*M. tuberculosis*		
Sulfonamides (including cotrimoxazole)	*M. pneumoniae*		
	Rickettsia species		
	Salmonella species		
NSAIDs, including COX-2 inhibitors and salicylates	*Staphylococcus* species		
	Streptococcus species		
Fenoprofen	*Y. pseudotuberculosis*		
Ibuprofen	**Viruses**		
Indomethacin	CMV		
Naproxen	EBV		
Phenylbutazone	Hantaviruses		
Piroxicam	HBV		
Tolmetin	HIV		
Zomepirac	HSV		
Anticonvulsants	Measles		
Phenytoin	Polyomaviruses		
Diuretics	**Parasites**		
Furosemide	*L. donovani*		
Thiazides	*T. gondii*		
Gastric antisecretory drugs			
Cimetidine			
Proton pump inhibitors			
Others			
Allopurinol			
Phenindione			

[a]Due to the fact that a very large number of drugs have been associated with acute interstitial nephritis, only drug classes and the most common individual offending medicines are listed here.

CMV, cytomegalovirus; COX-2, cyclooxygenase 2; EBV, Epstein–Barr virus; HBV, hepatitis B virus; HIV, human immunodeficiency syndrome; HSV, herpes simplex virus; NSAIDs, nonsteroidal anti-inflammatory drugs.

TABLE 13-6	VARIOUS CAUSES OF ACUTE INTERSTITIAL NEPHRITIS, THEIR CLINICAL AND LABORATORY FEATURES, AND DISEASE COURSES		
Inciting Agent	Signs and Symptoms	Laboratory Findings	Course
Drug-induced AIN, in general[a]	• Fever, 45%; rash, 42%; arthralgias, 12%; flank pain, 45%; oliguria, 40%; macroscopic hematuria, 17%; new or worsened hypertension, 20%	• Hematuria, 53%; pyuria, 50%; mild proteinuria, 58%; eosinophilia, 40%	• Mean 10-day exposure before presentation • Temporary dialysis required in 32%–50%; CKD persists in 36%–40%
Methicillin	• Hypersensitivity symptoms[b] common; macroscopic hematuria very common	• Hematuria, pyuria, and eosinophiluria in almost all; eosinophilia very common	• CKD persists in only 10%
NSAIDs	• Hypersensitivity symptoms[b] uncommon	• Nephrotic range proteinuria in 1/3 of cases • Renal biopsy may also show glomerular findings similar to minimal change	• Mean exposure 2–3 months prior to presentation; CKD persists in 1/2 of cases
Allopurinol	• Often occurs in setting of renal insufficiency as the causative metabolite accumulates • Hypersensitivity symptoms[b] are very common and robust with signs of vasculitis possible[42]	• Eosinophilia and hepatitis common • Renal biopsy may sometimes reveal immune complex deposition at tubular basement membrane	• Death occurs in as many as 1/4 of cases.

Rifampin	• Hypersensitivity symptoms[b] common and robust; oligoanuria in almost all	• Coombs-positive hemolysis, thrombocytopenia, and/or hepatitis occurs • Almost all have anti-rifampin antibodies	• Usually occurs with intermittent dosing • Dialysis is required in almost all cases, though CKD persists only rarely[43]
Leptospiral nephropathy	• Preceding exposure to animal excrement • Fever, jaundice, hepatomegaly, gingival and/or GI bleeding, and purpura very common; altered mental status in 1/2 of cases; oligoanuria in almost all	• Cholestatic hepatitis, hemolytic anemia, and thrombocytopenia very common; hyponatremia common with hypokalemia from renal potassium wasting in some cases • Positive blood/urine cultures or serology • Renal biopsy reveals inflammation predominating at proximal tubules early on, with interstitial hemorrhage possible	• Leptospiral nephropathy occurs in 1/2 of cases of leptospirosis • Death in 1/4 of cases; persistent tubular transport defects may remain in 1/3 of cases[44]
BK nephropathy	• Most often occurs in renal allografts within 1 year after transplant in the setting of aggressive immunosuppression; may occur in other immunosuppressed states as well (e.g., HIV)[45]	• "Decoy cells" (tubular cells with enlarged nucleus and intranuclear inclusions) in urine sediment very common • BK viremia by PCR, 100% sensitive/88% specific • Renal biopsy reveals SV40 stain-positive intranuclear inclusion bodies	• Acute or gradual deterioration in renal function evident • Often resolves with a decrease in immunosuppression

(continued)

TABLE 13-6 | VARIOUS CAUSES OF ACUTE INTERSTITIAL NEPHRITIS, THEIR CLINICAL AND LABORATORY FEATURES, AND DISEASE COURSES (Continued)

Inciting Agent	Signs and Symptoms	Laboratory Findings	Course
Sarcoidosis	• Most often occurs in young adults, with higher incidence in blacks • Extrarenal symptoms of sarcoidosis predominate with pulmonary, ocular, and skin symptoms most common	• Hypercalcemia or normocalcemia despite advanced renal failure may be present • Chest radiography with hilar adenopathy and/or infiltrates very common • Renal biopsy reveals interstitial noncaseating granulomas and giant cells	• Often a relapsing course responsive to pulse increase in steroids; CKD persists in 90%[46]
TINU	• 3:1 female predominance, with median age of onset 15 • Eye pain or redness, fever, and/or weight loss common	• Elevated serum IgG very common • Renal biopsy may uncommonly reveal granulomas in interstitium	• Uveitis may precede, follow, or coexist with the renal disease • Complete renal recovery often occurs spontaneously within 1 year, although uveitis recurs in 1/2[47]

[a]The general characteristics of *drug-induced* interstitial nephritis as a group, together with rates of occurrence, are given in the first row. Features that distinguish between specific causative agents are emphasized in the remaining rows.

[b]Fevers, rash, and/or arthralgias.

AIN, acute interstitial nephritis; CKD, chronic kidney disease; GI, gastrointestinal; HIV, human immunodeficiency virus; IgG, immunoglobulin G; NSAIDs, nonsteroidal anti-inflammatory drugs; PCR, polymerase chain reaction; SV40, simian virus 40; TINU, tubulointerstitial nephritis with uveitis syndrome.

than with Wright stain. Though the **positive predictive value of this test is low,** the test's performance characteristics might be improved if other causes of eosinophiluria, such as urinary tract infection and atheroembolic disease, can be excluded.[41,51]

- ○ **Mild proteinuria** is common, but sometimes it may be in the nephrotic range. Heavy proteinuria is classically associated with NSAIDs, occurring in a third of cases attributable to this drug class and associated with concomitant minimal-change glomerulopathy. NSAID-induced membranous nephropathy can also occur.[49,52]
- Signs of multiorgan dysfunction such as elevated transaminases and hemolysis can occasionally be seen.
- Renal imaging may occasionally reveal normal-to-large kidneys with increased echogenicity.
- Renal biopsy is the gold standard for definitive diagnosis and reveals an **edematous interstitium infiltrated mostly by T-cells and macrophages.** Neutrophils, eosinophils, and plasma cells can also be found and occasionally there may be granulomatous inflammation. There may be tubulitis or frank tubular necrosis in severe AIN. The glomeruli are usually normal, but electron microscopy may reveal foot process effacement in NSAID-associated AIN.

TREATMENT

- The most important therapeutic maneuver in AIN is **prompt removal of the inciting agent.** In those cases associated with infection or other systemic disease, treatment of the underlying cause is necessary.
- Though it is tempting to combat the hypersensitivity response with **corticosteroids,** the usefulness of this intervention remains uncertain.
  - ○ Retrospective studies, including a series of 42 cases, suggest no reduction in the incidence of chronic kidney disease with corticosteroids.[38] However, it might be argued that beneficial effects were not seen because patients with more severe disease were more likely to receive corticosteroids.
  - ○ The best data supporting the use of corticosteroids comes from a small series of 14 patients, all with methicillin-induced AIN. Corticosteroids were associated with complete renal recovery more often than withdrawal of methicillin alone, and the treated group recovered more quickly.[53]
  - ○ Positive observational data with corticosteroids in AIN from other etiologies exist, but are limited to small case series. In many reports, the most apparent effect of corticosteroids was a more rapid recovery of renal function.
- The literature is sparse regarding the use of other immunosuppressants and often describes cases associated with unusual etiologies. Successful treatment has been described using calcineurin inhibitors, cyclophosphamide, azathioprine, and mycophenolate mofetil.
- A reasonable treatment strategy in light of these data would be to **reserve corticosteroids for patients with idiopathic AIN, systemic diseases** for which corticosteroids have a proven role (e.g., sarcoidosis, Sjögren, vasculitides), **or cases with poor prognostic features.** Predictors of worse prognosis include delayed onset of improvement in renal function after withdrawal of the inciting agent (>1 week), prolonged exposure to the offending agent (>2 to 3 weeks), preexisting chronic kidney disease, and a renal histology characterized by

intense and diffuse interstitial infiltrate, granuloma formation, or significant fibrosis and tubular atrophy.

- ○ A frequently used regimen is oral prednisone (1 mg/kg), with the duration of therapy guided by the improvement in renal function. Most patients will improve in the first 1 to 2 weeks.
- ○ The presence of conditions that can be exacerbated by corticosteroid therapy (e.g., slow-healing wounds, brittle diabetes, or active infection) should dissuade the clinician from using this therapy.
- ○ Studies have suggested that corticosteroids do not alter the course of NSAID-induced AIN, though if poor prognostic features are present, treatment can still be considered.
- ○ Other immunosuppressants are occasionally used when corticosteroid therapy has failed.

OUTCOME/PROGNOSIS

- • AIN has a variable clinical course and response to treatment.
  - ○ In the previous prototype for the disease—methicillin-induced AIN—the prognosis was excellent with complete recovery of renal function noted in 90% of patients.[53]
  - ○ In nonmethicillin drug-induced AIN, chronic kidney disease persists in 35% to 40% of cases.[54]
  - ○ The prevalence of chronic kidney disease is even higher with NSAID-induced AIN, occurring in 55% of cases.
- • The prognosis for AIN may depend on the promptness of elimination of the inciting agent.
  - ○ The etiologies associated with milder symptoms, and therefore delayed diagnosis (e.g., NSAIDs, chronic infections, or sarcoidosis), have worse prognosis than those with more acute and dramatic presentations (e.g., methicillin, rifampin, or acute bacterial or viral infections).
- • Interestingly, the peak serum creatinine does not seem to correlate with the long-term renal prognosis.[41]

INFILTRATIVE MALIGNANCIES

GENERAL PRINCIPLES

- • Infiltration of the kidneys by malignant cells occurs commonly in lymphoid and myeloid leukemias and lymphomas.
- • The kidneys are the most common extramedullary organs involved by leukemic infiltration, with 63% of autopsies from leukemia patients displaying this finding.[55]
- • Renal dysfunction attributable to leukemic infiltration is rare.[56]

DIAGNOSIS

- • AKI from leukemic infiltration may be difficult to distinguish from spontaneous TLS, which occurs much more commonly and in similar settings.
  - ○ Hyperuricemia will be evident in both cases, as uric acid production is increased in leukemia, and renal failure from any cause leads to decreased uric acid excretion.

- ○ Further complicating this distinction is the fact that leukemic infiltration of the kidneys is a risk factor for TLS.
- Examination of the **urine sediment is not helpful,** as it usually reveals nonspecific pyuria and/or hematuria.
- The phenomenon is clinically silent in most cases, even though nephromegaly might be evident on imaging.
- **Definitive diagnosis requires renal biopsy.** Histology usually reveals tremendous numbers of malignant cells invading the interstitium, resulting in wide separation and distortion of the tubules.

TREATMENT

- Management involves **treatment of the underlying malignancy** while employing preventive strategies for TLS (see above).
- Recovery to near-normal renal function is possible, even in cases of profound renal dysfunction.

ACUTE PYELONEPHRITIS

GENERAL PRINCIPLES

Etiology
- AKI in the setting of acute pyelonephritis occurs most commonly from prerenal physiology, concomitant obstruction, or ATN from hypotension or nephrotoxic antibiotics.
- The edema and suppurative infiltration of the kidney parenchyma may alone cause AKI in rare cases.

Pathophysiology
- The inflammatory reaction may impinge on the vasa recta that tenuously support the medullary tubules, and frank **papillary necrosis** may occur in patients with vasculopathy such as diabetics.

Risk Factors
- Populations at risk for this form of AKI include patients with a single kidney, renal allograft recipients, and malnourished alcoholics.[57,58]

DIAGNOSIS

- Patients may present with fever, flank pain, or pain over the allograft, though these classic symptoms of pyelonephritis are absent in a significant proportion of patients.
- The urinalysis reveals bacteria and pyuria with or without white blood cell casts.
- Imaging studies may reveal increased renal size.
- Renal histology reveals edema, intense neutrophilic infiltration of the interstitium, and tubular lumens with microabscess formation. With concomitant papillary necrosis, there may be loss of collecting-duct epithelium.

TREATMENT

- Antibiotic therapy results in slow resolution of the renal dysfunction.
- Persistent mild-to-moderate impairment in renal function often occurs, as inflammation is replaced by sclerosis.

REFERENCES

1. Scolari F, Tardanico R, Zani R, et al. Cholesterol crystal embolism: a recognizable cause of renal disease. *Am J Kidney Dis.* 2000;36:1089–1109.
2. Scolari F, Ravani P, Gaggi R, et al. The challenge of diagnosing atheroembolic renal disease: clinical features and prognostic factors. *Circulation.* 2007;116:298–304.
3. Scolari F, Ravani P, Pola A. Predictors of renal and patient outcomes in atheroembolic renal disease: a prospective study. *J Am Soc Nephrol.* 2003;14:1584–1590.
4. Thadhani RI, Camargo CA Jr, Xavier RJ, et al. Atheroembolic renal failure after invasive procedures. Natural history based on 52 histologically proven cases. *Medicine.* 1995;74:350–358.
5. Mittal BV, Alexander MP, Rennke HG, et al. Atheroembolic renal disease: a silent masquerader. *Kidney Int.* 2008;73:126–130.
6. Modi KS, Rao VK. Atheroembolic renal disease. *J Am Soc Nephrol.* 2001;12:1781–1787.
7. Nochy D, Daugas E, Droz D, et al. The intrarenal vascular lesions associated with primary antiphospholipid syndrome. *J Am Soc Nephrol.* 1999;10:507–518.
8. Steen VD, Costantino JP, Shapiro AP, et al. Outcome of renal crisis in systemic sclerosis: relation to availability of angiotensin converting enzyme (ACE) inhibitors. *Ann Intern Med.* 1990;113:352–357.
9. Saftlas AF, Olson DR, Franks AL, et al. Epidemiology of preeclampsia and eclampsia in the United States, 1979–1986. *Am J Obstet Gynecol.* 1990;163:460–465.
10. Coomarasamy A, Honest H, Papaioannou S, et al. Aspirin for prevention of preeclampsia in women with historical risk factors: a systematic review. *Obstet Gynecol.* 2003;101:1319–1332.
11. Steen VD, Costantino JP, Shapiro AP, et al. Outcome of renal crisis in systemic sclerosis: relation to availability of angiotensin converting enzyme (ACE) inhibitors. *Ann Intern Med.* 1990;113:352–357.
12. Perazella MA. Crystal-induced acute renal failure. *Am J Med.* 1999;106:459–465.
13. Markowitz GS, Stokes MB, Radhakrishnan J, et al. Acute phosphate nephropathy following oral sodium phosphate bowel purgative: an under-recognized cause of chronic renal failure. *Am Soc Nephrol.* 2005;16:3389–3396.
14. Keeney RE, Kirk LE, Bridgen D. Acyclovir tolerance in humans. *Am J Med.* 1982;73:176–181.
15. Boubaker K, Sudre P, Bally F, et al. Changes in renal function associated with indinavir. *AIDS.* 1998;12:F249–F254.
16. Widemann BC, Balis FM, Kempf-Bielack B, et al. High-dose methotrexate-induced nephrotoxicity in patients with osteosarcoma. *Cancer.* 2004;100:2222–2232.
17. Becker K, Jablonowski H, Häussinger D. Sulfadiazine-associated nephrotoxicity in patients with the acquired immunodeficiency syndrome. *Medicine.* 1996;75:185–194.
18. Daudon M, Estépa L, Vicard JP, et al. Urinary stones in HIV-1 positive patients treated with indinavir. *Lancet.* 1997;349:1294–1295.
19. Simon DI, Brosius FC 3rd, Rothstein DM. Sulfadiazine crystalluria revisited. The treatment of toxoplasma encephalitis in patients with acquired immunodeficiency syndrome. *Arch Intern Med.* 1990;150:2379–2384.
20. Hande KR, Garrow GC. Acute tumor lysis syndrome in patients with high-grade non-Hodgkin's lymphoma. *Am J Med.* 1993;94:133–139.
21. Cairo MS, Bishop M. Tumor lysis syndrome: new therapeutic strategies and classification. *Br J Haematol.* 2004;127:3–11.

22. Cairo MS, Coiffier B, Reiter A, et al. Recommendations for the evaluation of risk and prophylaxis of tumor lysis syndrome (TLS) in adults and children with malignant diseases: an expert TLS panel consensus. *Br J Haematol.* 2010;149:578–586.
23. Goldman SC, Holcenberg JS, Finklestein JZ, et al. A randomized comparison between rasburicase and allopurinol in children with lymphoma or leukemia at high risk for tumor lysis. *Blood.* 2001;97:2998–3003.
24. Jacobsen D, Hewlett TP, Webb R, et al. Ethylene glycol intoxication: evaluation of kinetics and crystalluria. *Am J Med.* 1998;84:145–152.
25. Brent J. Fomepizole for ethylene glycol and methanol poisoning. *N Engl J Med.* 2009;360:2216–2223.
26. Sanders PW. Pathogenesis and treatment of myeloma kidney. *J Lab Clin Med.* 1994;124:484–488.
27. Sakhuja V, Jha V, Varma S, et al. Renal involvement in multiple myeloma: a 10-year study. *Ren Fail.* 2000;22:465–477.
28. Pasquali S, Zucchelli P, Casanova S, et al. Renal histological lesions and clinical syndromes in multiple myeloma. Renal Immunopathology Group. *Clin Nephrol.* 1987;27:222–228.
29. Solomon A, Weiss DT, Kattine AA. Nephrotoxic potential of Bence Jones proteins. *N Engl J Med.* 1991;324:1845–1851.
30. Rota S, Mougenot B, Baudouin B, et al. Multiple myeloma and severe renal failure: a clinicopathologic study of outcome and prognosis in 34 patients. *Medicine.* 1987;66:126–137.
31. Bladé J, Fernández-Llama P, Bosch F, et al. Renal failure in multiple myeloma: presenting features and predictors of outcome in 94 patients from a single institution. *Arch Intern Med.* 1998;158:1889–1893.
32. Korbet SM, Schwartz MM. Multiple myeloma. *J Am Soc Nephrol.* 2006;17:2533–2545.
33. Sanders PW, Booker BB. Pathobiology of cast nephropathy from human Bence Jones proteins. *J Clin Invest.* 1992;89:630–639.
34. Zucchelli P, Pasquali S, Cagnoli L, et al. Controlled plasma exchange trial in acute renal failure due to multiple myeloma. *Kidney Int.* 1998;33:1175–1180.
35. Leung N, Gertz MA, Zeldenrust SR, et al. Improvement of cast nephropathy with plasma exchange depends on the diagnosis and on reduction of serum free light chains. *Kidney Int.* 2008;73:1282–1288.
36. Clark WF, Stewart AK, Rock GA, et al. Plasma exchange when myeloma presents as acute renal failure: a randomized, controlled trial. *Ann Intern Med.* 2005;143:777–784.
37. Knudsen LM, Hjorth M, Hippe E. Renal failure in multiple myeloma: reversibility and impact on the prognosis. Nordic Myeloma Study Group. *Eur J Haematol.* 2000;65:175–181.
38. Clarkson MR, Giblin L, O'Connell FP, et al. Acute interstitial nephritis: clinical features and response to corticosteroid therapy. *Nephrol Dial Transplant.* 2004;19:2779–2783.
39. Baker RJ, Pusey CD. The changing profile of acute tubulointerstitial nephritis. *Nephrol Dial Transplant.* 2004;19:8–11.
40. Schubert C, Bates WD, Moosa MR. Acute tubulointerstitial nephritis related to antituberculous drug therapy. *Clin Nephrol.* 2010;73:413–419.
41. Rossert J. Drug-induced acute interstitial nephritis. *Kidney Int.* 2001;60:804–817.
42. Arellano F, Sacristán JA. Allopurinol hypersensitivity syndrome: a review. *Ann Pharmacother.* 1993;27:337–343.
43. Covic A, Goldsmith DJ, Segall L, et al. Rifampicin-induced acute renal failure: a series of 60 patients. *Nephrol Dial Transplant.* 1998;13:924–929.
44. Covic A, Goldsmith DJ, Gusbeth-Tatomir P, et al. A retrospective 5-year study in Moldova of acute renal failure due to leptospirosis: 58 cases and a review of the literature. *Nephrol Dial Transplant.* 2003;18:1128–1134.
45. Hirsch HH, Knowles W, Dickenmann M, et al. Prospective study of polyomavirus type BK replication and nephropathy in renal-transplant recipients. *N Engl J Med.* 2002;347:488–496.
46. Hannedouche T, Grateau G, Noël LH, et al. Renal granulomatous sarcoidosis: report of six cases. *Nephrol Dial Transplant.* 1990;5:18–24.

47. Mandeville JT, Levinson RD, Holland GN. The tubulointerstitial nephritis and uveitis syndrome. *Surv Ophthalmol.* 2001;46:195–208.
48. Kodner CM, Kudrimoti A. Diagnosis and management of acute interstitial nephritis. *Am Fam Physician.* 2003;67:2527–2534.
49. Clive DM, Stoff JS. Renal syndromes associated with nonsteroidal anti-inflammatory drugs. *N Engl J Med.* 1984;310:563–572.
50. Neilson EG. Pathogenesis and therapy of interstitial nephritis. *Kidney Int.* 1989;35:1257–1270.
51. Praga M, González E. Acute interstitial nephritis. *Kidney Int.* 2010;77:956–961.
52. Radford MG Jr, Holley KE, Grande JP, et al. Reversible membranous nephropathy associated with the use of nonsteroidal anti-inflammatory drugs. *JAMA.* 1996;276:466–469.
53. Galpin JE, Shinaberger JH, Stanley TM, et al. Acute interstitial nephritis due to methicillin. *Am J Med.* 1978;65:756–765.
54. Schwarz A, Krause PH, Kunzendorf U, et al. The outcome of acute interstitial nephritis: risk factors for the transition from acute to chronic interstitial nephritis. *Clin Nephrol.* 2000;54:179–190.
55. Barcos M, Lane W, Gomez GA, et al. An autopsy study of 1206 acute and chronic leukemias (1958 to 1982). *Cancer.* 1987;60:827–837.
56. Da'as N, Polliack A, Cohen Y, et al. Kidney involvement and renal manifestations in non-Hodgkin's lymphoma and lymphocytic leukemia: a retrospective study in 700 patients. *Eur J Haematol.* 2001;67:158–164.
57. Jones SR. Acute renal failure in adults with uncomplicated acute pyelonephritis: case reports and review. *Clin Infect Dis.* 1992;14:243–246.
58. Camilleri B, Wyatt J, Newstead C. Acute renal failure in a patient suffering from chronic alcoholism. *Nephrol Dial Transplant.* 2003;18:840–842.

Contrast Induced Nephropathy

14

Ethan Hoerschgen

GENERAL PRINCIPLES

- Acute decline in renal function can occur shortly after the administration of intravascular iodinated contrast.
- Contrast-induced nephropathy (CIN) is the third leading cause of hospital-acquired acute kidney injury (AKI).
- CIN is **usually reversible,** and in many cases preventable with appropriate management prior to exposure.
- CIN is associated with increased length of hospital stay, need for increased medical care, and mortality.[1]

Definition

- The definition of CIN varies amongst studies, with no absolute consensus reached.
- The most frequent definition of CIN used in literature and clinical practice is an **elevation of serum creatinine >0.5 mg/dL above baseline or increase of serum creatinine >25%, within 48 to 72 hours after administration of contrast media (CM).**
- Other etiologies of AKI must also be excluded.

Epidemiology

- The incidence of CIN varies significantly from study to study due to differences in definition of CIN, procedure performed, amount and type of contrast agent used, patient risk factors, and preventative measures used.
- The risk for significant CIN is extremely low in patients with normal renal function.
- One study showed that the risk of CIN was 2.5%, 22.4%, and 30.6% in patients with a serum creatinine of 1.2 to 1.9 mg/dL, 2.0 to 2.9 mg/dL, and >3.0 mg/dL, respectively.
- The need for hemodialysis from CIN is generally <1%, but increases in high-risk patients.

Etiology

- **Contrast media:**
  - The **osmolality, type, route of administration,** and **volume of contrast agent** used all can change its nephrotoxic potential.
  - The risk of CIN increases as volume of CM used increases, especially >100 mL.

○ **Repeated contrast exposure,** especially <72 hours apart, also increases the risk for CIN. It is preferred to allow 2 weeks between exposures if possible.

○ If there is a rise in serum creatinine after initial exposure to CM, it is preferable to allow the levels to return to baseline before repeat exposure.

○ Intraarterial CM administration has a higher risk for developing CIN than intravenous (IV) CM administration.

○ The use of **low-osmolar contrast agents** (osmolarity ranging from 570 to 900) have shown to be superior to high-osmolar agents (osmolarity >2000) in preventing CIN.

○ The use of isoosmolar CM (osmolarity of ~290) has been shown to be superior to low-osmolar CM in the prevention of CIN in the past in certain patient populations.[2]

○ However, recent studies, including Prospective Evaluation of Diabetic Ischemic heart disease by Computerized Tomography (PREDICT) and Cardiac Angiography in REnally impaired patients (CARE), have demonstrated no significant differences in the rate in CIN between nonionic low-osmolar and nonionic isoosmolar CM in higher-risk patients.[3,4]

Pathophysiology

• There are likely several mechanisms that lead to AKI from iodinated contrast exposure.

• Studies have consistently shown that administration of intravascular contrast leads to **reduced renal perfusion due to vasoconstriction.**[5]

○ Vasoconstriction is most pronounced at the outer medulla, an area highly susceptible to hypoxia and ischemia.

○ The likely mechanisms of vasoconstriction are **increases in vasoconstrictors** such as **endothelin and adenosine.** There is also a decreased production of nitric oxide, a potent vasodilator.

• Research has also demonstrated direct tubular toxic effects from exposure to CM.

• Iodinated contrast may also induce renal cellular injury through oxygen-free radicals and decreased antioxidant activity.

Risk Factors

• It is important to identify those patients at increased risk for CIN prior to exposing them to the potential harm of CM. Risk factors for developing CIN can be divided into those factors that are modifiable and those that are fixed risk markers (Table 14-1).

• Preexisting **renal insufficiency is the most important risk factor** for the development of CIN.

• A risk stratification score might be useful to identify the high-risk patients (Table 14-2).[6,7]

○ **Concomitant medications:**

■ Inhibitors of prostaglandins, such as nonsteroidal anti-inflammatory drugs or cyclooxygenase 2 inhibitors, should be avoided at least 24 to 48 hours prior to procedure, even though there are no randomized controlled trials to support this recommendation.

■ The **use of IV diuretics has been shown to be deleterious** if given prior to the procedure. There are no recommendations regarding oral diuretics, but they should be stopped if the patient appears to have a decreased effective circulatory volume or hypotension.

TABLE 14-1	RISK FACTORS FOR CONTRAST-INDUCED NEPHROPATHY

Nonmodifiable Risk Markers

- Advanced age (>75 y)
- Diabetic nephropathy
- CKD (SCr >1.5 mg/dL)
- CHF
- NYHA III–IV
- History of pulmonary edema
- Acute MI <24 h prior to CM
- IABP
- Proteinuria/ immunoglobulinopathies
- Peripheral vascular disease

Modifiable Risk Factors

- High volume of contrast agent (>100 mL)
- Osmolality of CM (high > low ≥ iso)
- Anemia/blood loss (Hct <39% for men, 36% for women)
- Short duration between CM exposure
- Hypertension/hypotension
- Hypovolemia
- Nephrotoxic agents
- Aminoglycosides
- NSAIDs
- Calcineurin inhibitors
- Diuretics
- ACE inhibitors
- Intraarterial injection of CM

ACE, angiotensin-converting enzyme; CHF, congestive heart failure; CKD, chronic kidney disease; CM, contrast media; Hct, hematocrit; IABP, intraaortic balloon pump; MI, myocardial infarction; NSAIDs, nonsteroidal anti-inflammatory drugs; NYHA, New York heart association classification; SCr, serum creatinine.

- Stable doses of **angiotensin-converting enzyme inhibitors** and **angiotensin receptor blockers** may be continued, as long as the patient is euvolemic and normotensive, as there is no data to support discontinuation of these medications. Initiation or titration of the medications probably should be avoided in the pericontrast period.

TABLE 14-2	RISK SCORE PREDICTION

Risk Factor	Points	Risk Score	Risk of RCIN
• Hypotension	5	0–5	7.5%
• IABP	5	6–10	14.0%
• CHF	5	11–15	26.1%
• SCr >1.5 mg/dL	4	16+	57.3%
• Age >75 y	4		
• Anemia	3		
• Diabetes	3		
• Volume of CM	1 point per 100 mL		

IABP, intraaortic balloon pump; CHF, congestive heart failure; SCr, serum creatinine; CM, contrast media.

Modified with permission from Elsevier—Mehran R, Aymong ED, Nikolsky E, et al. A simple risk score for prediction of contrast-induced nephropathy after percutaneous coronary intervention. *J Am Coll Cardiol.* 2004;44:1393–1399.

- The **calcineurin inhibitors,** cyclosporine and tacrolimus, have vasocon-strictive properties. However, they should not be stopped in the pericon-trast period because of increased risk of rejection in transplanted organs. Drug levels should be monitored and adjusted to appropriate levels in the pericontrast period.
- Exposure to CM should be avoided when possible while the patients are on other nephrotoxic medications such as **amphotericin B** and **amino-glycosides.**
- **Metformin** may increase risk of lactic acidosis in setting of renal insuffi-ciency. The U.S. Food and Drug Administration recommend that metfor-min should be held for **2 to 3 days after CM exposure,** to assure that the patient has not developed AKI.
- **HMG-CoA reductase inhibitors (statins) may have a beneficial effect** and should be continued if possible in the pericontrast period.

DIAGNOSIS

Clinical Presentation

- AKI from CM is characterized by a **rise in serum creatinine,** usually within the **first 24 to 48 hours after administration of the agent.**
- If serum creatinine elevation starts >72 hours after contrast exposure, then another etiology must be sought.
- The AKI is usually **nonoliguric** and patients are usually asymptomatic.
- The elevation in serum creatinine usually peaks ~3 to 5 days after exposure.
- Some patients may develop oliguric AKI, and these patients usually have underlying renal insufficiency or conditions that predispose them to other forms of renal injury.
- Approximately 1% of patients will require renal replacement therapy because of CIN. These patients usually have a longer recovery period.
- In general CIN is reversible, but persistent renal injury may occur in patients with significant renal insufficiency.
- Renal athroemboli that occur at the time of the procedure can also cause renal injury. Onset of renal failure may not occur for days to weeks, and usually has a prolonged course with less chance for renal recovery.[8]

History

- The likelihood that the etiology of AKI is caused by CIN is strongest if the individual has had an exposure to CM in the previous 24 to 72 hours.
- One should closely search for other etiologies of AKI such as hypotensive events or the presence of nephrotoxic medications.

Physical Examination

- The physical exam is mostly important in helping to differentiate other causes of AKI from CIN. Evidence of hypovolemia may support the diag-nosis of CIN.
- Physical exam may help to diagnose atheroemboli, if there is evidence of livedo reticularis in the lower extremities, "blue toes", or Hollenhorst plaques in the retina.

Differential Diagnosis

- Other possibilities for AKI must be explored even with a high likelihood of CIN.
- Other etiologies include, but not limited to, renal athroembolic disease, prerenal disease, interstitial nephritis, and other causes of tubular necrosis.

Diagnostic Testing

- **Fractional excretion of sodium is usually <1%,** due to the profound vasoconstriction that happens early in the disease process. However, this is not diagnostic.
- Urine sediment is usually bland and not conclusive, but essential to evaluate other causes of AKI. Rarely, granular casts are noted.
- CM may cause significantly elevated urine specific gravity.
- **Eosinophilia or low complement levels may suggest renal athroembolic disease.**
- Persistent contrast within the kidney on imaging, 24 hours after exposure to CM, may suggest CIN.
- A **kidney biopsy is not recommended** to evaluate for CIN, unless further evaluation for other etiologies is needed.

PREVENTION

Avoidance of Contrast

- The only way to completely prevent CIN is to avoid the contrast procedure if at all possible.[9]
- The use of noniodinated contrast agents such as gadolinium and carbon dioxide can be considered in some patients in order to prevent CIN.
- Carbon dioxide can give satisfactory imaging with digital extraction, but has a risk of neurotoxicity and is usually limited to imaging below the diaphragm.
- Gadolinium is associated with pseudocalcemia due to interference with the calcium assay; calcium replacement should not be routinely administered without checking an ionized calcium level.
- Gadolinium is also associated with nephrogenic systemic fibrosis, and extreme caution should be used before giving gadolinium to patients with renal insufficiency.

Volume Expansion

- IV volume expansion around the time of contrast exposure is believed to alleviate renal vasoconstriction and improve medullary blood flow.
- IV half-normal saline is shown to be superior to half-normal saline plus diuretics (i.e., furosemide and mannitol) in preventing CIN.
- Administration of normal saline has been shown to be superior to half-normal saline.
- IV isotonic sodium bicarbonate has been shown to be superior to isotonic saline in prevention of CIN after coronary interventions (1.7% in the sodium bicarbonate group, compared to 13.6% in the normal saline group).[10] Several studies have demonstrated that sodium bicarbonate is superior or equally effective as normal saline in preventing CIN in patients at higher risk.

- **IV normal saline** is typically administered at 75 mL/h for 10 hours prior to the procedure and after the procedure. Patients should be carefully monitored for signs of volume overload and appropriate urine output.
- Typical administration of **isotonic sodium bicarbonate** (150 mEq/L) is at a rate of 3 mL/kg for 1 hour prior to the procedure and at a rate of 1 mL/kg for 6 hours after the procedure.
- Oral hydration, when compared to IV solutions, was not effective in preventing CIN.

N-acetylcysteine

- *N*-acetylcysteine (NAC) is thought to prevent CIN by acting as a scavenger of oxygen free radicals. The side effect profile of NAC is also very favorable, which makes it an attractive prevention strategy.
- The ability of NAC to prevent CIN is controversial, but several randomized control trials have demonstrated NAC to be an effective therapy in preventing CIN when used with IV hydration in high-risk patients.
- The standard dose of NAC was 600 mg PO bid the day before procedure and the day of procedure.[11]
- **Patients undergoing percutaneous coronary intervention** (PCI) had significant reduction in CIN, with 1200 mg IV bolus of NAC plus 1200 mg PO bid for 48 hours, compared to 600 mg IV and PO dosing. This suggests a possible dose-dependent benefit with NAC.[12]
- Given conflicting studies regarding NAC, we cannot recommend the routine use of NAC. In high-risk patients, high-dose IV NAC can be considered.

Other Therapies

- **Ascorbic acid:**
  - Ascorbic acid may prevent CIN through its antioxidant properties, and it has a strong safety profile. Doses of 3 g prior to cardiac angiography, followed by 2 g twice after, showed a significant decrease in CIN.
  - In the renal insufficiency following contrast media administration (REMEDIAL) trial, treatment with normal saline plus ascorbic acid showed similar rates of CIN in high-risk patients when compared to normal saline plus NAC.[13]
- **Iloprost:**
  - Iloprost is a synthetic analog of prostacyclin PGI_2. Iloprost dilates systemic and pulmonary arterial vascular beds.
  - A recent study found that prophylactic periprocedural IV administration of the prostacyclin analog iloprost in patients with renal dysfunction undergoing a coronary procedure reduced the incidence of CIN by 70%.[14]
  - Iloprost may be limited by its blood-pressure-lowering effects.
  - The use of Iloprost for prevention of CIN is not recommended until further confirmation of effectiveness and safety.
- **Fenoldopam:**
  - Fenoldapam is a dopamine-1 receptor agonist, which promotes renal and systemic vasodilatation.
  - The CONTRAST **trial found no significant reduction** in CIN with the use of fenoldopam when compared to placebo.[15]
  - Fenoldapam is not recommended for routine use to prevent CIN.

- **Theophylline and aminophylline:**
  - ○ Theophylline and aminophylline block adenosine's vasoconstrictive effects.
  - ○ Both agents have **a narrow therapeutic window** and dangerous side effects.
  - ○ The studies looking at both agents for the prevention of CIN have yielded conflicting results.
  - ○ The use of these agents is **not recommended for the prevention of CIN.**
- **Hemofiltration:**
  - ○ The role of hemofiltration has been investigated in few studies.
  - ○ One group demonstrated that CIN occurred less in high-risk patients receiving hemofiltration when compared to IV volume expansion alone. In this study, CIN was defined by a rise in serum creatinine, and hemofiltration alone can alter serum creatinine levels. The hospital and 1-year mortality rates were significantly lower in the hemofiltration group.[16]
  - ○ Hemofiltration is **limited by its invasiveness, need for intensive care, and cost.**
  - ○ Hemodialysis has shown no benefit in preventing CIN.
  - ○ The use of hemofiltration and hemodialysis is **not recommended.**
  - ○ However, planning for renal replacement therapy and counseling of patients regarding potential need for post procedure dialysis should be included for those patients at extremely high risk for developing CIN.

TREATMENT

- There are currently no pharmacologic treatments for CIN.
- Treatment consists of **supportive care,** with focus on **avoiding any further nephrotoxic insults.**
- Close attention should be given to patient's volume status, urine output, and laboratory test results to evaluate for complication of AKI.
- Renal replacement therapy may be needed if patient has persistent complications from AKI, especially volume overload, hyperkalemia, and metabolic acidosis.

OUTCOME/PROGNOSIS

- CIN is usually reversible, but has both immediate and sustained effects.
- Patients who developed CIN had a higher rate of in-hospital and postdischarge mortality.
- Those patients who develop CIN are also susceptible to other in-hospital events, including myocardial infarction after PCI, bleeding, shock, and respiratory failure, and a significant increase in length of hospital stay.[17]
- CIN is potentially a preventable disease. Recognizing high-risk patients and providing adequate IV hydration and avoiding nephrotoxic agents prior to the procedure is essential in preventing AKI.

REFERENCES

1. Finn WF. The clinical and renal consequences of contrast-induced nephropathy. *Nephrol Dial Transplant.* 2006:(suppl 1):i2–i10.
2. Aspelin P, Aubry P, Sven-Goran F, et al. Nephrotoxic effects in high-risk patients undergoing angiography. *N Engl J Med.* 2003;348:491–499.

3. Solomon RJ, Natarajan MK, Doucet S, et al. Cardiac Angiography in Renally Impaired Patients (CARE) study: a randomized double-blind trial of contrast-induced nephropathy in patients with chronic kidney disease. *Circulation.* 2007;115:3189–3196.

4. Kuhn MJ, Chen N, Sahani DV, et al. The PREDICT study: a randomized double-blind comparison of contrast-induced nephropathy after low- or isoosmolar contrast agent exposure. *AJR Am J Roentgenol.* 2008;191:151–157.

5. Tumlin J, Fulvio S, Adam A, et al. Pathophysiololgy of contrast-induced nephropathy. *Am J Cardiol.* 2006;98(suppl):14K–20K.

6. Mehran R, Aymong ED, Nikolsky E, et al. A simple risk score for prediction of contrast-induced nephropathy after percutaneous coronary intervention. *J Am Coll Cardiol.* 2004; 44:1393–1399.

7. McCullough P, Adam A, Becker C, et al. Risk prediction of contrast-induced nephropathy. *Am J Cardiol.* 2006;98(suppl):27K–36K.

8. Morcos SK, Contrast-medium induced nephrotoxicity. In: Dawson P, Cosgrove DO, Grainger RG, eds. *Textbook of Contrast Media.* San Francisco, CA: Isis Medical Media; 1999:135–148.

9. Pannu N, Wiebe N, Marcello T. Prophylaxis strategies for contrast-induced nephropathy. *JAMA.* 2006;295:2765–2779.

10. Merten GJ, Burgess WP, Gray LV, et al. Prevention of contrast-induced nephropathy with sodium bicarbonate. *JAMA.* 2004;291:2328–2334.

11. Tepel M, van der Giet M, Schwarzfeld C, et al. Prevention of radiographic-contrast-agent-induced reductions in renal function by acetylcysteine. *N Engl J Med.* 2000;343:180–184.

12. Marenzi G, Assanelli E, Marana I, et al. N-acetylcysteine and contrast-induced nephropathy in primary angioplasty. *N Engl J Med.* 2006;354:2773–2782.

13. Ricciardelli B, Colombo A, Focaccio A, et al. A Randomized Comparison of 3 Preventive Strategies (REMEDIAL). *Circulation.* 2007;115:1211–1217.

14. Spargias K, Adreanides E, Demerouti E, et al. Iloprost prevents contrast-induced nephropathy in patients with renal dysfunction undergoing coronary angiography or intervention. *Circulation.* 2009;120:1793–1799.

15. Stone G, McCullough P, Tumlin J, et al. Fenoldopam mesylate for the prevention of contrast-induced nephropathy. *JAMA.* 2003;290:2284–2291.

16. Marenzi G, Lauri G, Campodonico J, et al. Comparison of hemofiltration protocols for prevention of contrast induced nephropathy in high-risk patients. *Am J Med.* 2006; 119(2):155–162.

17. Rihal CS, Textor SC, Grill DE, et al. Incidence and prognostic importance of acute renal failure after percutaneous coronary intervention. *Circulation.* 2002;105:2259–2264.

Renal Replacement Therapy in Acute Kidney Injury

15

Anitha Vijayan

GENERAL PRINCIPLES

- Renal replacement therapy (RRT) is required in patients with acute kidney injury (AKI) when the residual native function is insufficient to maintain volume, electrolyte, and acid–base balance, or uremic factors trigger systemic complications such as mental status changes, bleeding diathesis, pericarditis, and so forth.
- The timing of initiation of RRT in AKI remains controversial.
- RRT should be dosed appropriately based on evidence-based data.
- There are different modalities available to patients.
- RRT should be carefully supervised by the treating nephrologist, and every attempt should be done to minimize complications and adverse events. Patients should be carefully monitored for signs of renal recovery such as increasing urine output and downtrending of serum creatinine.

Indications

- The **conventional factors that trigger RRT** include:
  - metabolic acidosis
  - hyperkalemia
  - volume overload
  - uremia
- The exact definition of "uremia" is vague. Therefore, there is extensive variability in the timing of initiation from institution to institution and even among individual nephrologists at the same institution.[1,2]
- The important indications for initiation of hemodialysis in AKI are provided in Table 15-1.

Modalities of RRT

- The available modalities are:
  - **intermittent hemodialysis (IHD)**
  - **continuous RRT (CRRT)**
  - **sustained low-efficiency dialysis (SLED) or extended dialysis (ED)**
  - **peritoneal dialysis (PD)**
- The choice depends on the availability of therapies at the institution, physician preference, the patient's hemodynamic status, and the presence of comorbid conditions.[3]
- Patients with sepsis or hepatic failure may have potential benefits with continuous therapies.

TABLE 15-1   INDICATIONS FOR INITIATION OF RRT IN AKI

- Volume overload refractory to diuretics
- Hyperkalemia refractory to medical therapy
- Metabolic acidosis refractory to medical therapy
- "Uremic" syndrome
  - Anorexia, nausea, vomiting
  - Serositis
  - Seizures, confusion
  - Neuropathy
  - Bleeding
- Need to start total parenteral nutrition (volume/solute issues)
- Overdoses/intoxications (e.g., ethylene glycol, methanol, lithium, theophylline, barbiturates, and so forth)
- Refractory hypercalcemia
- Refractory hyperuricemia

RRT, renal replacement therapy; AKI, acute kidney injury.

- Small studies have shown that intracranial pressure is more stable with CRRT than with IHD in patients with hepatic encephalopathy.[4]
- High-flow CRRT has been shown to remove inflammatory cytokines in sepsis, but hard end points such as mortality, hospital length of stay, and renal recovery are yet to be studied.
- Intermittent modalities are generally accepted to cause greater fluctuations in blood pressure and produce greater fluid shifts in a short amount of time.
- Continuous modalities allow for the same solute clearance and fluid removal, but spread out over a 24-hour period, and thus are favored in hemodynamically unstable patients.
- In the United States, CRRT is performed in ~30% of patients with AKI and has almost completely replaced PD in the treatment of AKI.[5]
- CRRT has not shown improved survival over IHD in critically ill patients.[6,7]
- Likewise, randomized trials have not shown a difference in time to renal recovery or length of intensive care unit (ICU) or hospital stay between groups treated with IHD versus CRRT. Table 15-2 lists the advantages and disadvantages of the different modalities.
- The principles of hemodialysis and PD are discussed in other chapters. This section will focus primarily on CRRT, and how this modality compares with IHD in AKI.
- SLED will also be discussed briefly.

Dosing of RRT

- Evidence from end-stage renal disease patients suggests that a thrice-weekly regimen for IHD, a **urea reduction ratio (URR)** of ~65% to 68% per session, is considered adequate dialysis. This correlates to a **fractional urea clearance** ($Kt/Vurea$) of 1.2, where K is the dialyzer efficiency, t is the time of treatment, and V is the volume of distribution of urea.[8]
- Given the acuity of the AKI population, urea clearances are notoriously unreliable, with frequent volume shifts, sepsis, high catabolic state, and so forth.

| TABLE 15-2 | ADVANTAGES AND DISADVANTAGES OF DIFFERENT MODALITIES | |

Modality	Advantages	Disadvantages
IHD	• High-efficiency transport of solutes when rapid clearance of toxins or electrolytes is required • Allows time for off-unit testing	• Hemodynamic intolerance secondary to fluid shifts • "Saw-tooth" pattern of metabolic control between sessions
CRRT	• Gentler hemodynamic shifts than IHD • Steady solute control	• Continuous need for specialized nursing • Requires continuous anticoagulation (heparin vs. citrate)
SLED	• Fewer hemodynamic shifts compared to IHD • Less work for intensive care nursing staff compared to CRRT • Can be performed at night, avoiding cessation of therapy for procedures • No need for expensive dialysate and replacement fluids	• Needs to be performed 5–6 days per week to achieve adequate clearance • ICU nurses need to be trained to utilize regular HD machines • Need outcome data, in comparison to IHD and CRRT
PD	• Gentler hemodynamic shifts than IHD	• Requires invasion of peritoneal cavity, which may not be possible in postoperative patients • Less predictable fluid removal rates • Efficiency of urea removal low compared with other therapies

CRRT, continuous renal replacement therapy; HD, hemodialysis; ICU, intensive care unit; IHD, intermittent hemodialysis; PD, peritoneal dialysis; SLED, sustained low efficiency dialysis.

- The current acute dialysis quality initiative recommendation is to prescribe at least a single-pool *Kt/Vurea* of 1.3 for each dialysis treatment in AKI.
- This is based on the assumption that AKI patients should at least receive the dose recommended for end-stage renal disease patients.
- However, studies have shown that even this dose is rarely achieved in AKI.
- It has been proposed that benefit may be derived from increasing the renal replacement dose with higher treatment doses, more frequent treatments, or increasing flow rates in CRRT.
- A small study published in 2001 suggested that short daily dialysis improved mortality in AKI compared with three times per week dialysis (28% vs. 46%). However, the *Kt/Vurea* obtained per session was <1.0, suggesting inadequate dialysis.[9]

- In CRRT, one single-center study demonstrated a survival advantage in critically ill patients who underwent intensive CRRT (35 mL/kg/h vs. 20 mL/kg/h).[10]
- Two large multi-center trials addressing the question of dosing of RRT in AKI have recently been published.
  - The acute renal failure trial network (ATN) study published in 2008 demonstrated no survival benefit in AKI with more intensive therapy (IHD six times per week with Kt/Vurea of 1.3 per session or continuous venovenous hemodiafiltration (CVVHDF) at 35 mL/kg/h) compared to less intensive therapy (IHD three times per week or CVVHDF at 20 mL/kg/h).[11]
  - The randomized evaluation of normal versus augmented level replacement therapy (RENAL) study evaluated CVVHDF with effluent flow rates of 40 mL/kg/h in the high-dose group versus 25 mL/kg/h in the low-dose group. There was no difference in 90-day mortality between the two arms.[12]
- On the basis of the existing data, the current recommendation is to prescribe CRRT at 20 to 25 mL/kg/h.
- If prescribed therapy is not being delivered at least 80% of the time because of interruptions (machine malfunction, catheter malfunction, patient interruption for procedures), then the prescription dose can be increased to take this into account.
- IHD should be prescribed to achieve a URR of 70% (Kt/Vurea of 1.3) per treatment, three times per week.
- URR should be performed during each treatment, and subsequent dialysis treatment should be adjusted (change of duration, dialysis filter, blood flow, and so forth, to improve adequacy) accordingly.

CONTINUOUS RRT

Principles of CRRT

- CRRT utilizes the principles of **diffusion, convection,** or **both,** depending on the modality.
- **Diffusion:**
  - This involves the same principles as dialysis and drives solutes such as urea across the dialysis membrane from the blood (higher concentration) to the dialysate (lower concentration), which is running countercurrent to the blood.
  - The dialysate flow rate is ~15 to 40 mL/min compared with dialysate flow rate in IHD of 300 to 450 mL/min.
  - This process is called **CVVHD.**
- **Convection:**
  - During *convection,* solute movement across the membrane is driven by solvent drag.
  - The plasma water is pushed across the membrane by filtrating pressure and takes solutes with it, similar to glomerular ultrafiltration.
  - This large volume loss has to be restored with necessary solutes, and therefore convection requires the addition of **replacement fluid solution** to the CRRT setup.
  - This is called **CVVH.**
- **Diffusion and convection:**
  - The *combination* of the two processes utilizes both dialysate and replacement fluid solutions and is termed **CVVHDF.**

TABLE 15-3	NOMENCLATURE OF CONTINUOUS RENAL REPLACEMENT THERAPY MODALITIES

Abbreviations

A	Arterio-
V	Venous
C	Continuous
HD	Hemodialysis
H	Hemofiltration
HDF	Hemodiafiltration
UF	Ultrafiltration

Modalities

CVVH/CAVH	Continuous venovenous/arteriovenous hemofiltration
CVVHD/CAVHD	Continuous venovenous/arteriovenous hemodialysis
CVVHDF/CAVHDF	Continuous venovenous/arteriovenous hemodiafiltration
SCUF	Slow continuous ultrafiltration
SLED	Slow low-efficiency dialysis

- **Ultrafiltration:**
  - CRRT also can be used without dialysate or replacement fluid to treat volume overload with minimal solute clearance. This process is called *slow continuous ultrafiltration.* The nomenclature of CRRT is outlined in Table 15-3.
- Some of the membranes used for CRRT also have adsorptive properties, but it is unclear to what extent this results in significant clearance of substances.
- Studies have suggested that adsorption with polysulfone membranes might result in clearance of cytokines, but, to date, this has not been demonstrated to have clinical benefit.

Fluids in CRRT

- **Bicarbonate-based solutions** have essentially replaced lactate-based solutions in CRRT.
- Bicarbonate-based solutions are either prepared at individual institutions by the pharmacy or supplied premixed by various manufacturers.
- Even if they are provided by manufacturers, the final constitution of the fluid is conducted by the local pharmacy as various products have different compositions and mixing instructions.
- **The typical concentrations of solutes** in the solution is given below:
  - Bicarbonate concentration is ~35 mEq/L.
  - Sodium is 140 mEq/L.
  - Chloride is ~106 to 109 mEq/L.
  - Magnesium is ~1.0 to 1.5 mEq/L.
  - Potassium concentrations vary and the prescription should reflect the patient's serum levels.
  - Calcium concentration should be zero if citrate anticoagulation is used and calcium should be replaced through a central venous catheter.

Anticoagulation in CRRT

- Slow continuous blood flow through extracorporeal circulation mandates the use of anticoagulation to prevent platelet activation and thrombosis of the circuit.
- The primary goal of anticoagulation is to prevent clotting of the tubes and filters, thereby ensuring the delivery of prescribed therapy.
- Currently, the **two primary methods of anticoagulation** utilized in the United States are:
  - **Intravenous heparin** (either provided through the circuit or systemically) to maintain partial thromboplastin time (PTT) between 60 and 80 seconds.
  - **Citrate anticoagulation:**
    - There are different ways of administering citrate, but the principles remain the same.
    - Citrate administered prefilter chelates the ionized calcium extracorporeal circuit.
    - Calcium is an essential cofactor for the coagulation cascade and its deficiency prevents coagulation in the circuit.
    - To counteract the effect of citrate in the systemic circulation, calcium is given via a **central venous catheter** to maintain blood-ionized calcium in the normal range.
    - It is of utmost importance to closely monitor ionized calcium levels during citrate anticoagulation.
- Other methods of anticoagulation used include argatroban and bivalirudin, usually reserved for patients who develop heparin-induced thrombocytopenia (HIT).

Typical Regimen for CRRT

- An example of CRRT orders for a 70-kg patient, assuming 20 mL/kg/h of replacement fluid and dialysate, serum potassium of 4 mEq/L, is given below:
  - **Blood flow 180 mL/min**
  - **Dialysate flow rate 700 mL/hour—Replacement fluid flow rate 700 mL/hour**
  - **Heparin bolus** xx^* units loading dose IV, then infusion (1000 units/mL) at xx mL/h
    - Heparin should be individualized for the patient. Patients at high risk for bleeding should not receive heparin or target PTT should be lower.
  - **Dialysate** (bicarbonate-based solution), 0 K, 3.5 Ca—add KCl to make the final concentration of K 3 mEq/L
  - **Replacement fluid** (bicarbonate-based solution), 0 K, 3.5 Ca—add enough KCl to make the final concentration of K 3 mEq/L

Drug Dosing in CRRT

- Total clearance of any compound depends on its elimination by nonrenal route, residual renal function, and CRRT.
- Unlike IHD, the clearance of medications is continuous, controlled, and somewhat predictable if the patients remain on continuous therapy.
- Patient, drug, and dialysis characteristics determine appropriate dosing schedules to be used.
- Generally, the nonrenal clearance is taken to be constant, although in critically ill patients with multiorgan system failure, this component may be less than predicted.
- The CRRT clearance relies on convection, diffusion, and adsorption.

TABLE 15-4	DOSING OF COMMON ANTIMICROBIAL AGENTS DURING CONTINUOUS RENAL REPLACEMENT THERAPY (ultrafiltration rates of 20 to 30 mL/min)
Medication	**Dosing in CRRT**
Vancomycin	500 mg once daily or bid
Cefepime	2000 mg once daily or bid
Ceftazidime	500–1000 mg bid
Cefotaxime	2000 mg bid
Ceftriaxone	2000 mg once daily
Imipenem	250–500 mg tid or qid
Ciprofloxacin	200 mg once daily or bid
Metronidazole	500 mg tid
Piperacillin	4000 mg tid
Amikacin	250 mg once daily or bid
Tobramycin	100 mg once daily
Fluconazole	100–200 mg once daily
Acyclovir	3.5 mg/kg once daily

CRRT, continuous renal replacement therapy.

- *Convective* elimination is determined primarily by the protein-bound fraction of the drug.
- In *diffusive* elimination, the saturation of the drug in the dialysate (and filtrate) becomes important, and decreases as flow rates increase.
- By taking these guidelines into consideration, therapeutic doses have been calculated for a variety of drugs used in the ICU. The recommended doses of some of the more commonly prescribed antibiotics are listed in Table 15-4.

Complications of CRRT

- As with any procedure, there are certain complications and adverse events that can be associated with renal replacement therapies.
- Vigilance for such complications and their immediate rectification are essential to prevent life-threatening situations, especially in the vulnerable population of the ICU.
- Some are related to the procedure itself, whereas others are a result of fluid removal or electrolyte and acid–base disturbances.
- In addition, the necessity for a central venous catheter places the patient at risk for infection complications.
- **Hypotension:**
  - Hypotension can occur in all clinical settings with all modalities, although it is more commonly seen with IHD and its rapid fluid shifts.
  - Volume-depleted and septic patients are at heightened risk; careful attention to the physical examination and invasive hemodynamic monitoring when indicated can help ensure adequate volume resuscitation prior to initiating the dialysis session.
  - A target central venous pressure of 8 to 12 mm Hg can be used in these settings and may dictate a reduction or stoppage of fluid ultrafiltration.

- Alternatively, if pulmonary edema or acute lung injury is complicating the picture, then pressor support can be used to maintain blood pressure while continuing ultrafiltration with CRRT. However, this must be done with extreme caution given the risk of peripheral ischemia.
- **Arrhythmias:**
  - Cardiac arrhythmias can occur in the setting of RRT and electrolyte shifts.
  - Although generally seen with IHD, arrhythmia can also be seen in CRRT.
  - **Potassium, magnesium, and calcium levels must be monitored every 12 to 24 hours during CRRT.** If 0 or 1 mEq/L of potassium concentration is being used, then potassium should be monitored every 6 to 8 hours to ensure stable potassium plasma concentration.
  - Patients on digitalis are especially sensitive to hypokalemia. Potassium competes with digitalis for binding at the Na^+/K^+-ATPase pump, and reduced serum levels can enhance the medicine's toxicity.
  - Supraventricular arrhythmias can also be triggered during the placement of the dialysis catheter or by a malpositioned dialysis catheter.
  - If the arrhythmia is resulting in hemodynamic compromise, then therapy is discontinued immediately and appropriate measures to treat the arrhythmia should be started.
- **Central venous catheter problems:**
  - CRRT requires the insertion of a nontunneled, large-bore, dual-lumen, central venous catheter into either the internal jugular, subclavian, or femoral veins.
  - Nontunneled catheters are typically placed at the bedside into a central vein and **ultrasound guidance is strongly recommended** to reduce complications such as bleeding and infections.
  - Sterile precautions should be mandatory during placement of central venous catheters.
  - Immediate risks include bleeding, injury to other organs or vessels (e.g., pneumothorax, carotid artery injury), and malposition of the catheter.
  - Infection risks increase after 3 weeks for internal jugular vein catheters and after 1 week for femoral vein catheters in bed-bound patients.[13]
  - When infection and bacteremia occur, prompt catheter removal is generally recommended, unless vascular access is especially difficult. Persistent bacteremia, fever, or an elevated white blood cell count should prompt a search for bacterial endocarditis in this particularly susceptible population.
  - Thrombus or fibrin sheaths can form around or inside the catheters, causing inadequate blood flows for dialysis. Although heparin is usually instilled into the hub of the catheter after each dialysis, this does not necessarily prevent clot formation. An attempt at clot lysis can be made by the local instillation of alteplase (2 mg). Alteplase should not be administered systemically for this purpose.
  - If the catheter malfunctions, then it may be changed over a guidewire or replaced, preferably at a different site.
  - In patients with chronic kidney disease, subclavian veins are not used for dialysis catheters, as there is a high risk of subclavian venous stenosis, which can prevent the future placement of an arteriovenous fistula for dialysis in that extremity.
  - Tunneled catheters maybe more beneficial in reducing infection rates, but nontunneled catheters are considered first line due to the ease of placement.

Tunneled catheters are typically used in patients with multiple malfunctioning temporary catheters, or in those with poor chance for early renal recovery, or in those being transferred out of the institution to a different facility.

○ Interventional radiology or nephrology consultation is required to perform endoluminal brushing to dislodge thrombi and fibrin sheaths in malfunctioning tunneled catheters.[14]

• **Electrolyte disturbances:**

○ Standard CRRT solutions do not contain phosphate, and uninterrupted CRRT can cause dramatic **hypophosphatemia**, especially during high-dose therapy.[11]

■ This problem is aggravated by an intracellular shift that occurs during dialysis secondary to alkalemia.

■ Hypophosphatemia can be corrected by intravenous or oral repletion. Alternatively, phosphorus can be added to the dialysate solution, although this technique is not employed widely at this time.

○ **Hypokalemia and hypomagnesemia** can also result from CRRT, and serum electrolytes need to be monitored at least twice a day to avoid such complications.

■ Hypomagnesemia is usually replaced intravenously or orally.

■ Hypokalemia can be treated by increasing the concentration of potassium in the dialysate and replacement fluid. The typical concentration of potassium in the solution is 2 mEq/L. However, potassium can be added by the pharmacist to make the final concentration 3 or 4 mEq/L, depending on serum potassium levels.

• **Anticoagulation problems:**

○ The use of anticoagulant increases the risk for hemorrhagic episodes.

○ Studies have shown higher incidence with heparin compared with citrate; therefore, citrate should be used preferentially in patients who are at higher risk for bleeding.

○ If a major bleed occurs, then use of heparin or other systemic anticoagulants should be immediately discontinued. Citrate anticoagulation can be continued, with close attention to bleeding parameters and ionized calcium levels.

○ Heparin can also be associated with HIT. If HIT is suspected, heparin should be discontinued and alternative agents such as argatroban, bivalirudin, or citrate should be used. The direct thrombin inhibitor, argatroban, can be initiated at 2 μg/kg/min and adjusted to maintain an activated partial thromboplastin time of 1.5 to 3 times the baseline value.

○ Citrate anticoagulation can result in metabolic alkalosis, and in the setting of hepatic dysfunction, can lead to life-threatening hypocalcemia. The titration protocol for addressing changes in serum and machine-ionized calcium levels must be closely followed to prevent adverse events.

○ Metabolic alkalosis can be treated by changing the replacement fluid to sodium chloride from a bicarbonate-based product, and hypocalcemia is treated by adjusting the calcium rates.

• **Hypothermia:**

○ Hypothermia is a frequent complication of CRRT, especially at higher flow rates of dialysate and replacement fluid, with an incidence as high as 60% to 70%.

○ Significant amounts of heat are lost from the slow-flowing extracorporeal circuit and can cause decreases in body temperature of 2 to 5°C.

○ Hypothermia can result in cardiac arrhythmias, hemodynamic compromise, increased risk for infections, and coagulation problems.

○ This can be **addressed by encasing the venous tubing** (blood returning to the patient) **with specialized warming devices** that can be attached to the machine.

SUSTAINED LOW-EFFICIENCY DIALYSIS

- SLED (slow ED) combines the benefits of CRRT and IHD.
- The **dialysate flow rates** are usually ~100 to 200 mL/min, similar to the blood flow rates, and the procedure lasts anywhere from 10 to 12 hours.
- SLED is performed by the dialysis nursing staff and utilizes a modified dialysis machine. It typically does not require replacement fluids or special filters or machines. However, it can also be performed by certain machines that are typically considered as CRRT machines. In these cases, bicarbonate-based solutions are used as dialysate.
- Anticoagulation is usually required, although in our experience, during SLED therapy with NxStage®, anticoagulation is not required in ~75% of the cases.
- The therapy is **associated with fewer hemodynamic alterations compared with IHD,** and because the procedure can be performed at night in the ICU, it leaves the day for various procedures such as imaging studies or surgeries. This is a clear advantage over CRRT, where stopping the therapy for various reasons prevents adequate delivery of dialysis.
- SLED has been shown to provide adequate urea clearance and has been successfully used in critically ill patients with AKI.[15] More centers are using this option in addition to CRRT and IHD in the treatment of critically ill patients with AKI.
- The clearances of various drugs during SLED have not been established. It is recommended to give drugs after the procedure, and levels, whenever available, should be monitored closely.

REFERENCES

1. Mehta RL. Indications for dialysis in the ICU: renal replacement vs. renal support. *Blood Purif.* 2001;19(2):227–232.
2. Palevsky PM. Renal replacement therapy I: indications and timing. *Crit Care Clin.* 2005; 21(2): 347–356.
3. O'Reilly P, Tolwani A. Renal replacement therapy III: IHD, CRRT, SLED. *Crit Care Clin.* 2005;21(2):367–378.
4. Davenport A, Will EJ, Davison AM, et al. Changes in intracranial pressure during haemo-filtration in oliguric patients with grade IV hepatic encephalopathy. *Nephron.* 1989;53 (2):142–146.
5. Overberger P, Pesacreta M, Palevsky PM. Management of renal replacement therapy in acute kidney injury: a survey of practitioner prescribing practices. *Clin J Am Soc Nephrol.* 2007;2(4):623–630.
6. Vinsonneau C, Camus C, Combes A, et al. Continuous venovenous haemodiafiltration versus intermittent haemodialysis for acute renal failure in patients with multiple-organ dysfunction syndrome: a multicentre randomised trial. *Lancet.* 2006;368(9533):379–385.

7. Kellum JA, Angus DC, Johnson JP, et al. Continuous versus intermittent renal replacement therapy: a meta-analysis. *Intensive Care Med.* 2002;28(1):29–37.

8. National Kidney Foundation I. NKF-K/DOQI clinical practice guidelines for hemodialysis adequacy: update 2000. *Am J Kidney Dis.* 2001;37(1 suppl 1):S7–S64.

9. Schiffl H, Lang SM, Fischer R. Daily hemodialysis and the outcome of acute renal failure. *N Engl J Med.* 2002;346(5):305–310.

10. Ronco C, Bellomo R, Homel P, et al. Effects of different doses in continuous veno-venous haemofiltration on outcomes of acute renal failure: a prospective randomised trial. *Lancet.* 2000;356(9223):26–30.

11. Palevsky PM, Zhang JH, O'Connor TZ, et al. Intensity of renal support in critically ill patients with acute kidney injury. *N Engl J Med.* 2008;359(1):7–20.

12. Bellomo R, Cass A, Cole L, et al. Intensity of continuous renal-replacement therapy in critically ill patients. *N Engl J Med.* 2009;361(17):1627–1638.

13. Oliver MJ, Callery SM, Thorpe KE, et al. Risk of bacteremia from temporary hemodialysis catheters by site of insertion and duration of use: a prospective study. *Kidney Int.* 2000;58 (6):2543–2545.

14. Vijayan A. Vascular access for continuous renal replacement therapy. *Semin Dial.* 2009;22 (2):133–136.

15. Marshall MR, Golper TA, Shaver MJ, et al. Sustained low-efficiency dialysis for critically ill patients requiring renal replacement therapy. *Kidney Int.* 2001;60(2):777–785.

Overview and Approach to the Patient with Glomerular Disease

16

Syed A. Khalid

GENERAL PRINCIPLES

- **Glomerular diseases** are a heterogeneous collection of inflammatory and/or noninflammatory insults to the filtering unit of the kidney.[1]
- The hallmark of glomerular disease is an alteration in glomerular permeability and selectivity, resulting in proteinuria and/or hematuria.
- Glomerular diseases **occurring in the absence of a known systemic process** are called *primary.*
- *Secondary* glomerular diseases are **caused by systemic disease processes.** Examples include diabetes mellitus, systemic lupus, certain cancers, or vasculitis.
- Secondary glomerular diseases often present in a similar fashion to primary glomerular diseases and their pathological and clinical picture may be indistinguishable (e.g., primary focal segmental glomerulosclerosis (FSGS) vs. FSGS caused by obesity).[2]
- Sometimes glomerular pathology may be the first manifestation of systemic disease (membranous nephropathy in cancers). Many systemic diseases may be diagnosed on renal biopsy (amyloidosis, drug reactions, sarcoidosis), and in some, the biopsy results indicate disease activity and guide treatment (lupus nephritis). Table 16-1 illustrates the primary pathology and secondary causes of glomerular diseases.

CLASSIFICATION OF GLOMERULAR DISEASES

- Glomerular diseases are diagnosed by their clinical presentation and histomorphological appearance.
- Classification of glomerular diseases is **based on histological injury patterns,** with evaluation by light microscopy, immunofluorescence, and electron microscopy (EM).
- One pattern can have multiple etiological causes such as membranoproliferative glomerulonephritis (MPGN), and one etiology can give different histological patterns (e.g., hepatitis B- and C-associated glomerular diseases, lupus nephritis); hence, all histologies must be evaluated with clinical correlations.

Light Microscopy

- Light microscopy is useful for determining pattern of disease, cellularity, and assessment of interstitium and vessels.
- Standard slide preparation includes staining with hematoxylin and eosin, periodic acid-Schiff, trichrome, and a silver stain.
- The glomerulus consists of four regions: Bowman's capsule and space, arterioles, the mesangium, and the glomerular capillary wall (Fig. 16-1A).

TABLE 16-1	PRIMARY GLOMERULAR DISEASES AND THEIR SECONDARY CAUSES

Name of Primary Disease	Secondary Causes
IgA nephropathy	• Liver disease • Henoch–Schönlein purpura • Celiac sprue • Inflammatory bowel disease • Dermatitis herpetiformis • Seronegative spondyloarthropathy • Mycosis fungoides
Membranous nephropathy	• Malignancy (lung, colon, breast, leukemia, non-Hodgkin lymphoma) • Drugs (NSAIDs, penicillamine, gold, captopril) • Infectious diseases (hepatitis B, hepatitis C, syphilis, malaria) • Diabetes mellitus • Autoimmune diseases (lupus nephritis, autoimmune thyroiditis)
Minimal change disease	• Malignancy (Hodgkin disease, leukemia, solid tumors) • Heavy metals (lead, mercury) • Drugs (NSAIDs, ampicillin/penicillin, trimethadione, lithium, gold, rifampicin, interferon-α) • Infections (mononucleosis, HIV)
Focal segmental glomerulosclerosis	• HIV • IV drug use (heroin) • With glomerulomegaly (morbid obesity, sickle-cell disease, cyanotic congenital heart disease, hypoxic pulmonary disease) • With reduced renal mass (unilateral renal agenesis, postnephrectomy, reflux nephropathy, postfocal cortical necrosis) • Drug toxicity (lithium, pamidronate, interferon-α) • Genetic (podocin, α–actinin-4, nephrin mutations)
MPGN	• Infections (hepatitis C, infective endocarditis, malaria, mycoplasma, visceral abscess, schistosoma) • Cryoglobulinemia • Lupus nephritis • Malignancy (leukemia and lymphoma) • Rheumatologic disorders (SLE, scleroderma, Sjögren's syndrome, sarcoidosis)

MPGN, membranoproliferative glomerulonephritis; NSAID, nonsteroidal anti-inflammatory drug; HIV, human immunodeficiency virus; IV, intravenous; SLE, systemic lupus erythematosus.

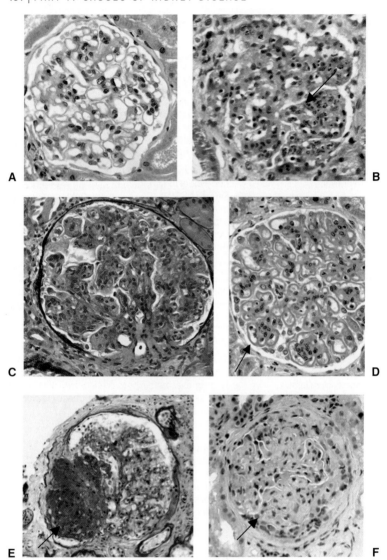

FIGURE 16-1. Pathology of glomerular disease—light microscopy. (**A**) Normal glomerulus in minimal change disease. (**B**) Diffuse hypercellularity, infiltration with neutrophils (*arrow*) in poststreptococcal glomerulonephritis. (**C**) Lobular accentuation due to expansion of mesangial matrix and mesangial hypercellularity in membranoproliferative glomerulonephritis. (**D**) Capillary loop thickening (*arrow*) in membranous nephropathy (class V lupus nephritis). (**E**) Segmental sclerosis (*arrow*) in focal segmental glomerulosclerosis. (**F**) Crescent formation (*arrow*) in Wegener's granulomatosis. (Courtesy of Dr. H. Liapis.)

- The latter consists of endothelium, basement membrane, epithelium, and podocytes.
- A **normal glomerulus** has **entire loops that are patent** and approximately **two to three mesangial cells per capillary tuft.**
- The basement membrane is about the same thickness as a proximal tubule basement membrane. Bowman's capsule has one layer of cells and Bowman's space is empty.
- The lesions in glomerular diseases can be *diffuse* (affecting the majority of glomeruli) or *focal* (only some of the glomeruli).
- They also can be *segmental* (only part of a glomerulus involved) or *global* (affecting all regions of any given glomerulus). The best example of a segmental disease would be FSGS (Fig. 16-1E).
- Lesions also can be *hypercellular* or *proliferative* due to mesangial proliferation (IgA nephropathy) or *infiltrative* due to inflammatory cells (leukocytes, monocytes, neutrophils) (Fig. 16-1B and 16-1C).
- The **mesangium** is composed of cells and matrix. It may expand because of mesangial cell proliferation (hypercellularity), as seen in IgA nephropathy or systemic lupus erythematosus (SLE).
- Matrix expansion can be seen in diabetic nephropathy or be due to matrix infiltration by abnormal proteins (amyloidosis, fibrillary glomerulonephritis).
- **Crescent formation** refers to cellular or fibrous crescents formed by invasion of cells (proliferating parietal epithelial cells, invading inflammatory cells, and fibrous products of those cells) into Bowman's space, resulting from severe glomerular injury with capillary leak of cells and proteins (Fig. 16-1F).
- **Basement membrane** proliferation can be assessed by the **silver stain.** Thickening of the glomerular basement membrane (GBM) is seen in membranous nephropathy or class V lupus nephritis (Fig. 16-1D).
- Tubulointerstitial inflammation usually accompanies acute glomerular injury. Interstitial fibrosis is usually a poor prognostic sign and is consistent with irreversible damage.

Immunofluorescence

- Immunofluorescence studies include staining for deposition of IgG, IgA, IgM, and components of classic and alternative complement pathways (C3, C4, and C1q).
- Staining patterns are *linear* (continuous staining along the glomerular capillary wall) or *granular* (discontinuous staining along the capillary wall or in the mesangium) (Fig. 16-2).
- Putative antigens are not known in most cases, but there are some exceptions (e.g., anti-GBM disease).
- Several glomerular diseases are diagnosed primarily by immunofluorescent staining. Examples are IgA nephropathy and C1q nephropathy.

Electron Microscopy

- EM can detect GBM thickness, duplication, infiltration, and podocyte foot process effacement.
- Precise localization of immune deposits that appear to be homogeneous and electron dense (subepithelial, subendothelial, mesangial, or within the GBM) is critical for the classification of most primary glomerular renal diseases.

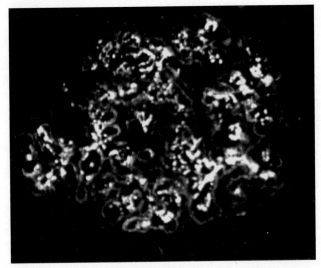

FIGURE 16-2. Pathology of glomerular disease—immunofluorescence microscopy. Postinfectious glomerulonephritis showing granular staining. (Courtesy of Dr. H. Liapis.)

- **Thin basement membrane disease** and Alport's syndrome (hereditary nephritis) can be diagnosed by demonstration of abnormally thin areas of basement membrane.
- Fibrillary glomerulopathies and amyloidosis can be diagnosed by EM, depending on the fibrils that are seen.

PRESENTATION OF GLOMERULAR DISEASES

Clinical Presentations

Patients with glomerular diseases generally present with one of the following clinical syndromes. Often there is significant overlap between the proteinuric and hematuric disorders (Fig. 16-3).

Asymptomatic Hematuria

- This syndrome is **defined as >2 to 3 red blood cells (RBCs) per high-power field** in spun urine (microscopic), or painless brown/red macroscopic hematuria without clots in patients who have normal renal function and no evidence of systemic diseases known to affect kidneys.
- The **differential diagnosis** is broad and urological problems (bladder, prostate, urethra, stones, and renal tumors) account for up to 80% of all cases of hematuria.
- The presence of RBC casts and/or dysmorphic RBCs indicates a glomerular cause for the hematuria.
- The **most common diseases** presenting as asymptomatic hematuria are thin basement membrane disease, IgA nephropathy, hereditary nephritis, and sickle-cell disease.

Clinical/laboratory features suggestive of glomerular disease:
- Proteinuria
- Microscopic/macrocopic hematuria in absence of urologic cause
- Dysmorphic RBCs and RBC casts
- Nephrotic syndrome: edema, proteinuria >3g/day, hypoalbuminemia, hypercholesterolemia
- Hypertension
- Acute oliguria

Laboratory evaluation in all patients:
- Urinalysis, microscopic evaluation of urine sediment
- Serum Cr, BUN, eGFR calculation
- Spot protein to spot creatinine ratio for proteinuria calculation
- Renal ultrasound

Etiology of glomerular disease is readily identifiable (biopsy may not be needed):
- Children with features typical for MCD who respond to steroids
- Longstanding DM with retinopathy with typical diabetic nephropathy features
- Precedings streptococcal infection with typical poststreptococcal GN presentation
- Mild asymptomatic urine abnormalities in setting of normal renal function

Additional laboratory evaluation required (biopsy usually indicated):
- ANA, anti-dsDNA: SLE
- Cryoglobulins, RF: cryoglobulinemia
- Anti-GBMAb: anti GBM disease
- ANCA:
  c-ANCA: Wegener's granulomatosis
  p-ANCA: PAN
- ASO, anti-DNASe-B: poststrep GN
- Hep B Ag, HCV ab: MPGN
- HIV ab: HIVAN
- SPEP/UPEP: amyloid, LCDD

Appropriate treatment

Renal biopsy
Appropriate treatment

FIGURE 16-3. Spectrum of glomerular diseases with nephrotic and nephritic features. FSGS, focal segmental glomerulosclerosis; GBM, glomerular basement membrane; GN, glomerulonephritis; strep, streptococcal.

- Kidney biopsy is usually not done to evaluate asymptomatic hematuria, unless there is concern for an unexplained systemic process that might warrant therapy.[3,4]

Asymptomatic Proteinuria
- **Proteinuria in the range of 150 mg to 3 g/d** (in 24-hour urine collection) or as measured as **spot protein-to-creatinine ratio ranging from 0.2 to 3 g protein per gram creatinine** is usually asymptomatic. It is sometimes referred to as *nonnephrotic proteinuria.*

- It may occur with glomerular or nonglomerular diseases such as tubulointerstitial diseases or orthostatic proteinuria (usually <1 g/d).
- Any type of glomerular disease can cause proteinuria in this range with FSGS, membranous nephropathy, and diabetic nephropathy being common examples.[3,4]

Nephrotic Syndrome
- This syndrome is a clinical pentad of **proteinuria >3 g/d, hypoalbuminemia <3.5 g/dL, edema, hypercholesterolemia, and lipiduria** (most specific finding is presence of oval fat bodies in urinalysis). **Complications** of nephrotic syndrome include:
  - **Hypercoagulability** due to loss of hemostasis control proteins such as antithrombin III and increased hepatic synthesis of protein C, fibrinogen, and von Willebrand factor. Venous thrombosis is more common than arterial thrombosis.
  - **Infection** due to loss of immunoglobulins and immunosuppressive drugs
  - **Hyperlipidemia** and **atherosclerosis**
- The **most common glomerular diseases** presenting as nephrotic syndrome are primary diseases such as minimal change disease, membranous nephropathy, and FSGS, as well as secondary forms such as diabetic nephropathy, amyloidosis, and light-chain deposition disease.[4,5]

Nephritic Syndrome
- This syndrome **presents gross or microscopic hematuria with dysmorphic RBCs and/or RBC casts, hypertension, and reduction in glomerular filtration rate with or without oliguria.** Proteinuria (usually nonnephrotic) and edema may also be present.
- Distinction between nephrotic and nephritic syndromes is usually based on clinical and laboratory evaluation.
- The **most common diseases** presenting as nephritic syndrome are poststreptococcal glomerulonephritis, other postinfectious diseases (endocarditis, abscess), IgA nephropathy, vasculitis, and lupus nephritis.
- Generally, diseases presenting with nephritic syndrome tend be acute and rapidly progressive, and time is of essence in diagnosis and early treatment, so as to avoid chronic renal damage.[3,6]

Rapidly Progressive Glomerulonephritis
- This presentation is **the most severe form of the nephritic syndromes.**
- In this case, glomerular injury is so acute that renal failure develops over the course of a few days to weeks.
- Rapidly progressive glomerulonephritis (RPGN) usually presents as proteinuria <3 g/d and hematuria with dysmorphic RBCs and/or red cell casts, with or without signs of systemic vasculitis.
- A specific finding on kidney biopsy is **crescent formation.** RPGN can progress to end-stage renal disease in most untreated patients within a period of weeks to months.
- RPGN is usually due to one of the following disorders, which reflect different mechanisms of glomerular injury. It is classified into four types.
  - **Type 1:** Anti-GBM disease
    - Type 1 refers to anti-GBM antibody disease.
    - Anti-GBM antibody disease in the setting of pulmonary involvement is known as Goodpasture's syndrome.

- The immunofluorescence pattern shows positivity with antibody to IgG and has a smooth, diffuse, linear pattern (ribbon-like appearance).
- Serologic testing for anti-GBM in patient serum is often positive.
  ○ **Type 2:** Immune complex glomerulonephritis
  - Type 2 refers to immune complex RPGN.
  - Examples include mesangial IgA deposits in IgA nephropathy, antistreptococcal antibodies and subepithelial humps in postinfectious glomerulonephritis, antinuclear antibodies and subendothelial deposits in lupus nephritis, and circulating cryoglobulins and intraluminal "thrombi" in mixed cryoglobulinemia.
  ○ **Type 3:** Pauci-immune
  - Type 3 refers to pauci-immune RPGN, in which there is a necrotizing glomerulonephritis but few or no immune deposits by immunofluorescence or EM.
  - The majority of patients with renal-limited vasculitis are antineutrophil cytoplasmic antibody (ANCA) positive, with 75% to 80% having myeloperoxidase-ANCA, and many have or will develop the systemic symptoms of a vasculitis.
  - Patients with ANCA-negative, pauci-immune RPGN are also considered part of this spectrum.
  ○ **Type 4:** Double–antibody-positive disease
  - Type 4 has features of both types 1 and 3. This is also called "double–antibody"-positive disease.

Chronic Glomerulonephritis

- This terminology is sometimes **used to describe patients thought to have some form of previous glomerular disease presenting with hypertension, chronic kidney disease (CKD), proteinuria >3 g/d, and small, atrophic, smooth kidneys on ultrasound.**
- Any glomerulonephritis can slowly progress to kidney failure; hence, chronic glomerulonephritis may be the presumptive diagnosis when patients present with shrunken kidneys and biopsy is not appropriate.

History and Physical Examination

- Patients with **nephrotic syndrome** usually complain of pitting edema (especially periorbital) and foamy urine.
- Physical examination may reveal xanthelasma, Muehrke bands (white bands in fingernails from chronic hypoalbuminemia), and elevated blood pressure, along with signs of volume overload.
- Patients with **nephritic syndrome** may complain of decreased urine output and uremic symptoms that are often vague (nausea, vomiting, fatigue, headaches, and anorexia).
- Other findings in nephritic syndrome include elevated blood pressure, gross hematuria ("tea-colored urine"), and generalized edema.
- If the patient has a **RPGN**, he may have systemic symptoms of vasculitis—rash, fevers, and pulmonary symptoms (pulmonary-renal syndrome).
- **Timing of recent infections** can be very helpful. In a patient with hematuria, it is important to know about timing of recent infections. **IgA nephropathy** patients will have hematuria **within 1 to 3 days after onset of upper respiratory tract infection** (synpharyngitic hematuria). In contrast, **hematuria from**

postinfectious glomerulonephritis will develop **1 to 2 weeks after** the streptococcal upper respiratory tract infection or up to 6 weeks after a skin infection.

- **Family history** of renal failure and deafness may suggest Alport's syndrome. Family history of thin basement membrane disease, IgA nephropathy, FSGS, and hemolytic-uremic syndrome is important because those diseases may be inherited.
- **Medications** should be evaluated. Prescriptions, over-the-counter medications, and herbal preparations should be reviewed. Particular attention should be paid to the use of nonsteroidal anti-inflammatory drugs and antibiotics.
- **Malignancies** (Hodgkin disease; graft-versus-host disease after bone marrow transplant; solid tumors of lung, breast, and colon) are also associated with glomerular disease, and renal disease may be the initial presentation.[3]

Laboratory Evaluation

- The routine initial evaluation of patients with suspected glomerular disease should include the following tests:
  - *Urinalysis:* The presence of protein and/or RBCs on microscopic exam of the urine sediment is helpful. RBC casts or dysmorphic RBCs are specific for glomerular disease and always warrant further testing. The presence of other formed elements in urine (e.g., granular casts, WBCs, WBC casts) is less specific. Oval fat bodies, fatty casts, and hyaline casts may be seen in the urine sediment of patients with nephrotic syndrome.
  - *Serum creatinine* (Cr) and *blood urea nitrogen* should be measured. Prior values may be important to determine the duration of disease.
  - *Urine protein quantification:* Spot urine protein-to-creatinine ratio provides a rough estimation of 24-hour urine protein excretion in g/d. A 24-hour urine collection for protein and Cr can provide more precise quantification of both protein excretion and estimation of Cr clearance (see Chap. 4).
  - *Urine culture:* Patients with hematuria should have a urine culture to rule out cystitis or prostatitis.
  - *Renal ultrasound:*
    - Patients with hematuria should undergo kidney ultrasound to evaluate for anatomical abnormalities such as polycystic kidney disease, cysts, renal masses, stones, and kidney size.
    - The presence of atrophic smooth kidneys (<9 cm) suggests CKD, which is usually irreversible. This finding should limit use of aggressive diagnostic workup (including renal biopsy, which carries greater risk with small, scarred kidneys) and aggressive immunosuppressive therapies.
    - Large kidneys (>13 cm) can be associated with diabetes nephropathy, amyloid or lymphoma infiltration, human immunodeficiency virus (HIV) associated nephropathy, or other glomerulonephritis or interstitial nephritis.[3]

Specialized Laboratory Evaluation

- Several serologic studies should be considered in all nephritic presentations, nephrotic syndrome, and in selected patients with proteinuria and/or hematuria.
- The decision as to which of these tests to order in a particular patient depend on the age, gender, and features of the presentation.

- A "shot-gun" approach, in which all the laboratory studies are ordered with no regard to clinical findings, is not recommended, as it can lead to further inappropriate testing and significantly increase the healthcare costs.
  - Antinuclear antibody and anti–double-stranded-DNA antibody tests evaluate the presence of SLE.
  - Cryoglobulins and rheumatoid factor should be measured to support a diagnosis of cryoglobulinemia.
  - Anti-GBM antibodies support a diagnosis of Goodpasture's disease.
  - ANCAs: Cytoplasmic ANCA (C-ANCA)/Proteinase 3 (PR3) are typically positive in Wegener's granulomatosis, and perinuclear-ANCA/myeloperoxidase are often present in microscopic polyangiitis and Churg–Strauss syndrome.
  - Antistreptolysin-O antibody and Anti-DNAse B in poststreptococcal glomerulonephritis. Other streptococcal antibodies are also available.
  - Hepatitis B and C serologies: Infections with these viruses have been associated with MPGN, membranous nephropathy, vasculitis, and cryoglobulinemia.
  - HIV antibodies for HIV-associated nephropathy should also be measured.
  - Serum protein electrophoresis/urine protein electrophoresis and immunofixation can detect light-chain or heavy-chain paraproteins that are commonly seen in amyloidosis, multiple myeloma, or light-chain deposition disease.
  - Complement levels (C3, C4, and CH50) are decreased in a limited spectrum of diseases and can be useful in limiting the differential diagnosis (Table 16-2).[3,4]

Kidney Biopsy

- A kidney biopsy is required to establish diagnosis and treatment of most glomerular diseases. Figure 16-4 gives a broad algorithm to the management of patient with glomerular disease.
- Biopsy is usually not required in the following special patient groups:
  - Children who present with features typical of minimal change disease and who respond appropriately to steroid trial.

TABLE 16-2	COMPLEMENT LEVELS IN VARIOUS GLOMERULAR DISEASES		
	C3	C4	CH50
Lupus nephritis	Low	Low	Low
Mixed essential cryoglobulinemia	Low	Low	Low
MPGN type 1	Low	Low	Low
Poststreptococcal GN	Low	Normal	Low
Infectious GN (endocarditis, shunt nephritis, Hepatitis B-related GN)	Low	Normal	Low
MPGN type II	Low	Normal	Low

GN, glomerulonephritis; MPGN, membranoproliferative glomerulonephritis.

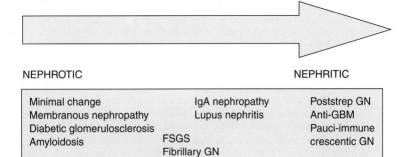

NEPHROTIC		**NEPHRITIC**
Minimal change	IgA nephropathy	Poststrep GN
Membranous nephropathy	Lupus nephritis	Anti-GBM
Diabetic glomerulosclerosis		Pauci-immune
Amyloidosis	FSGS	crescentic GN
	Fibrillary GN	

FIGURE 16-4. Algorithm for initial evaluation of the patient with suspected glomerular renal disease. Ab, antibody; Ag, antigen; ANA, antinuclear antibody; ANCA, antineutrophil cytoplasmic antibody; ASO, antistreptolysin-O; BUN, blood urea nitrogen; Cr, creatinine; DM, diabetes mellitus; ds, double stranded; eGFR, estimated glomerular filtration rate; GBM, glomerular basement membrane; GN, glomerulonephritis; HCV, hepatitis C virus; Hep, hepatitis; HIV, human immuno-deficiency virus; HIVAN, HIV-associated nephropathy; LCDD, light-chain deposition disease; MCD, minimal change disease; MPGN, membranoproliferative glomerulonephritis; PAN, polyarteritis nodosa; p-ANCA, perinuclear-ANCA; RBC, red blood cell; RF, rheumatoid factor; RPGN, rapidly progressive glomerulone-phritis; SLE, systemic lupus erythematosus; SPEP, serum protein electrophoresis; strep, streptococcal; UPEP, urine protein electrophoresis.

○ Longstanding diabetes with evidence of microvascular complications of diabetes (e.g., retinopathy, peripheral neuropathy) and other features typical of diabetic nephropathy.

○ History of preceding streptococcal infection, with features typical of post-streptococcal glomerulonephritis with confirmatory serological findings such as positive antistreptolysin antibody, antihyalurinidase antibody, or anti-DNAase.

○ Mild, asymptomatic urine abnormalities (microscopic hematuria, nonnephrotic proteinuria) with preserved renal function. These patients have excellent prognosis, and biopsy results would be unlikely to alter management.

TREATMENT

• Treatment consists of **disease-specific treatment** and **symptomatic and supportive** treatment of proteinuria, hypertension, hyperlipidemia, and control of edema.

• Patients with **proteinuria** should be treated with angiotensin-converting enzyme inhibitors and/or angiotensin-2 receptor blockers (ARBs) to reduce proteinuria to <1 g/d. Use caution with these agents in patients with accelerating renal failure or a tendency toward hyperkalemia. Serum chemistries, including potassium and Cr, should be monitored within 1 to 2 weeks of initiation of therapy. Creatinine increases of up to 30% from baseline are acceptable after initiation of these agents.

- **Control of blood pressure** is essential in order to preserve kidney function. Blood pressure should be controlled, with a goal of <135/80 mm Hg. In patients with proteinuria, ACE inhibitors or ARBs should be the first-line therapy.
- Control of edema or volume overload requires the use of **dietary salt and water restriction** in conjunction with diuretics. **Loop diuretics are the most effective agents.**
- Treatment of **hyperlipidemia** usually consists of hydroxymethylglutaryl coenzyme-A reductase inhibitors (statins). Most patients with nephrotic syndrome should be on statin therapy to prevent coronary and other atherosclerotic long-term complications.
- Disease-specific therapy is most often guided by results of renal biopsy and by supplemental laboratory evaluation.
- A final decision regarding the initiation and intensity of immunosuppressive therapy and use of other potentially toxic agents must include consideration of the patient's age and comorbid conditions, the likelihood of reversibility of the kidney disease, and compliance with the medical regimen. These therapies will be discussed in the next several chapters on primary and secondary glomerular diseases.

PREVENTION OF COMPLICATIONS OF IMMUNOSUPPRESSIVE REGIMENS

Infection

- It is clear that the risk of infections is increased with immunosuppressive therapies.
- Much of the data for prevention of infection during immunosuppression are derived from the solid organ transplant literature. The following options should be considered when treating glomerular diseases.
- The intensity of immunosuppression and other patient risk factors should also be factored into the decision, when deciding on **prophylaxis.**
  - Trimethoprim/sulfamethoxazole (80 mg/400 mg) one tablet daily for prophylaxis against *Pneumocystis jiroveci*
  - Low-dose acyclovir, 200 mg daily for prevention of herpes zoster
  - Vaccination for *Pneumococci* and influenza is advised to prevent fatal infections.[7]
  - Monitoring for the development of oropharyngeal thrush, which is usually treatable with nystatin oral suspension.

Other Medical Complications

- Histamine-2 blockers to prevent steroid-induced **gastritis.**
- Calcium supplementation and vitamin D therapy for the prevention of **osteoporosis** in patients requiring prolonged courses of corticosteroids. Bisphosphonates may be required in patients with osteopenia, but has to be used with caution in the setting of CKD.
- Gonadotropin-releasing hormone agonists (leuprolide) to suppress **gonadal function** (to protect against gonadal failure before treatment with cytotoxic agents) where indicated.

- Although patients with hypoalbuminemia due to nephrotic syndrome are at much higher risk to develop **thromboembolic events,** prophylactic anticoagulation is controversial. If there is documented thrombosis, the patient should receive long-term anticoagulation during the course of the disease.[8]
  - **Adverse effects** of disease-specific therapy should be considered in all patients receiving aggressive immunosuppressive regimens for the treatment of glomerular diseases.
    - Some adverse effects of **high-dose corticosteroids** include:
    - Steroid-induced osteoporosis
    - Glucose intolerance
    - Worsening diabetic control
    - Opportunistic infections
    - Change in body fat distribution, striae, and cushingoid facies
  - **Cyclosporin** carries the following adverse effects:
    - Nephrotoxicity requires monitoring of serum Cr. Trough levels of cyclosporine A between 70 and 120 ng/mL may reduce the chances of nephrotoxicity.
    - Glucose intolerance, hypertension, and dyslipidemia
    - Multiple drug interactions
  - Use of **cyclophosphamide** may cause the following effects:
    - Leukopenia is common with some therapies, and the WBC count should be monitored every 1 to 2 weeks.
    - During therapy with cyclophosphamide, the dose should be held if the absolute neutrophil count falls to <2000 per μL and restarted at a lower dose when leukocyte counts recover.
    - Hemorrhagic cystitis incidence can be reduced by aggressive hydration with a daily urine output of >2000 mL/d and with 2-mercaptoethane sulfonate sodium given concomitantly with cyclophosphamide. This agent binds toxic metabolites in the bladder and may be used to reduce cystitis risk.
    - Irreversible gonadal failure incidence may be reduced with pretreatment with leuprolide to suppress gonadal function.
    - Hair thinning
    - Increased risk of bladder cancer
    - Nausea and vomiting
  - **Mycophenolate mofetil** use places the patient at risk for the following:
    - Increased risk of lymphoma or other malignancies
    - Neutropenia
    - Gastrointestinal distress, diarrhea
  - **Azathioprine** use carries the following risks:
    - Leukopenia
    - Malignancies, especially skin cancer and lymphoma
  - **Rituximab** is associated with the following adverse effects:
    - Severe infusion reactions within the first 24 hours after start of the infusion, including angioedema and bronchospasm
    - Lymphopenia
    - Neutropenia
    - Prolonged pancytopenia

REFERENCES

1. Clarkson M, Brenner B. *Pocket Companion to Brenner & Rector's The Kidney.* 7th ed. London: WB Saunders; 2005.
2. Couser WG. Glomerulonephritis. *Lancet.* 1999;353:1509.
3. Johnson RJ, Feehally JF. *Comprehensive Clinical Nephrology.* 2nd ed. London: Harcourt; 2003.
4. Greenberg A, *Primer on Kidney Diseases.* 4th ed. London: WB Saunders; 2005.
5. Orth SR, Ritz E. The nephrotic syndrome. *N Engl J Med.* 1998;338:1202–1211.
6. Hricik DE, Chung-Park M, Sedor JR. Glomerulonephritis. *N Engl J Med.* 1998;339: 888–899.
7. Dinits-Pensy M, Forrest GN, Cross AS, et al. The use of vaccines in adult patients with renal disease. *Am J Kidney Dis.* 46;2005:997–1011.
8. Sarasin FP, Schifferli JA. Prophylactic oral anticoagulation in nephrotic patients with idiopathic membranous nephropathy. *Kidney Int.* 1994;45:578–585.

Primary Glomerulopathies

17

Ying Chen

GENERAL PRINCIPLES

- **Primary glomerular diseases** are a group of disorders in which the main manifestations of disease are directly related to kidney involvement rather than as part of a systemic disease process. Systemic diseases associated with glomerular disease are discussed in a separate chapter.
- Primary glomerular diseases can present with **nephrotic syndrome, asymptomatic proteinuria,** isolated **hematuria,** or **a nephritic picture.** In many cases, they are described as being idiopathic without known association or cause. For each of the primary glomerulopathies, secondary causes are also discussed. For instance, medications, infections, and malignancies are all associated with glomerular pathology that is otherwise indistinguishable from the idiopathic forms.
- Proper diagnosis and management of the primary glomerulopathies requires an understanding of patient characteristics, risk of progressive kidney disease, and safe use of immunosuppressive agents.
- These cases should be managed in conjunction with a physician experienced in the evaluation and management of glomerular kidney disorders.

FOCAL SEGMENTAL GLOMERULOSCLEROSIS

- Focal segmental glomerulosclerosis (FSGS) has become **the most important form of primary glomerular disease,** both because of increasing incidence and because of its contribution to the growth of end-stage renal disease (ESRD).
- In the United States, FSGS is the **most common cause of idiopathic nephrotic syndrome** in adult African Americans. Idiopathic FSGS is also the most common primary glomerular disease detected on renal biopsy that leads to ESRD in all races.
- FSGS is a group of disorders that shares several histologic features. Renal biopsy shows some glomeruli (focal) with sclerosis in part of the glomerular tuft (segmental). Patients with these abnormalities often present with nephrotic syndrome, but may also have asymptomatic proteinuria.
- Several means of **categorizing FSGS** are in use.
  - **FSGS can be described as a primary or secondary disorder** associated with a range of causes and potential differences in treatment. For instance, primary FSGS is usually treated with corticosteroids or immunosuppressive regimens, whereas secondary disease typically does not respond to this regimen.

TABLE 17-1	HISTOLOGIC VARIANTS OF FOCAL SEGMENTAL GLOMERULOSCLEROSIS	
Name	Histology	Comments
FSGS (not otherwise specified)	At least one glomerulus with segmental increase in matrix obliterating capillary loop. Excludes other variants	Most common form
Perihilar variant	Perihilar hyalinosis and sclerosis in >50% of affected glomeruli	Seen in primary and secondary FSGS
Cellular variant	Endocapillary proliferation involving at least 25% of the tuft and occluding the lumen	Fairly responsive to immunosuppressive therapy
Collapsing variant	At least one glomerulus with segmental or global collapse and overlying podocyte hyperplasia	More aggressive with rapid progression to ESRD. Associated with secondary FSGS
Tip variant	At least one segmental lesion involving the outer 25% of the glomerulus next to the origin of the proximal tubule	May correlate with better prognosis and increased responsiveness to steroids

FSGS, focal segmental glomerulosclerosis; ESRD, end-stage renal disease.

○ **Histologic variants** have been described that take into account subglomerular localization of the sclerotic lesion, presence of proliferation, and presence of glomerular capillary collapse. The value of this system is thought to arise from better prediction of causation and outcomes.[1]

- ■ **The collapsing FSGS variant** is associated with human immunodeficiency virus (HIV) and some drug-associated diseases. Of all the histologic variants, collapsing FSGS is **notable for a poor renal prognosis.**[2]
- ■ Patients with the tip lesion pattern of FSGS have the most favorable outcome.
- ■ Table 17-1 summarizes the histologic variants and some of their associations.
- ■ In addition, a variant of FSGS has been termed **C1q nephropathy.**

PRIMARY IDIOPATHIC FSGS

Clinical Features

- FSGS is responsible for ~25% of kidney disease in a series of adults with ≥2 g of protein per 24 hours, and up to 35% if patients present with nephrotic syndrome.

- The disease is markedly **more common in African Americans** and the mean age of onset in adults is 40 years.
- Proteinuria is typically nonselective.
- Secondary forms of FSGS typically have lower levels of proteinuria than classic idiopathic FSGS.
- Other **common features on presentation** are **hypertension (30% to 50%), microscopic hematuria (25% to 75%), and renal insufficiency (20% to 30%).**
- Serologic testing and complement levels should be normal.

Outcomes of Primary FSGS

- Spontaneous remission of proteinuria is unusual (5% to 25%).[3]
- **Poor prognostic indicators** are nephrotic range proteinuria or massive proteinuria, elevated serum creatinine, greater degree of tubulointerstitial fibrosis, and presence of collapsing lesions at the time of biopsy, black race, and failure to achieve partial or complete remission.
- FSGS has a **significant risk of progression to ESRD,** with 5- and 10-year renal survival rates of 76% and 57% in those initially presenting with nephrotic syndrome.[4]
- Nonnephrotic proteinuria is associated with >90% 10-year kidney survival.

Treatment of Primary FSGS

- There is still considerable debate over the appropriate treatment for patients with FSGS.[5]
- **All nephrotic FSGS patients and those at risk of progressive disease should be treated with corticosteroids.**
  - ○ **Standard therapy** is initiated with **high-dose daily corticosteroids** (prednisone, 1 mg/kg of ideal body weight per day to maximum dose of 80 mg/d or 2 mg/kg alternate-day treatment).
  - ○ Treatment with high-dose daily or alternate-day steroids should be continued for 2 to 4 months with a prolonged course (6 to 9 months).[6]
  - ○ The median duration of steroid treatment to achieve complete remission is **3 to 4 months,** with most patients responding by 6 months. However, potential morbidities associated with steroid-related side effects need to be considered if this approach is planned.
  - ○ If remission occurs, the steroids may be tapered slowly. Longer courses may be used in patients who achieve only partial remission or who relapse with steroid tapering.
- **Cyclosporine** (3.5 mg/kg ideal body weight per day in two divided doses) and low dose (10 to 15 mg/d) prednisone for 6 months **for steroid-resistant FSGS** have been studied by the North American Collaborative Study of Cyclosporine in Nephrotic Syndrome.
  - ○ The remission rate in this trial was >70% (complete and/or partial) in steroid-resistant patients.
  - ○ In addition to reduction in proteinuria, slower progression of kidney disease was found.
  - ○ Given the lesser toxicity profile, many clinicians believe that cyclosporine or tacrolimus are better second-line agents than are cytotoxic agents such as cyclophosphamide and chlorambucil.
  - ○ However, relapse is common after cyclosporine is discontinued and patients need to be followed closely for recurrence of nephrotic syndrome.[7]

- **Cyclophosphamide and chlorambucil** can be added to the corticosteroid regimen in patients with recurrent disease. These drugs have not been tested in randomized controlled studies. About 15 to 20% of steroid-resistant patients respond to these drugs.
- **Mycophenolate mofetil (MMF)** is being investigated in a large multicenter National Institutes of Health trial in the United States comparing cyclosporine and a regimen of oral MMF plus dexamethasone for steroid-resistant patients with FSGS.
- Recurrence of FSGS after renal transplantation is common (up to 30%) and is associated with decreased graft survival. **Plasmapheresis** has been used with limited success in the management of posttransplant FSGS recurrence.[8]

SECONDARY FSGS

Etiology

FSGS represents a common phenotypic expression of diverse clinicopathologic syndromes with distinct etiologies.

- **Genetic causes of FSGS:**
  - Several genetic mutations are associated with FSGS. Most have been related to defects in structural proteins of podocytes and slit diaphragms.
  - Mutations in the *NHPS1* gene, which codes for nephrin, are responsible for the autosomal recessive congenital nephrotic syndrome of the Finnish type. Compound heterozygous mutations in small numbers of tested adults have been linked to steroid-resistant FSGS.[9,10]
  - Mutations in the *NPHS2* gene, which codes for podocin, are responsible for autosomal recessive steroid-resistant FSGS in children and rarely in adults.
  - Autosomal dominant FSGS in children or adults is associated with mutations in *ACTN4*, which encodes the podocyte cytoplasmic protein α-actinin-4 as well as a mutation in the transient receptor potential cation 6 channel (*TRPC6* channel).[11,12]
- **Viral infection:**
  - **HIV-associated nephropathy** may occur at any time during the course of HIV infection, although it is usually diagnosed when CD4 count falls below 200.[13]
    - The glomerular disease appears to result from **direct infection of podocytes,** leading to podocyte proliferation and dedifferentiation.
    - Up to 95% of HIV-associated nephropathy cases occur in **young African-American men** with HIV infection contracted by any route (mean age, 33 years; male-to-female ratio, 10:1).
    - The clinical presentation includes nephrotic or nonnephrotic proteinuria, progressive azotemia, and the relative rarity of hypertension.
    - Laboratory evaluation reveals HIV seropositivity, normal C3, normal C4, and CD4 count usually <200.
    - **Renal ultrasound** typically **shows enlarged kidneys** with increased echogenicity.
    - The pathology of HIV-associated nephropathy includes collapsing FSGS, mesangial proliferation, hypertrophied podocytes with protein resorption

droplets, microcystic dilated tubules, and endothelial cell tubuloreticular inclusions.
  ○ **Parvovirus B19** infection has also been associated with collapsing FSGS.
- **Drugs:**
  ○ Drugs associated with FSGS include pamidronate, heroin, lithium, and **interferon-α.**
  ○ **Pamidronate** has been associated with the collapsing form.
  ○ Secondary FSGS was attributed to heroin use in older studies. These cases presented with nephrotic syndrome and with rapid progression to ESRD. More recent studies have shown that the incidence of heroin-associated disease has declined markedly.
- **Sickle-cell nephropathy:**
  ○ Kidney disease can occur in persons with sickle-cell disease.
  ○ The prevalence of proteinuria was 26% in one series.
  ○ Chronic kidney disease has been seen in 7% to 30% of patients with long-term follow-up.
  ○ Hyperfiltration and increased glomerular pressure are thought to be the mechanism for injury.
  ○ The most common lesion on kidney biopsy is FSGS, although other histology can sometimes be found (e.g., membranoproliferative glomerulonephritis [MPGN]).
- **Other:**
  ○ **Reduced renal mass** (unilateral renal agenesis, surgical renal ablation, chronic allograft nephropathy, and chronic vesicoureteral reflux).
  ○ Secondary FSGS may also be seen in the setting of **chronic hypoperfusion and ischemia to the kidney.** Some examples are hypertension, morbid obesity, congenital cyanotic heart disease, obstructive sleep apnea (OSA) and atheroemboli.

Treatment of Secondary FSGS

- **Therapy for the underlying disorder** is first-line management. Lesions of FSGS may regress with management of the underlying condition (e.g., treatment of obesity with bariatric surgery or continuous positive airway pressure for OSA).
- Nonspecific therapy to reduce edema and proteinuria with diuretics, dietary sodium restriction, and angiotensin-converting enzyme (**ACE**) **inhibitor/angiotensin receptor blocker (ARB) therapy** should be aggressively pursued.
- Steroid treatment as for idiopathic FSGS can be considered in refractory cases, but limited data do not support the use of aggressive immunosuppressive or cytotoxic agents.

OTHER FSGS VARIANTS: C1q NEPHROPATHY

- Distinctive features of C1q nephropathy are a predominance of **C1q staining in the glomerulus and mesangial electron-dense deposits.**[14]
- It is predominant in males and African Americans are commonly affected.
- Proteinuria is usually in the nephrotic range and hematuria is present in ~20% of the patients.

- The best treatment for this lesion is unclear but should include antiproteinuric strategies, such as ACE inhibitors.

MINIMAL CHANGE DISEASE

- Minimal change disease (MCD) is the **most common cause of nephrotic syndrome in children** (~65%) and in up to 10% to 15% of cases in adults. The peak incidence of MCD is in children aged 2 to 7 years, but the disease may occur at any age.

Clinical Presentation

- The typical presentation of MCD is **nephrotic syndrome.** Clinical presentation is usually characterized by rapid onset of edema, often with periorbital edema, marked weight gain, pleural effusions, and ascites.
- **Children** presenting with typical features of nephrotic syndrome usually **undergo empiric steroid therapy** without a definitive diagnosis by renal biopsy. Steroid responsiveness in this group is equated with a diagnosis of MCD.
- **Acute kidney injury can occur in up to 18% of adults.** Major risk factors for this presentation are male, older and hypertensive with lower serum albumin and more proteinuria.[15]
- **Other complications** of MCD include sepsis, peritonitis in ascitic fluid, and thromboembolism.
- The pathogenesis remains unknown but may be related to a disorder of T-lymphocytes. There is a postulated circulating factor acting on podocytes. The majority of cases are idiopathic.

Secondary Causes of MCD

- **Drugs** can cause MCD, with the most common culprit being nonsteroidal anti-inflammatory drugs (**NSAIDs**) or interferon-α.
- Hematologic malignancies, most notably Hodgkin disease, can present with MCD and this should be kept in mind in the older age group. However, it is not recommended to screen these patients extensively for malignancy.
- Heavy metals (mercury, lead) are rare causes of MCD.
- Systemic allergic reactions to environmental allergens or vaccines may rarely trigger MCD.

Diagnostic Testing

Laboratory Evaluation

- **Hypoalbuminemia** and **elevated cholesterol** are frequently noted.
- In children, the **urine sediment** may show **Maltese-cross oval fat bodies** under polarized light.
- In adults, **microscopic hematuria** is present in >30% of the cases.
- Complement levels and other serologic markers are normal.
- A urine protein electrophoresis will show that the negatively charged protein albumin predominates. This has been termed **selective proteinuria.**
- **Renal biopsy** is required for diagnosis in children unresponsive to steroids and in all adults presenting with nephrotic syndrome.

Pathology
- Light microscopy is typically normal, although mild mesangial hypercellularity may be found. Tubular and interstitial structures are normal.
- Immunofluorescence may reveal IgM and C3 trapped in damaged capillary loops and mesangium. Heavy mesangial deposits of IgM are associated with worse prognosis and poor response to treatment (so-called IgM nephropathy).
- Electron microscopy reveals **diffuse podocyte foot process fusion,** but this is a nonspecific finding.

Treatment
- The initial treatment of **adults** with MCD is **corticosteroids.**
  - Typical regimens are daily dosing with **prednisone** 1 mg/kg (to maximum of 80 mg/d) or alternate-day dosing with 2 mg/kg every other day. These approaches appear to have similar initial response rates.
  - Treat for not less than 12 to 16 weeks at first presentation. Almost all children respond rapidly by 8 weeks; however, adults may take longer, with 75% to 80% achieving remission by 12 to 16 weeks of therapy.
  - Adults who initially respond to corticosteroids will experience at least one relapse around 70% of the time. Relapses are usually treated with a second course of corticosteroids.
- In **children,** nephrotic syndrome is often treated with **empiric treatment.**
  - As in adults, the mainstay of therapy is **corticosteroids** (prednisone, 1 mg/kg of ideal body weight per day, not to exceed 80 mg/d).
  - This regimen is usually continued for 4 weeks after resolution of proteinuria and then tapered by 10 mg on an alternate-day regimen every 2 weeks (total course of 3–4 months in steroid responders).
  - The typical course is remitting and relapsing, with ~75% of patients who initially achieve remission on steroids relapsing within 5 years.
  - Shorter courses of prednisone (6 to 10 weeks) can generally be used to treat relapses.
- **Frequent relapsing** (four or more relapses within 1 year), **steroid-dependent** (relapse upon tapering steroid therapy or within 2 weeks of discontinuing steroids and need for long-term maintenance steroids), or **steroid-resistant** (failure to reach remission within 4 months of steroid treatment) patients should be treated with second-line agents. Options for management include:
  - Oral **cyclophosphamide** (2 mg/kg of ideal body weight per day) for 8 to 12 weeks with tapering dose of prednisone. Although there are no satisfactory studies comparing 8- and 12-week courses in adults, a 12-week course may be logical by extension of the pediatric experience.[16]
  - For patients who relapse after cyclophosphamide treatment, **cyclosporine** (4 to 5 mg/kg/d, target trough levels of 125 to 175 ng/mL) or tacrolimus (target trough levels of 5 to 7 ng/mL) is also effective.
  - **MMF** has been used as an effective alternative therapy in small case series.
  - Steroid-resistant patients are most susceptible to complications of steroid therapy (osteoporosis, avascular necrosis, abnormal fat deposition).
- A small percentage of adults initially thought to have MCD will progress to ESRD. Repeat histology will typically reveal FSGS in these patients.

MCD VARIANT: IgM NEPHROPATHY

- The term **IgM nephropathy** is used by some to describe patients presenting with nephrotic syndrome and with the findings of mesangial deposits of IgM, often with a minor degree of mesangial hypercellularity on renal biopsy.
- Controversy exists regarding whether to include this constellation of findings as a variant of minimal disease or FSGS or as part of a continuum related to both entities.
- Patients are more likely to have microscopic hematuria and are less likely to respond to corticosteroids. In one series, 23% progressed to ESRD over 15-year follow-up.

MEMBRANOUS NEPHROPATHY

Epidemiology

- Membranous nephropathy (MN) is a common cause of nephrotic syndrome due to primary glomerular disease in adults with an incidence that roughly equals that of FSGS (~35%).
- It is the most common cause of nephrotic syndrome in white adults aged >60 years, and has a male predominance (~2 to 3:1).
- It is distinctly uncommon in children and adolescents.
- Most cases (two-thirds) are idiopathic.

Pathogenesis

- The pathogenesis of MN is still not completely known. It is thought to be due to autoimmunity via specific nephritogenic autoantibodies.
- Heymann nephritis is a rat model of MN that is induced by inoculation with megalin, a large (516-kDa) glycoprotein extracted from rat cortical nephrons. Formation of antigen–antibody complexes are seen at the podocyte level, with complement activation and formation of the membrane attack complex (C5b–9). This leads to destruction of the glomerular base membrane (GBM) and shedding of the immune complexes to form the characteristic subepithelial deposits.[17]
- Recently, experimental studies have advanced the understanding of the pathogenesis of human membranous glomerulonephritis.
  - Identification of neutral endopeptidase (NEP) as the target antigen on the glomerular podocyte in alloimmune MN resulting from fetomaternal immunization in NEP-deficient mothers.[18]
  - A recent study demonstrated the presence of circulating antibodies to the M-type phospholipase A2 receptor, a transmembrane protein located on podocytes.[19]

Clinical Presentation

- MN presents as **nephrotic syndrome in 80% of patients.**
- **Microscopic hematuria** may be found in 50% of cases, but red blood cell casts are unusual.
- As with the other causes of nephrotic syndrome, a renal biopsy is necessary to make the diagnosis.

- Plasma complement levels are normal in the idiopathic form. Decreased C3 or C4 should prompt further evaluation for systemic lupus erythematosus (SLE) or other systemic disorders associated with hypocomplementemia.
- There is an increased incidence of **thromboembolism,** especially **renal vein thrombosis.** Thromboembolism has been reported in up to 30% of patients with MN.
- MN is characterized by **slow progression of renal insufficiency** (<20% of patients have renal insufficiency at time of presentation).
- **Hypertension** develops only with advancing renal insufficiency and is usually not characteristic of MN at earlier stages.

Secondary Causes of MN

- A diagnosis of MN should prompt a thorough evaluation for other related diseases. It is associated with a variety of autoimmune, infectious, and malignant diseases, as well as with toxic or drug exposures.
- **Autoimmune diseases** associated with MN include SLE (WHO class V), type 1 diabetes mellitus, rheumatoid arthritis, mixed connective tissue disease, Sjögren's syndrome, Hashimoto's thyroiditis, and myasthenia gravis.
- **Associated infectious diseases** are hepatitis B, hepatitis C (HCV), syphilis, malaria, and schistosomiasis.
- The **most common associated cancers** are those of the lung, breast, kidney, and gastrointestinal tract, but cases of MN have been reported with most forms of cancer. Nephrotic syndrome may precede clinical evidence of malignancy by 12 to 18 months.[20]
- **Drugs** such as NSAIDs, gold, penicillamine, hydrocarbons, mercury, formaldehyde, and captopril have been reported in association with MN.

Diagnostic Testing

Pathology

- **Light microscopy:**
  - Normal at early stages and later progresses to thickened glomerular capillary wall with **epithelial "spikes"** seen by methenamine silver staining.
  - Absence of leukocyte infiltration with no evidence of hypercellularity or proliferative lesions. **The presence of significant mesangial hypercellularity** suggests immune deposit formation in the mesangium and is more consistent with a secondary MN such as class V lupus nephritis.
- **Immunofluorescence:**
  - Characteristic IgG granular subepithelial staining in all portions of the glomerular capillary loop. In idiopathic MN, staining is exclusively IgG. The predominant IgG subclass in idiopathic MN is IgG4. Presence of IgM or IgA staining, particularly in the mesangium, as well as tubuloreticular structures seen by electron microscopy suggests class V lupus nephritis.
  - Complement C3 and light chains are also present with similar localization to IgG in ~50% of cases.
- **Electron microscopy** demonstrates the **diagnostic subepithelial electron-dense deposits** in stages:
  - **Stage I:** subepithelial dense deposits without adjacent projections of GBM; normal light microscopy.
  - **Stage II:** adjacent GBM projections forming spikes around immune deposits.

○ **Stage III:** GBM projections surrounding deposits completely.
○ **Stage IV:** markedly thickened GBM with electron-lucent zones replacing the dense deposits.

These stages reflect the severity and duration of disease but do not correlate well with prognosis. The finding of **extensive mesangial electron-dense deposits should prompt consideration of MN secondary to lupus.**

Treatment

- All patients with MN should be managed with **blood pressure control** (goal, <130/80 mm Hg), **dietary sodium restriction, ACE inhibition or angiotensin receptor blockade,** and **lipid-lowering therapy.**
- Patients with documented renal vein or other venous thrombosis should be **anticoagulated** with warfarin.
  ○ At present, there is no consensus for anticoagulation for primary prevention, although patients with hypoalbuminemia of <2.0 g/dL are considered to be at high risk for thrombosis and may be considered for anticoagulation as primary prevention.
  ○ Once anticoagulation is started for a thrombotic event, the patient should remain on therapy until nephrotic syndrome has resolved and should be restarted if there is recurrence.
- **Aggressive cytotoxic therapy is reserved for patients considered to be at higher risk for kidney disease progression,** as the natural history can be relatively benign in up to one-half of affected patients. The higher risk group has decreased kidney function and/or has proteinuria in excess of 8 g/d for >6 months despite maximal therapy to reduce proteinuria.[21]
  ○ **Ponticelli protocol** for the treatment of MN (10-year follow-up study by Italian group)[22]:
    ▪ **Months 1, 3, and 5:** Methylprednisolone, 1 g given intravenously for 3 days, followed by prednisone, 0.5 mg per kg of ideal body weight PO daily for the remainder of the 4 weeks.
    ▪ **Months 2, 4, and 6:** Chlorambucil, 0.2 mg per kg of ideal body weight PO daily for 4 weeks.
    ▪ At 10-year follow-up, 88% of patients treated with this protocol had partial or complete remission compared with 47% of controls.[23] The original study reported using chlorambucil (0.2 mg/kg). However, these doses are limited by bone marrow toxicity of chlorambucil and lower doses may be a more prudent course.
  ○ In the United States, more popular protocol has been **cyclophosphamide and corticosteroids.** Cyclophosphamide, 1.5 to 2 mg/kg of ideal body weight per day PO daily, plus prednisone, 0.5 mg/kg of ideal body weight per day PO daily, can be given for 3 to 6 months. This regimen has been found to be comparable to the original Ponticelli protocol in smaller studies.[24]
  ○ In both regimens, **white blood cell (WBC) counts should be carefully monitored.** Typically, the WBCs are monitored weekly with both chlorambucil and cyclophosphamide use.
  ○ **Prophylaxis against opportunistic infections** such as cytomegalovirus, herpes zoster virus, *Pneumocystis jiroveci* should be considered in the setting of immunosuppressive medications.

○ **Alternative regimens** include:

- **Cyclosporine,** 3.5 to 5 mg/kg of ideal body weight per day (trough levels of 125 to 225 mg/L) in two divided doses with low-dose prednisone, which usually requires a more prolonged course (1 to 2 years) to sustain remission.
- **MMF plus steroids** had shown some promise in small case series, but a recent controlled trial **did not show any significant benefit** over conservative management with blood pressure control, use of ACE inhibitors and statins. It is not recommended in the treatment of MN.
- **Rituximab,** a monoclonal anti-CD20 antibody, has been used with success in resistant MN.

Outcomes/Prognosis

- **Factors associated with poor prognosis** include male gender, age >50 years, presence of hypertension, decreased glomerular filtration rate (plasma creatinine >1.2 mg/dL in women, >1.4 mg/dL in men), nephrotic syndrome of >6-month duration, focal sclerosis, and >20% interstitial fibrosis on renal biopsy specimen.
- Spontaneous, partial, or complete remission is seen in up to 50% of patients with MN within 3 to 5 years of diagnosis.
- Up to one-fourth of patients who remit may experience a relapse of nephrotic range proteinuria that may require disease-specific therapy.

MEMBRANOPROLIFERATIVE GLOMERULONEPHRITIS

MPGN is a pathologic diagnosis based on the finding of diffuse mesangial proliferation, thickening of the capillary wall, subendothelial immune deposits, and hypercellularity. Most cases are associated with circulating immune complexes and hypocomplementemia.

Classification

Type I MPGN

- **Pathology:**
  ○ Type I MPGN is defined by **subendothelial and mesangial immune deposits** seen on electron microscopy at renal biopsy.
  ○ Light microscopy reveals expanded mesangium with increased matrix and cellularity, with a classic lobular appearance to the glomeruli. Using the methenamine silver stain, a double contouring of the GBM can often be appreciated ("**tram tracks**").
  ○ Immunofluorescence usually shows discrete, granular staining of the peripheral capillary wall for IgG and C3.
  ○ Type I MPGN is frequently idiopathic but is also often associated with cryoglobulinemia, chronic HCV infection, chronic hepatitis B viral infection, endocarditis, or malarial infection.
  ○ Cryoglobulinemic MPGN may histologically appear similar to MPGN type 1. However, intracapillary hyaline-like deposits (cryoprecipitates) can be found by light microscopy occasionally. Electron microscopy may also show the highly organized tubular or finely fibrillar structures consistent with cryoglobulins.

- **Pathogenesis:**
  - Type I MPGN is most likely associated with chronic immune-complex diseases.
  - The pathogenesis includes glomerular deposition of immune complexes that preferentially localize to the mesangium and subendothelial space, with subsequent **complement activation via classic pathway** with resultant inflammation, leukocyte infiltration, and cellular proliferation.
  - Type I MPGN can also be associated with hereditary complement deficiencies (C1q, C2, C4, or C3) or with impaired reticuloendothelial system, as occurs with liver or splenic disease.
  - C3, C4, and CH_{50} are reduced in most cases.

Type II MPGN (Dense Deposit Disease)

- **Pathology:**
  - Type II MPGN is defined by the presence of **electron-dense deposits within the mesangium and the GBM** on electron microscopy.
  - The immunofluorescence staining is positive for C3 but is negative for both classic complement pathway components and for immunoglobulins.
- **Pathogenesis:**
  - Type II MPGN is associated with **C3 nephritic factor** (a circulating autoantibody that binds to C3 convertase and prevents its inactivation by factor H) or the dysfunction of a constitutive inhibitor **factor H**, which leads to constitutive **activation of the alternate pathway of complement** and damage to the GBM.
  - The condition is associated with **partial lipodystrophy** in up to 25% of pediatric patients, leading to marked reduction in subcutaneous fat tissues, especially in the face and upper body.
  - **C3 and CH_{50} are reduced** in most cases; C4 is usually normal.

Type III MPGN

- **Pathology:**
  - Type III MPGN is defined by diffuse **subendothelial deposits** and electron-dense **deposits within the GBM and in the subepithelial spaces.**
  - The immunofluorescence pattern of MPGN type III is similar to MPGN type I.
- **Pathogenesis:**
  - Type III MPGN includes activation of the classic or terminal pathway of complement activation.
  - The nephritic factor of the terminal pathway may be present in this form. It activates terminal components and requires properdin.
  - C3 and the terminal complement components (C5 through C9) are reduced, and C5b to C9 membrane attack complex levels are elevated.

Clinical Presentation of MPGN

- Clinical presentation of patients with MPGN types 1 and 2 can range from **nephrotic syndrome** and **microscopic or gross hematuria** to **acute nephritic syndrome** with rapid decline of kidney function.
- MPGN type I is frequently associated with **cryoglobulinemia and HCV** infection in older adults (aged >30 years). MPGN type II is most often seen in children.
- Hypertension is present in a majority of cases.

- Diagnosis of MPGN should prompt investigation for underlying causes, including blood cultures to rule out infective endocarditis; serologies for hepatitis B, HCV, and HIV; evaluation for malignancy; chronic liver disease; or SLE.

Laboratory Findings

- **Type I and cryoglobulinemic MPGN:** low C3, low C4, low CH_{50}
- **Type II:** low C3, normal C4, low CH_{50}, C3 nephritic factor present in ~60% of cases
- **Type III:** low C3, low C5 to C9
- **Cryoglobulinemia:**
  - Cryoglobulins are immunoglobulins that precipitate in the cold.
  - **Type 1 cryoglobulinemia** is a monoclonal immunoglobulin (IgG, IgA, or IgM), associated with lymphoproliferative disease (multiple myeloma, chronic lymphocytic leukemia, Waldenström's macroglobulinemia).
  - **Type II (mixed essential cryoglobulinemia)** is monoclonal IgM, usually **IgM-κ**, with polyclonal IgG. This monoclonal IgM autoantibody is a **rheumatic factor**, that is, directed against the Fc portion of other immunoglobulins.
  - **Type III** is polyclonal IgM directed against polyclonal IgG.
  - Types II and III are most commonly associated with MPGN. They have also been strongly related to chronic HCV infection.
  - **Systemic cryoglobulinemia,** in patients who usually have chronic HCV infection, may present with the **triad of weakness, arthralgias, and painless, palpable, nonpruritic purpura.** The vasculitic lesions classically involve the lower extremities and buttocks. Other manifestations may include Raynaud's phenomenon, digital necrosis, peripheral neuropathy, and hepatomegaly.

Treatment

- Always **exclude causes of secondary MPGN** before planning treatment.
- General measures to reduce proteinuria, control blood pressure, and treat dyslipidemia are indicated for all types.
- **For patients with normal renal function and asymptomatic nonnephrotic range proteinuria, no specific therapy is necessary.** Close follow-up every 3 to 4 months is recommended.[25]
- In patients with nephrotic syndrome or progressive renal failure, **corticosteroids** (tapering prednisone started at 1 mg/kg/d) **with or without cytotoxic agents for 3 to 6 months** may be prescribed.
- Treatment with **cyclosporine, tacrolimus, or MMF** can be considered if there is no response to steroids within 3 months.
- Other therapies:
  - **Antiplatelet therapies,** such as aspirin or dipyridamole, have been studied in several trials. Although proteinuria was reduced in the treatment group, no differences in renal function were observed.
  - Systemic anticoagulation with warfarin has also been studied in the MPGN population and is of unclear benefit with substantial bleeding risks.
- **HCV-associated cryoglobulinemia** has been successfully treated with pegylated interferon-α plus ribavirin in the setting of stable renal function. If renal function is rapidly deteriorating (commonly termed **fulminant cryoglobulinemia**), high-dose steroid therapy is indicated, with or without cytotoxic therapy and plasma exchange.[26]

Natural History

- Untreated MPGN progresses to death or ESRD in 50% of adults within 5 years and up to 90% in 20 years.
- The factors associated with outcome include: the severity of crescents (regardless of pathologic type), the tubulointerstitial lesions, and interstitial fibrosis.
- The disease can recur after renal transplantation, especially types II and III and MPGN associated with HCV.

IgA NEPHROPATHY AND HENOCH–SCHÖNLEIN PURPURA

Epidemiology

- IgA nephropathy (also known as **Berger's disease**) is the **most common form of glomerular disease diagnosed worldwide.**
- The incidence in the United States and Canada is substantially lower than that in Europe and Asia. This discrepancy may be due to rates of routine urinalysis in the United States compared with Asian countries and due to attitudes toward doing kidney biopsies in patients with asymptomatic hematuria.
- In populations of Caucasian descent, the male-to-female ratio is 3:1, whereas the ratio approaches 1:1 in most Asian populations.
- **Henoch–Schönlein purpura** is a syndrome associated with IgA deposition in the kidney with other systemic features. This disorder is seen predominantly in children and adolescents.

Clinical Presentation

- **Microscopic or gross hematuria** is almost always part of the initial presentation of IgA nephropathy.
  - Asymptomatic microscopic hematuria with variable degrees of proteinuria is found in 30% to 40% of cases.
  - Acute macroscopic hematuria concurrent with upper respiratory tract infection is seen in roughly 50% of patients. The timing of the hematuria after the infection is usually **within 1 to 2 days.** This is **in contrast to poststreptococcal glomerulonephritis,** in which the hematuria (often associated with nephritic syndrome) **occurs 10 to 14 days** after pharyngitis.
- Occasionally, patients will present with nephrotic syndrome, acute kidney injury, or rapid progressive course with glomerular epithelial crescents on biopsy (<5%).
- Progressive renal insufficiency and hypertension are seen in a minority of patients.
- Laboratory evaluation demonstrates normal complement levels and increased plasma IgA levels in approximately one-third of patients.
- Diagnosis is made by renal biopsy.
- **Henoch–Schönlein purpura** is a syndrome with IgA nephropathy associated with systemic vasculitis caused by IgA deposition. It is usually seen in children and adolescents and presents with arthralgias, purpuric skin rash (buttocks, abdomen, lower extremities), abdominal pain, ileus, or gastrointestinal bleeding. Renal involvement may be transient.

Secondary Causes of IgA Nephropathy

- IgA deposition associated with mesangial cell proliferation can appear **secondary to systemic diseases** associated with decreased IgA clearance or increased IgA production.[27]
  - Celiac sprue
  - Inflammatory bowel disease
  - Ankylosing spondylitis
  - Dermatitis herpetiformis
  - IgA monoclonal gammopathy
  - HIV

Diagnostic Testing

Pathology

- Light microscopy reveals global or segmental **mesangial hypercellularity** with normal-appearing peripheral GBMs.
- Immunofluorescence demonstrates mesangial IgA deposition, codeposition of C3, and, less commonly, IgG and IgM codeposition.
- Electron microscopy shows mesangial electron-dense deposits and focal thinning of GBM in up to one-third of patients.

Treatment

- Little controversy exists in the general management of patients with IgA nephropathy.
- **Blood pressure control with ACE inhibitor or ARB** is indicated in all hypertensive patients with IgA nephropathy and may be of some benefit despite normal blood pressure at presentation.
- **If proteinuria is <1 g/d, no specific treatment is indicated.**
- The treatment of IgA nephropathy with proteinuria >1 g/d remains controversial.
  - The effect of **fish oil containing omega-3 fatty acids** has been studied by several groups. One group found that the patients receiving fish oil (12 g daily) had a significantly lower rate of progression of renal insufficiency and lower rate of progression to ESRD compared with placebo.[28] Other studies have shown no benefit. It remains unclear if certain subgroups would benefit from this therapy.
  - **Immunosuppressive therapy:**
    - If proteinuria is still >1 g/d on maximal supportive therapy and renal function is not stabilized, consider a trial of steroids for 6 months.
    - In IgA nephropathy, when MCD with nephrotic syndrome coincides, a trial of high-dose corticosteroid therapy is justified.
    - If there is crescentic IgA nephropathy, treat aggressively to save renal function: prednisone 0.5 to 1 mg/kg/d plus cyclophosphamide 2 mg/kg/d for 8 to 12 weeks of induction, followed by tapering prednisone and azathioprine for maintenance. Treatment has often combined plasma exchange with steroids and cyclophosphamide.
    - In sum, the use of immunosuppressive regimens needs to be tailored to the severity (and thus prognosis) of disease.
  - Mesangial IgA deposition occurs in up to 60% of patients receiving a renal transplant for ESRD secondary to primary IgA nephropathy, but the majority of recurrences do not worsen graft outcome and have a benign course.

Natural History

- The majority of patients with IgA nephropathy do not progress to ESRD and experience a benign disease course.
- Several **markers predicting a better outcome** are minimal proteinuria, normal blood pressure, and normal renal function on presentation. In addition, lack of fibrosis of glomeruli and tubulointerstitium are good prognostic signs.
- Approximately 30% of patients with IgA nephropathy will experience progressive disease. These patients often have **poor prognostic features** including poorly controlled hypertension, older age at diagnosis, persistent proteinuria >1 g/d, reduced renal function at diagnosis, and tubulointerstitial fibrosis or more advanced glomerular lesions on renal biopsy.[27]

REFERENCES

1. Thomas DB, Franceschini N, Hogan SL, et al. Clinical and pathologic characteristics of focal segmental glomerulosclerosis pathologic variants. *Kidney Int.* 2006;69:920–926.
2. Schwimmer JA, Markowitz GS, Valeri A, et al. Collapsing glomerulopathy. *Semin Nephrol.* 2003;23:209–218.
3. Korbet SM. Clinical picture and outcome of primary focal segmental glomerulosclerosis. *Nephrol Dial Transplant.* 1999;14(Suppl 3):68–73.
4. Rydel JJ, Korbet SM, Borok RZ, et al. Focal segmental glomerular sclerosis in adults: presentation, course, and response to treatment. *Am J Kidney Dis.* 1995;25:534–542.
5. Matalon A, Valeri A, Appel GB. Treatment of focal segmental glomerulosclerosis. *Semin Nephrol.* 2000;20:309–317.
6. Banfi G, Moriggi M, Sabadini E, et al. The impact of prolonged immunosuppression on the outcome of idiopathic focal-segmental glomerulosclerosis with nephrotic syndrome in adults. A collaborative retrospective study. *Clin Nephrol.* 1991;36:53–59.
7. Cattran DC, Appel GB, Hebert LA, et al. A randomized trial of cyclosporine in patients with steroid-resistant focal segmental glomerulosclerosis. North America Nephrotic Syndrome Study Group. *Kidney Int.* 1999;56:2220–2226.
8. Matalon A, Markowitz GS, Joseph RE, et al. Plasmapheresis treatment of recurrent FSGS in adult renal transplant recipients. *Clin Nephrol.* 2001;56:271–278.
9. Ruf RG, Lichtenberger A, Karle SM, et al. Patients with mutations in NPHS2 (podocin) do not respond to standard steroid treatment of nephrotic syndrome. *J Am Soc Nephrol.* 2004;15:722–732.
10. Weber S, Gribouval O, Esquivel EL, et al. NPHS2 mutation analysis shows genetic heterogeneity of steroid-resistant nephrotic syndrome and low post-transplant recurrence. *Kidney Int.* 2004;66:571–579.
11. Kaplan JM, Kim SH, North KN, et al. Mutations in ACTN4, encoding alpha-actinin-4, cause familial focal segmental glomerulosclerosis. *Nat Genet.* 2000;24:251–256.
12. Winn MP, Conlon PJ, Lynn KL, et al. A mutation in the TRPC6 cation channel causes familial focal segmental glomerulosclerosis. *Science.* 2005;308:1801–1804.
13. Weiner NJ, Goodman JW, Kimmel PL. The HIV-associated renal diseases: current insight into pathogenesis and treatment. *Kidney Int.* 2003;63:1618–1631.
14. Markowitz GS, Schwimmer JA, Stokes MB, et al. C1q nephropathy: a variant of focal segmental glomerulosclerosis. *Kidney Int.* 2003;64:1232–1240.
15. Waldman M, Crew RJ, Valeri A, et al. Adult minimal-change disease: clinical characteristics, treatment, and outcomes. *Clin J Am Soc Nephrol.* 2007;2:445–453.
16. Cyclophosphamide treatment of steroid dependent nephrotic syndrome: comparison of eight week with 12 week course. Report of arbeitsgemeinschaft fur padiatrische nephrologie. *Arch Dis Child.* 1987;62:1102–1106.
17. Ronco P, Debiec H. Molecular pathomechanisms of membranous nephropathy: from Heymann nephritis to alloimmunization. *J Am Soc Nephrol.* 2005;16:1205–1213.

18. Debiec H, Guigonis V, Mougenot B, et al. Antenatal membranous glomerulonephritis due to anti-neutral endopeptidase antibodies. *N Engl J Med*. 2002;346:2053–2060.
19. Beck LH, Jr., Bonegio RG, Lambeau G, et al. M-type phospholipase a2 receptor as target antigen in idiopathic membranous nephropathy. *N Engl J Med*. 2009;361:11–21.
20. Lefaucheur C, Stengel B, Nochy D, et al. Membranous nephropathy and cancer: epidemiologic evidence and determinants of high-risk cancer association. *Kidney Int*. 2006; 70:1510–1517.
21. Lai KN. Membranous nephropathy: when and how to treat. *Kidney Int*. 2007;71:841–843.
22. Ponticelli C, Zucchelli P, Passerini P, et al. Methylprednisolone plus chlorambucil as compared with methylprednisolone alone for the treatment of idiopathic membranous nephropathy. The Italian Idiopathic Membranous Nephropathy Treatment Study Group. *N Engl J Med*. 1992;327:599–603.
23. Ponticelli C, Zucchelli P, Passerini P, et al. A 10-year follow-up of a randomized study with methylprednisolone and chlorambucil in membranous nephropathy. *Kidney Int*. 1995;48: 1600–1604.
24. Ponticelli C, Altieri P, Scolari F, et al. A randomized study comparing methylprednisolone plus chlorambucil versus methylprednisolone plus cyclophosphamide in idiopathic membranous nephropathy. *J Am Soc Nephrol*. 1998;9:444–450.
25. Levin A. Management of membranoproliferative glomerulonephritis: evidence-based recommendations. *Kidney Int*. 1999;70(Suppl):S41–S46.
26. Kamar N, Rostaing L, Alric L. Treatment of hepatitis c-virus-related glomerulonephritis. *Kidney Int*. 2006;69:436–439.
27. D'amico G. Natural history of idiopathic IgA nephropathy: role of clinical and histological prognostic factors. *Am J Kidney Dis*. 2000;36:227–237.
28. Donadio JV, Jr., Grande JP, Bergstralh EJ, et al. The long-term outcome of patients with IgA nephropathy treated with fish oil in a controlled trial. Mayo Nephrology Collaborative Group. *J Am Soc Nephrol*. 1999;10:1772–1777.

Secondary Glomerular Diseases

18

Tingting Li

RENAL DISEASE IN SYSTEMIC LUPUS ERYTHEMATOSUS

GENERAL PRINCIPLES

- Renal disease is a common manifestation of systemic lupus erythematosus (SLE) and may be associated with substantial morbidity and mortality.
- Renal involvement is extremely diverse, ranging from asymptomatic urinary findings to fulminant renal failure or florid nephrotic syndrome.
- Renal manifestations may be the initial presentation of SLE or may emerge later in the disease course.

Epidemiology

- The incidence and prevalence of SLE vary with age (more common in those aged <55 years),[1] gender (female >> male), and ethnicity (African-American and Hispanics > Caucasians).[2]
- Men, non-European Americans, and patients younger than <33 years of age are more likely to develop nephritis.[3]
- Of the unselected patients with SLE, ~25% to 50% will have clinical evidence of lupus nephritis (LN) at disease onset, whereas up to 60% of adults and 80% of children may develop renal disease later in their course.[4]

DIAGNOSIS

Clinical Presentation

- LN is usually accompanied by extrarenal manifestations of lupus, but in some patients this might be the initial presentation of SLE.
- Proteinuria is present in virtually every patient with renal involvement.
- Nephrotic syndrome is present in 45% to 65% of patients with proteinuria.[4]
- Microscopic hematuria is very common; macroscopic hematuria is rare.
- Red blood cell (RBC) casts, white blood cell (WBC) casts, and granular casts can all be seen.
- Renal insufficiency may be rapidly progressive.
- Renal tubular dysfunction (type I and IV renal tubular acidosis) is also seen, and is associated with hypokalemia or hyperkalemia.
- Hypertension can be present, especially in those with severe nephritis.
- Clinical findings do not necessarily correlate with histologic findings on biopsy.

TABLE 18-1	THE 1982 REVISED CRITERIA FOR CLASSIFICATION OF SLE[7]

Malar rash
Discoid rash
Photosensitivity
Oral ulceration
Nonerosive arthritis
Serositis (pleuritis, pericarditis)
Renal involvement (proteinuria, hematuria, or the presence of cellular casts)
Neurologic disorder (seizures and psychosis without other etiologies)
Leukopenia, hemolytic anemia, and/or thrombocytopenia
Positive LE cell preparation, anti–double-stranded DNA antibody, anti-Smith antibody, or false-positive antitreponemal test
Positive anti-nuclear antibody (ANA)

Diagnostic Criteria

- Diagnosis of SLE can usually be made based on the 1982 **revised criteria of the American College of Rheumatology** (Table 18-1).[5] The presence of ≥ 4 criteria gives a sensitivity and specificity of 96% for SLE. The criteria were subsequently revised in 1997 with addition of "positive finding of antiphospholipid antibodies."[6]
- **Hypocomplementemia** is found in >70% of untreated patients with SLE, and is more common in active nephritis.[4] C4 tends to be more depressed than C3.
- Although a presumptive diagnosis of LN can be made in SLE patients with proteinuria, hematuria, cellular casts, and/or renal insufficiency, **renal biopsy is absolutely necessary** for diagnostic confirmation, therapy guidance, and prognostic information, as prognosis and treatment options depend on the histologic subtype. Also, recurrence of LN, even after years of remission, occurs in 50% of patients. Transformation from one class of LN to another can occur at any time in the disease course, spontaneously or during therapy. Commonly, class III progresses to class IV nephritis, and class IV nephritis transitions into class V nephritis.
- Renal biopsy is usually recommended in all patients with SLE who have proteinuria, hematuria, active urinary sediment, and/or reduced renal function.

Diagnostic Testing

Renal Pathology
- LN can affect all parts of the kidney—glomerulus, microvasculature, interstitium, and the tubules.
- The 2003 International Society of Nephrology/Renal Pathology Society (ISN/RPS) classification of LN is based on the degree of glomerular involvement (Table 18-2).[8]
- On immunofluorescence (IF) microscopy, IgG is the predominant immunoglobulin (especially IgG1 and IgG3). Complements are usually present. The presence of all three isotypes of immunoglobulin, C3, C4, and C1q, is called a "full house" and is highly suggestive of LN.

TABLE 18-2	ABBREVIATED ISN/RPS CLASSIFICATION OF LUPUS NEPHRITIS[9]
I	Minimal mesangial lupus nephritis
II	Mesangial proliferative lupus nephritis
III	Focal lupus nephritis (<50% of glomeruli)
IV	Diffuse segmental or global lupus nephritis (≥50% of glomeruli)
V	Membranous lupus nephritis
VI	Advanced sclerosing lupus nephritis (≥90% globally sclerosed glomeruli without residual activity)

- Thrombotic microangiopathy (TMA) involving intrarenal vessels and glomeruli may be associated with the presence of antiphospholipid antibodies.

TREATMENT

- Significant advances have been made over the last few decades in the treatment of LN, with improvement in both patient and renal survival. However, adverse effects of treatment remain a significant contributor to morbidity and mortality.
- The goal of treatment is to maximize clinical efficacy and minimize therapy-related complications.
- In all classes of LN, **blockade of renin–angiotensin–aldosterone system** and **treatment of dyslipidemia** should be implemented. **Blood pressure** should be well controlled, with **goal of <130/80 mm Hg.**
- Females should be counseled on **appropriate contraception** during therapy, as pregnancy during flares can have adverse maternal and fetal outcomes due to the disease itself, as well due to the teratogenic effects of some medications. Given potential for gonadal toxicity from treatment regimens, fertility preservation should be discussed prior to initiation.
- We also recommend **pneumococcal vaccination** for all patients with SLE, especially prior to starting immunosuppressive therapy.
- **Prophylaxis against** *Pneumocystis carinii* (**jiroveci**) should be considered prior to initiation of therapy.

Classes I and II

- Patients with mesangial LN have an **excellent renal prognosis** and **do not require specific treatment directed at the kidney.** Conservative management should include optimal blood pressure control and blockade of the renin–angiotensin–aldosterone system.
- One should be aware that transformation into a different class can occur at any time.

Classes III and IV

- The therapy for **Class III** LN remains controversial. The treatment is generally based on percentage of involved glomeruli, severity of renal histology findings, and clinical manifestations such as the severity of proteinuria, hypertension, and renal dysfunction. In milder cases of Class III LN, glucocorticoids alone might be sufficient, but patients have to be closely monitored. If the clinical manifestations deteriorate, then additional immunosuppressive therapy should be considered.

- Patients with more **severe form of focal proliferative and Class IV diffuse proliferative** LN require aggressive treatment, as these patients are at high risk for progressive renal failure. Treatment regimens are generally divided into **induction and maintenance phases.**

- **Induction therapy:** The goal of induction therapy is to **achieve complete remission.** The definition of complete remission is controversial, but includes reduction or stabilization of serum creatinine (SCr), reduction in proteinuria (at least <500 mg per 24 hour), and reduction in microscopic hematuria to less than five RBCs per high power field. Induction therapy usually consists of corticosteroids (pulse methylprednisolone 500 to 1000 mg intravenously (IV) daily for 3 days followed by prednisone 0.5 to 1.0 mg/kg PO daily, with tapering beginning at 8 weeks) and other immunosuppressive agents listed below.

  ○ **Cyclophosphamide:** Both oral and IV forms have been used for induction. The **IV route** involves a lower cumulative dose and is associated with **less complications** and better compliance. The following regimens have been used:

    ■ Monthly IV cyclophosphamide 0.5 to 1 gm/m² for 6 months, followed by maintenance therapy[10,11] (see below).

    ■ Fixed dose of cyclophosphamide (500 mg) IV every 2 weeks, for a total of 6 doses,[12] followed by maintenance therapy. This regimen should be used for Caucasians with less severe renal disease.

    ■ Others have used oral cyclophosphamide (1.5 to 2.5 mg/kg/d PO) for 3 to 6 months, followed by maintenance therapy.

  ○ **Mycophenolate mofetil (MMF;** 2 to 3 gm PO per day for 6 months followed by maintenance therapy) has been shown to be equally efficacious as, or better than, cyclophosphamide as induction therapy.[13–15]

- **Maintenance therapy:** After achieving remission, maintenance therapy with MMF (1 to 2 g/d PO) or azathioprine (2 mg/kg PO daily) with low-dose prednisone is generally continued for at least 24 months with a subsequent slow taper. This maintenance approach appears to be safer and perhaps more effective than using maintenance IV cyclophosphamide.

- In patients unresponsive to standard therapies, less well-studied treatments such as rituximab and IV immunoglobulin are administered to achieve induction.

- The addition of plasmapheresis to cyclophosphamide and corticosteroid regimen did not improve outcome in one randomized controlled trial and is generally not recommended.

Class V

- There is no well-defined treatment strategy for those with subnephrotic proteinuria.

- In patients with nephrotic range proteinuria, MMF, cyclosporine, and cyclophosphamide have all shown efficacy.[11,16] Cyclosporine may be associated with higher rates of relapse.

- Patients with concurrent proliferative features have a worse long-term renal outcome and may do better with combination therapy with MMF and tacrolimus as induction therapy.[17]

PAUCI-IMMUNE GLOMERULONEPHRITIS: WEGENER'S GRANULOMATOSIS, CHURG–STRAUSS SYNDROME, AND MICROSCOPIC POLYANGIITIS

GENERAL PRINCIPLES

- **Pauci-immune glomerulonephritis (GN)** is characterized by necrotizing crescentic GN with minimal or no immune complex deposits in vessel walls.
- Pauci-immune GN share the common feature of a spectrum of systemic necrotizing small vessel vasculitides that includes Wegener's granulomatosis (WG), microscopic polyangiitis (MPA), renal-limited vasculitis, and less frequently Churg–Strauss syndrome (CSS).
- These disorders are associated with the presence of circulating antineutrophil cytoplasmic antibodies (ANCAs) in 80% to 90% of the cases.

EPIDEMIOLOGY

- Pauci-immune small vessel vasculitides are the most common cause of rapidly progressive GN (RPGN) in adults.
- They may occur at any age, but are more frequent in older adults aged >50 years.
- There is no gender difference, and the incidence is higher in Caucasians than African-Americans.
- The disease is only limited to the kidney in about one-third of cases.[1]

DIAGNOSIS

Clinical Presentation

- The clinical presentation of WG, MPA, and CSS can be quite diverse. The extent of systemic organ involvement may differ. Generalized, nonspecific signs and symptoms of systemic inflammation are common (malaise, anorexia, fever, arthralgia, myalgia, and so forth).
- **WG** is characterized by necrotizing, granulomatous inflammation that typically involves the upper and lower respiratory tracts and the kidneys, although almost any other organ can be involved.
- **CSS**, like WG, is characterized by necrotizing granulomatous inflammation. In addition, patients with CSS have asthma and peripheral blood eosinophilia.
- **MPA** is generally a diagnosis of exclusion in the presence of pauci-immune GN and systemic vasculitis, and the absence of granulomas, eosinophilia, and asthma.
- Renal involvement can develop in 80% of patients with WG, 90% of patients with MPA, and 45% patient's with CSS.[18] Patients typically present with a nephritic urine sediment, variable degrees of proteinuria, hypertension, and often a rapid decline in renal function. Some patients, however, follow a more subacute renal course.

Diagnostic Testing

- The diagnosis of small-vessel vasculitides should be made promptly so that appropriate therapy can be initiated. Clinical presentation and urinalysis are often suggestive.

- **ANCA** is a useful diagnostic marker and should be obtained if there is pre-test suspicion for ANCA-associated GN.
- **Indirect immunofluorescence microscopy** (IIF) should be performed as a screening test cytoplasmic or C-ANCA vs. perinuclear or P-ANCA, followed by **ELISA,** which identifies the specific autoantigen (**myeloperoxidase** [MPO] vs. **proteinase 3** [PR3]).
- The sensitivity and specificity of combined testing (IIF + ELISA) is 72.5% and 98.4%, respectively.[19] The positive and negative predicative values of ANCA testing are determined not only by the sensitivity and specificity of ANCA but also by the prevalence of the disease in a given population. The prevalence of pauci-immune GN varies greatly with the clinical presentations of patients, most frequent in those with clinical evidence of severe glomerular disease.[20]
- A **negative ANCA test does not exclude the diagnosis,** as 10% to 20% of patients with pauci-immune vasculitis do not test positive for ANCA.
- cANCA most often has specificity for PR3, and pANCA most often has specificity for MPO. **WG is associated with PR3-ANCA, whereas MPA, CSS, and renal-limited vasculitis are primarily associated with MPO-ANCA.**
- Renal biopsy is often necessary to confirm the diagnosis of pauci-immune GN, given the potential toxicity associated with treatment, unless there is an absolute contraindication to undergoing a biopsy.

Renal Pathology
- Segmental fibrinoid necrosis, crescent formation, and a lack of immunoglobulin staining by IF or electron microscopy (EM) are the main features. Granulomatous inflammation is rarely seen in the kidney.

TREATMENT

- **Induction therapy:**
  - Combination therapy with **cyclophosphamide and corticosteroids.**
    - Cyclophosphamide at 1.5 to 2.0 mg/kg/d PO, or 15 mg/kg IV at monthly intervals (adjusted for renal function and age) can be given.
    - PO and IV form have similar efficacy but total drug exposure is less in the IV form, which may translate into less toxicity.[21] There is a trend toward higher relapses in the IV-treated patients.
    - Cyclophosphamide should be continued until clinical remission (usually 3 to 6 months) before switching to maintenance therapy.
    - Prednisone at 1 mg/kg/d (pulse methylprednisolone 250 to 1000 mg IV daily for 3 days prior to starting prednisone can be given in severe disease). Prednisone can be tapered at 4 weeks if clinical improvement is observed, with the goal of discontinuing corticosteroids by 6 to 9 months (if there are no extrarenal manifestations).
  - For patients who are unable to take cyclophosphamide, **rituximab** is an effective alternative therapy.[22,23]
  - **Plasmapheresis** (1 to 1.5 plasma volume exchanges for 5 to 7 days) should be considered in patients with life-threatening disease who are dialysis-dependent at presentation, have pulmonary hemorrhage, or manifest concomitant anti-glomerular basement membrane (anti-GBM) antibodies.[22]
  - For those patients who are dialysis-dependent, but there are no signs of renal recovery after 2 to 3 months of induction therapy, continued immunosuppressive therapy should be dictated by extrarenal involvement.

- **Maintenance therapy:**
  - ○ **Azathioprine** (2 mg/kg PO daily) and **methotrexate** (20 to 25 mg/wk maximum, along with folic acid) are equally efficacious in preventing relapses.
  - ○ MMF is less effective than azathioprine for maintaining disease remission.[23]
  - ○ Corticosteroids play very little role in maintenance therapy and should be used only for extrarenal manifestations.
  - ○ The optimal duration of maintenance therapy is unknown. Most recommend 12 to 18 months to reduce the risk of relapse.

PROGNOSIS

- Without treatment, 1-year mortality is ~80%. With aggressive immunosuppressive therapy, 5-year survival is ~65% to 75%.[24] Older age, dialysis dependence, and presence of pulmonary hemorrhage are all risk factors for poor outcome. The presence of irreversible, dialysis-dependent renal failure reduces the 5-year patient survival to 30% to 35%.[24]
- The best predicator of renal outcome is the SCr at the time of presentation and the extent of renal injury on biopsy. About 25% of patients progress to end-stage renal disease.
- About 40% of patients relapse after achieving remission. Patients with PR3-ANCA have higher relapse rate and carry a worse prognosis.
- Renal transplantation remains a good option in patients who have quiescent disease for at least 6 months prior to transplant. The presence of circulating ANCA without clinical disease activity is not a contraindication to transplantation.

ANTI-GLOMERULAR BASEMENT MEMBRANE ANTIBODY DISEASE

GENERAL PRINCIPLES

- Anti-GBM antibody disease is characterized by necrotizing crescentic GN in association with circulating antibodies against the noncollagenous-1 domain of the $\alpha 3$-chain of type IV collagen.
- Goodpasture's disease refers to the triad of RPGN, pulmonary hemorrhage, and presence of anti-GBM antibodies.

Epidemiology

- Anti-GBM antibody disease is a very rare condition, accounting for 1% to 2% of all glomerular diseases.
- The disease can occur at any age but usually peaks in the second to third decade, with a smaller peak later in the sixth decade. There tends to be a male predominance in the younger age group and female predominance in elderly patients.
- About **70% of patients have pulmonary hemorrhage.** Pulmonary involvement is more common in young males, whereas older patients are more likely to have isolated RPGN. Those with pulmonary hemorrhage are usually cigarette smokers.

DIAGNOSIS

Clinical Presentation

- **Renal disease** typically presents as **RPGN with rapid decline in renal function** (over days to weeks), oliguria, and active urinary sediment. Hypertension and edema can also be present. Occasionally, patients may have a subacute course with slower decline in renal function.
- **Pulmonary disease** presents with hemoptysis, cough, and dyspnea with alveolar infiltrates on chest x-ray.
- Up to **30% of patients with anti-GBM antibody disease have a positive ANCA,** typically **MPO-ANCA,** and may have other features of systemic vasculitis such as fever, malaise, or weight loss.
- In X-linked **Alport syndrome,** patients can develop *de novo* anti-GBM antibody disease after renal transplantation, with the antibodies targeting primarily against the α5-chain of type IV collagen.

Diagnostic Criteria

- The diagnosis is suspected when one presents with the above-mentioned clinical features, and confirmed by the presence of circulating anti-GBM antibodies and findings on the renal biopsy specimen. Renal histology will also provide prognostic information.

Diagnostic Testing

Renal Pathology

- Light microscopy (LM) reveals focal and segmental proliferative GN, with areas of fibrinoid necrosis and crescent formation.
- IF reveals the classic pattern of linear IgG deposition along the GBM. IgA, IgM, and C3 staining can occasionally be seen as well.

TREATMENT

- **Plasmapheresis** is aimed at removal of circulating anti-GBM antibodies. It is performed daily or on alternate days for 14 days, with monitoring of clinical response and anti-GBM antibody titers (typically, 4 L exchanges with 5% albumin as replacement solution, or fresh frozen plasma if recent biopsy or pulmonary hemorrhage is present).[25] Adverse effects of plasma exchange, including hypocalcemia, coagulopathy, metabolic alkalosis, and thrombocytopenia, must be closely monitored.
- **Cyclophosphamide** (2 mg/kg/d PO for 3 months) and **corticosteroids** (pulse methylprednisolone 500 to 1000 mg/d for 3 days, followed by prednisone 1 mg/kg/d PO, with taper to 20 mg/d by 6 weeks and slow taper to off by 6 months) are used to suppress production of anti-GBM antibodies. Monitoring of anti-GBM antibody level can help determine the duration of therapy.
- Patients who do not have pulmonary disease and are dialysis dependent at diagnosis, particularly those with crescents in all glomeruli, have a very poor renal prognosis and may not benefit from aggressive immunosuppression.

PROGNOSIS

- Patients who are **untreated** have a fulminant course with **mortality rate of >90%**, thus emphasizing the need for a high level of suspicion for this disease to enable early diagnosis and treatment. **With prompt treatment, mortality decreases to <10%.**[1]
- In those who are dialysis dependent at the time of presentation, patient and renal survival are only 65% and 8%, respectively, at 1 year with appropriate treatment. Conversely, the 1-year renal survival rate in those not requiring dialysis at presentation is 95% if creatinine was <5.7 mg/dL and 82% if creatinine was >5.7 mg/dL.[26]
- Clinical relapses are uncommon.

The prognosis of patients with both positive ANCA and positive anti-GBM antibody parallels that of the anti-GBM antibody disease (although data are controversial).

POSTSTREPTOCOCCAL GN

GENERAL PRINCIPLES

- Poststreptococcal GN (PSGN) is an immune–complex-mediated GN that is caused by certain nephritogenic strains of group A streptococci. PSGN can occur as sporadic cases or during a streptococcal epidemic. The nature of the nephritogenic antigen and the mechanisms that lead to renal immune complex deposition are not clearly understood.

Epidemiology

- PSGN is primarily a disease of children and the peak incidence is in the first decade (rare before the age of 3 years). However, PSGN has been increasingly reported in older patients (especially those aged >60 years). There is a male predominance.
- The incidence of PSGN is on the decline in industrialized nations, but remains high in the developing world.[26]

Prevention

- The risk is minimized by early treatment of streptococcal infection with antibiotics.
- Family members and close contacts should receive prophylactic antibiotics.

DIAGNOSIS

Clinical Presentation

- Typically, there is a sudden onset of **hematuria** (typically described as **tea or coca-cola colored**), **elevated SCr, hypertension,** and **edema** that occurs ~1 to 3 weeks after pharyngitis or a skin infection (latency period may be longer). Oliguria and, less commonly, anuria may occur.
- Subclinical forms of PSGN manifested by microscopic hematuria may occur and may be more common than overt nephritis.
- There is usually a recent history of streptococcal throat infection or skin infection.

Diagnostic Testing

Laboratories

- **Urine sediment** usually reveals **dysmorphic RBCs,** RBC casts, granular casts, and sometimes WBC casts.
- **Proteinuria is variable;** nephrotic range is more common in adults.
- Throat and skin cultures are infrequently positive.
- **Antistreptolysin-*O* (ASO)** and **antideoxyribonuclease B (anti-DNAse B)** titers are frequently elevated, the latter being more specific for skin infection. The streptozyme test, which measures antibodies to five different antigens—ASO, anti-DNAse B, antihyaluronidase, antistreptokinase, and anti-nicotinamide adenine dinucleotide (NAD)—is more sensitive.
- **Serum complement levels,** especially C3 and CH50, are almost always depressed during an acute episode and generally normalize by 6 weeks after diagnosis.
- Diagnosis can generally be made based on the clinical history and laboratory data. Renal biopsy should be performed if the diagnosis is in question or if renal disease fails to improve spontaneously.

Renal Pathology

- On LM, a diffuse endocapillary proliferative GN is seen. Neutrophils are abundant. Monocytic infiltrate can be present. The presence of crescents indicates a poor prognosis.
- IF microscopy reveals granular staining of IgG and C3 along the glomerular capillary walls and in the mesangium. IgA and IgM deposits have also been reported.
- On EM, large, dome-shaped subepithelial electron-dense deposits ("subepithelial humps") are characteristic; smaller mesangial and subendothelial deposits are also seen.

TREATMENT

- Treatment is generally supportive, including salt restriction, diuretics for edema, and blood pressure control.
- Antibiotics should be given if there is evidence of a persistent infection.
- For those patients who do not improve spontaneously (especially those with crescentic GN), pulse corticosteroids may be tried but the benefits are not well established.

NATURAL HISTORY AND PROGNOSIS

- Resolution of acute symptoms occurs within a few weeks.
- Microscopic hematuria may persist for up to 6 months, while mild proteinuria can be seen for years.
- In general, the prognosis of PSGN is excellent in children.
- Adults are more likely to have persistent proteinuria (22%), renal insufficiency (49%), and hypertension (30%) on long-term follow up.[27]
- Nephrotic proteinuria and presence of extensive crescents on renal biopsy predict a worse outcome. Progression to ESRD is uncommon.

THROMBOTIC MICROANGIOPATHIES: THROMBOTIC THROMBOCYTOPENIC PURPURA–HEMOLYTIC UREMIC SYNDROME

GENERAL PRINCIPLES

- TMA describes the histologic lesions that are characteristic of several clinically diverse disorders, with thrombotic thrombocytopenic purpura (TTP) and hemolytic uremic syndrome (HUS) being the most common. Other disorders, such as malignant hypertension, scleroderma, and the antiphospholipid antibody syndrome, will not be discussed here.
- TMA is the result of pathologic processes that affect the systemic microvasculature, leading to platelet aggregation and intraluminal thrombi formation.
- TTP and HUS are diseases of multiple etiologies associated with potentially different pathogenic mechanisms. They are characterized by the clinical syndrome of thrombocytopenia, microangiopathic hemolytic anemia (MAHA), and variable degree of organ damage, with the kidney and the central nervous system being the most affected.

Definition

- The current **diagnostic criteria for TTP** include otherwise **unexplained thrombocytopenia and MAHA.** The criteria are much less stringent compared to the classic pentad of thrombocytopenia, MAHA, fever, neurologic changes, and acute renal failure.[28]
  - ○ It applies usually to adults.
  - ○ Traditionally, neurologic symptoms dominate, although some patients present with both neurological abnormalities and renal failure.
  - ○ Most cases of TTP are acquired; a small proportion has hereditary deficiency of a disintegrin and metalloprotease with thrombospondin-1-like domains (ADAMTS-13).
- **HUS is defined by the same criteria as TTP plus the presence of renal failure.**
  - ○ It applies usually to children.
  - ○ Typical (diarrhea positive, D+): associated with Shiga toxin-producing *E. coli* O157:H7 (90%).
  - ○ Atypical (diarrhea negative, D–): associated with genetic mutations leading to dysregulation of complement system (10%).
- Given the overlapping features, some prefer to use the term TTP–HUS to refer to the syndrome of thrombocytopenia and MAHA without a clear etiology.

Etiology and Pathogenesis

Thrombotic Thrombocytopenic Purpura

- TTP is often idiopathic but may be familial or related to pregnancy, collagen vascular diseases such as SLE, malignancy, infections (HIV, parvovirus), bone marrow transplantation, or medications. Oral contraceptives, ticlopidine (and less commonly clopidogrel), mitomycin C, gemcitabine, and multiple other chemotherapeutics, calcineurin inhibitors, interferon-α, and quinine have all been associated with TTP.
- The pathogenesis of TTP is linked to inherited or acquired deficiencies of von Willebrand factor (vWF)-cleaving protease, which is normally responsible for

cleaving and clearing large vWF multimers that promote platelet aggregation and microvascular thrombosis. An inhibitory autoantibody to vWF-cleaving protease has been found in patients with acquired TTP.

Hemolytic Uremic Syndrome
- Classic childhood Shiga toxin-mediated HUS, or **D+ HUS,** is caused by **certain *E. coli* strains (usually O157:H7) and Shigella.** Transmission is from contaminated food (e.g., undercooked meat) or secondary person-to-person contact. The Shiga toxin triggers the microangiopathic process by entering the circulation via inflamed colonic tissue and causing endothelial damage and platelet activation.
- **D– HUS** is less well understood. **Mutations in genes for complement proteins** (such as C3, membrane cofactor protein, and factors I, H, and B) are seen in many cases. Excessive complement activation is thought to induce endothelial injury.

DIAGNOSIS

Clinical Presentation
Hemolytic Uremic Syndrome
- D+ HUS occurs most commonly in young children (aged <5 years) in the summer and is preceded by an acute hemorrhagic diarrheal illness. D+ HUS accounts for >90% of HUS.
- **Clinical features** of HUS include **sudden onset of oligoanuric renal failure,** pallor, and, in some cases, mental status changes (lethargy, confusion, coma, seizures) preceded by 1 week of diarrheal illness. Hypertension, purpuric rash, jaundice, and pancreatitis can be seen in some patients.
- **Laboratory features** include **schistocytes** on peripheral blood smear, **elevated lactate dehydrogenase, thrombocytopenia, elevated blood urea nitrogen and SCr,** and normal PT and PTT. Most patients have microscopic hematuria on urinalysis and proteinuria of varying degree. Evidence of *E. coli* O157:H7 infection may be present.

Thrombotic Thrombocytopenic Purpura
- TTP is not preceded by a diarrheal illness and is a disease generally occurring in adults, disproportionately affecting African-American women.
- The **classic pentad is not often seen in TTP.** Renal involvement is less common than HUS and may be less severe. The diagnosis of TTP is a clinical one, and the measurement of ADAMTS-13 activity is not required.

Diagnostic Testing
Renal Pathology
- Renal histology in TTP–HUS reveals TMA with fibrin and platelet thrombi in glomerular capillaries, arterioles, and arteries. Arterioles and arteries demonstrate endothelial swelling and intimal thickening, causing luminal narrowing. Capillary wall double contours may be seen due to widening of the subendothelial space. Ischemic glomeruli may have wrinkled, partially collapsed capillaries. Acute cortical necrosis may occur in severe cases of TTP–HUS.
- IF demonstrates diffuse fibrinogen staining in capillary and arterial walls.
- On EM, swelling of glomerular endothelial cells and widened subendothelial spaces are seen.

TREATMENT AND PROGNOSIS

Classic D+ HUS

- **Treatment is supportive only** and includes attention to fluid-electrolyte imbalances, bowel rest, RBC transfusion, and renal replacement therapy if needed.
- The role of plasma exchange has not been adequately evaluated by randomized, controlled studies. Some recommend a trial of plasma exchange in severe cases.
- **Antibiotics and antimotility agents are not recommended.** In fact, there are several epidemiological and retrospective studies showing increased incidence of HUS in patients treated with antibiotics and antimotility agents for diarrheal illnesses.
- Up to 90% have a partial recovery, although up to 40% may have reduced GFR and residual proteinuria. Adults tend to do worse than children.

Thrombotic Thrombocytopenic Purpura

- With the exception of TTP related to chemotherapeutic agents and hematopoietic stem cell transplantation, **plasma exchange is life saving and should be initiated promptly,** with consecutive daily treatments until platelet count is normal.[29] Twice-daily exchanges may be required initially.
- Patients with normal ADAMTS-13 activity who clinically have TTP appear to benefit from plasma exchange as much as those with low ADAMTS-13 activity.
- For those with inadequate or no response to plasma exchange, **corticosteroids** can be used as an adjunctive therapy.[30] Other therapies such as **intravenous immunoglobulin infusion, rituximab, and splenectomy** have been used with variable efficacy.
- The prognosis of TTP varies with the underlying etiology. Mortality has decreased from 90% before availability of plasma exchange to 20% with plasma exchange. Relapses are rare.

RENAL AMYLOIDOSIS

GENERAL PRINCIPLES

- Amyloidosis refers to a group of diseases characterized by extracellular deposition of insoluble fibrils, leading to organ dysfunction.
- Amyloidosis is classified based on the type of precursor protein that forms the amyloid fibrils. These precursor proteins are capable of adopting an antiparallel β-pleated sheet configuration.
- Renal involvement occurs most commonly in **primary (AL) amyloidosis and secondary (AA) amyloidosis,** but can also be seen in some hereditary forms of amyloidosis.
- The fibrils of AL amyloid derive from monoclonal light chains. Multiple myeloma or another lymphoproliferative disorder will be found in 20% of patients with AL amyloidosis.
- AA amyloid results from deposition of serum amyloid A (SAA) protein in chronic inflammatory states such as rheumatoid arthritis and familial Mediterranean fever.

DIAGNOSIS

Clinical Presentation

- Most patients present with varying degree of **proteinuria** (nephrotic range in <50%) and **renal insufficiency.** In AL amyloidosis, monoclonal light chains are present and are usually detected by serum (SPEP) or urine protein electrophoresis (UPEP) with immunofixation. (SIF or UIF). Serum free light chain assay is more sensitive for detecting light chains.
- Urine analysis is usually bland, but microscopic hematuria is occasionally observed.
- Renal tubular defects such as **renal tubular acidosis** and nephrogenic **diabetes insipidus** can be seen with tubular deposits of amyloid.
- Renal ultrasound usually reveals **enlarged kidneys.**
- Deposits in **other organs** can cause restrictive cardiomyopathy, hepatosplenomegaly, orthostatic hypotension, macroglossia, and gastrointestinal motility and absorption problems.
- **Prognosis of AL amyloidosis** is poor with median **survival of <2 years.** With the development of ESRD, survival for most patients is <1 year.
- Prognosis of AA amyloidosis is good if the underlying inflammatory process can be halted. If untreated, progression to ESRD is rapid.

Diagnostic Testing
Renal Pathology

- LM demonstrates eosinophilic, amorphous hyaline deposits in the mesangium, along the GBM, and sometimes in the blood vessels. Subepithelial deposits may give "spikes" similar to membranous nephropathy. The lesions are nonproliferative. **Congo red staining demonstrates apple-green birefringence** under polarized light.
- IF is positive for light chain staining in AL amyloidosis, usually lambda. In AA amyloidosis, staining for SAA protein is usually positive.
- On EM, **amyloid fibrils** are noted to be 8 to 15 nm in diameter and are randomly oriented and nonbranching.

TREATMENT

- Treatment regimens for AL amyloidosis, with or without myeloma, consist of **melphalan and glucocorticoids.** Selected patients may be candidates for high-dose melphalan and **hematopoietic cell transplantation.**[31] Bortezomib has shown to be beneficial in small trials and phase III study is underway. Renal response is directly related to the hematologic response.
- Treatment of AA amyloidosis involves targeting the underlying inflammatory process. Eprodisate, which interferes with the interaction between amyloid fibrils and glycosaminoglycans, may have some benefit in slowing renal progression in AA amyloidosis.[32] Familial Mediterranean fever, which is prevalent in Sephardic Jews, is an autosomal recessive cause of AA amyloidosis. Colchicine is beneficial in treating this disease.

LIGHT CHAIN DEPOSITION DISEASE

- Light chain deposition disease (LCDD) typically manifests as proteinuria with renal insufficiency and is not associated with Congo red staining on biopsy.

- In 50% to 60% of cases, LCDD is associated with a lymphoproliferative disorder, most commonly multiple myeloma. Unlike AL amyloidosis, the light chain in LCDD is usually of the kappa subtype. Up to 30% of patients may have a negative UPEP and SPEP. Like amyloidosis, light chain infiltration of the heart and liver can occur.
- On renal pathology, nodular mesangial matrix expansion with hypercellularity is seen. By IF, monoclonal light chain staining is seen in the GBM, the mesangium, and along tubular basement membranes. No fibrillar structures are seen on EM.
- Treatment regimens have been based on melphalan and prednisone. Bortezomib has also shown efficacy in small trials.
- Prognosis is better in patients with LCDD than in those with AL amyloidosis. The 4-year patient and renal survival rates are 52% and 40%, respectively.[33] LCDD recurs frequently in renal allografts.

REFERENCES

1. Appel GB, Radhakrishnan J, D'Agati V. Secondary glomerular disease. In Brenner BM, ed. *Brenner & Rector's The Kidney.* 8th ed. Philadelphia, PA: Saunders Elsevier; 2008:1067–1106.
2. Bastian HM, Roseman JM, McGwin G Jr, et al. Systemic lupus erythematosus in three ethnic groups. XII. Risk factors for lupus nephritis after diagnosis. *Lupus.* 2002;11(3):152–160.
3. Seligman VA, Lum RF, Olson JL, et al. Demographic differences in the development of lupus nephritis: a retrospective analysis. *Am J Med.* 2002;112:726–729.
4. Cameron JS. Lupus nephritis. *J Am Soc Nephrol.* 1999;10:413–424.
5. Tan EM, Cohen AS, Fries JF, et al. The 1982 revised criteria for the classification of systemic lupus erythematosus. *Arthritis Rheum.* 1982;25:1271–1277.
6. Hochberg MC. Updating the American College of Rheumatology revised criteria for the classification of systemic lupus erythematosus. *Arthritis Rheum.* 1997;40:1725.
7. Tan EM, Cohen AS, Fries JF, et al. The 1982 revised criteria for the classification of systemic lupus erythematosus. *Arthritis Rheum.* 1982;25:1271.
8. Weening JJ, D'Agati VD, Schwartz MM, et al. The classification of glomerulonephritis in systemic lupus erythematosus revisited. *J Am Soc Nephrol.* 2004;15(2):241–250.
9. Weening JJ, D'Agati VD, Schwartz MM, et al. The classification of glomerulonephritis in systemic lupus erythematosus revisited. *J Am Soc Nephrol.* 2004;15(2):241–250.
10. Gourley MF, Austin HA, Scott D, et al. Methylprednisolone and cyclophosphamide, alone or in combination, in patients with lupus nephritis. A randomized, controlled trial. *Ann Intern Med.* 1996;125:549–557.
11. Contreras G, Pardo V, Leclercq B, et al. Sequential therapies for proliferative lupus nephritis. *N Engl J Med.* 2004;350(10):971–980.
12. Houssiau FA, Vasconcelos C, D'Cruz D, et al. Immunosuppressive therapy in lupus nephritis; the Euro-Lupus Nephritis Trial, a randomized trial of low-dose versus high-dose intravenous cyclophosphamide. *Arthritis Rheum.* 2002;46(8):2121–2131.
13. Chan TM, Li FK, Tang CS, et al. Efficacy of mycophenolate mofetil in patients with diffuse proliferative lupus nephritis. Hong Kong-Guang-Zhou Nephrology Study Group. *N Engl J Med.* 2000;343:1156–1162.
14. Ginzler EM, Dooley MA, Aranow C, et al. Mycophenolate mofetil or intravenous cyclophosphamide for lupus nephritis. *N Engl J Med.* 2005;353:2219–2228.
15. Appel GB, Contreras G, Dooley MA, et al. Mycophenolate mofetil versus cyclophosphamide for induction treatment of lupus nephritis. *J Am Soc Nephrol.* 2009;20:1103–1112.
16. Austin HA III, Illei GG, Braun MJ, et al. Randomized, controlled trial of prednisone, cyclophosphamide, and cyclosporine in lupus membranous nephropathy. *J Am Soc Nephrol.* 2009;20:901–911.
17. Bao H, Liu ZH, Xie HL, et al. Successful treatment of class V+IV lupus nephritis with multitarget therapy. *J Am Soc Nephrol.* 2008;19(10):2001–2010.

18. Jennette JC, Falk RJ. Small-vessel vasculitis. *N Engl J Med.* 1997;337(21):1512–1523.

19. Hagen EC, Daha MR, Hermans J, et al. Diagnostic value of standardized assays for anti-neutrophil cytoplasmic antibodies in idiopathic systemic vasculitis. *Kidney Int.* 1998;53: 743–753.

20. Jennette, JC, Wilkman AS, Falk RJ. Diagnostic predicative value of ANCA serology. *Kidney Int.* 1998;53:796–798.

21. de Groot K, Harper L, Jayne DR, et al. Pulse versus daily oral cyclophosphamide for induction of remission in antineutrophil cytoplasmic antibody-associated vasculitis: a randomized trial. *Ann Intern Med.* 2009;150(10):670–680.

22. Jayne DR, Gaskin G, Rasmussen N, et al. Randomized trial of plasma exchange or high-dosage methylprednisolone as adjunctive therapy for severe renal vasculitis. *J Am Soc Nephrol.* 2007;18(7):2180–2188.

23. Hiemstra TF, Walsh M, Mahr A, et al. Mycophenolate mofetil vs azathioprine for remission maintenance in antineutrophil cytoplasmic antibody-associated vasculitis: a randomized controlled trial. *JAMA.* 2010;304(21):2381–2388.

24. Little MA, Pusey CD. Glomerulonephritis due to antineutrophil cytoplasmic antibody-associated vasculitis: an update on approaches to management. *Nephology.* 2005;10:368–376.

25. Levy JB, Turner AN, Rees AJ, et al. Long-term outcome of anti-glomerular basement membrane antibody disease treated with plasma exchange and immunosuppression. *Ann Intern Med.* 2001;134:1033–1042.

26. Rodriguez-Iturbe B, Musser JM. The current state of post-streptococcal glomerulonephritis. *J Am Soc Nephrol.* 2008;19:1855–1864.

27. Sesso R, Pinto SWL. Five-year follow-up of patients with epidemic glomerulonephritis due to *Streptococcus zooepidemicus. Nephrol Dial Transplant.* 2005;20(9):1808–1812.

28. George JN. The thrombotic thrombocytopenic purpura and hemolytic uremic syndromes: evaluation, management, and long-term outcomes experience of the Oklahoma TTP-HUS registry, 1989–2007. *Kidney Int.* 2008;75(suppl 112):S52-S54.

29. Rock GA, Shumak KH, Buskard NA, et al. Comparison of plasma exchange with plasma infusion in the treatment of thrombotic thrombocytopenic purpura. *N Engl J Med.* 1991; 325(6):393–397.

30. George JN. Thrombotic thrombocytopenic purpura. *N Engl J Med.* 2006;354(18)1927–1935.

31. Skinner M, Sanchorawala V, Seldin DC, et al. High-dose melphalan and autologous stem-cell transplantation in patients with AL amyloidosis: an 8-year study. *Ann Intern Med.* 2004;140:85–93.

32. Dember LM, Hawkins PN, Hazenberg BP, et al. Eprodisate for the treatment of renal disease in AA amyloidosis. *N Engl J Med.* 2007;356(23):2349–2360.

33. Pozzi C, D'Amico M, Fogazzi GB, et al. Light chain deposition disease with renal involvement: clinical characteristics and prognostic factors. *Am J Kidney Dis.* 2003;42: 1154–1163.

Diabetic Nephropathy

19

Steven Cheng

GENERAL PRINCIPLES

Diabetic nephropathy (DN) is a result of diabetes mellitus and is the most common cause of kidney disease in the United States.

Definition

DN is a clinical syndrome characterized by a progressive loss of kidney function resulting from diabetes. The development of albuminuria is a hallmark of this condition and is used to screen patients for DN. Although definitive evidence of diabetic kidney disease requires a kidney biopsy, clinical characteristics are usually sufficient to make the diagnosis.

Epidemiology

- DN is the most common cause of end-stage renal disease (ESRD) in the United States.
- Although both type 1 and type 2 diabetes can result in progressive kidney disease, the majority of diabetic patients at ESRD have type 2 diabetes, likely reflecting the greater prevalence of this form of the disease.
- DN imparts a significant increase in both morbidity and mortality, and the diabetic dialysis patient has a mortality rate that is 50% higher than that of nondiabetics. Early detection and aggressive intervention is crucial for the optimal management of this population.

Pathophysiology

- **Hyperglycemia** plays a central role in the development of DN by mediating hemodynamic and structural changes in the kidney.
  - The direct exposure to sustained high blood glucose concentrations results in glycosylation of mesangial proteins, leading to mesangial expansion and injury.
  - Furthermore, the hyperglycemic mileu induces several overlapping biochemical pathways that are injurious to renal architecture. These include the generation of advanced glycosylation end products and reactive oxygen species, the stimulation of transforming growth factor-β and proinflammatory cytokines.[1-3]
- **Hemodynamic changes** also likely contribute to the progression of renal disease.
  - Hyperfiltration at the glomerulus can be seen preceding the onset of microalbuminuria, reflecting impaired autoregulation and increasing glomerular pressures.[4]

Risk Factors

- Among modifiable risk factors, **control of blood glucose level** is perhaps the most obvious and most important.
  - A number of large studies, including the United Kingdom Prospective Diabetes Study (UKPDS) and the Diabetes Control and Complications Trial, have shown that poor glycemic control is associated with an increased risk of developing microalbuminuria and other microvascular complications of diabetes, such as retinopathy and neuropathy.[5,6]
  - The risk is increased for all hemoglobin A1C levels above the nondiabetic range, and greatest at levels >12%.
- **Hypertension** is also clearly associated with the development of nephropathy.
  - A number of factors may contribute to the development of hypertension in these patients, including hyperinsulinemia, fluid retention, increased arterial stiffness, and the development of nephropathy.
  - Blood pressure measurements consistently higher than the current goal of 130/80 mm Hg expose diabetic patients to an increased risk for the development or progression of DN.
- **Obesity** further increases this risk, although it is uncertain whether this effect is independent of diabetic and glycemic control.
- **Nonmodifiable risk factors** are also well documented.
  - Some have suggested that certain variations of the gene encoding the angiotensin-converting enzyme (ACE) are associated with the aggravation of proteinuria and overt nephropathy.[7]
    - A genetic predisposition is also supported by the fact that certain ethnicities are at greater risk for DN; particularly those of Mexican-American, African-American, and Pima Indian descent.[8]
  - Age, in conjunction with duration of diabetes, was associated with an increased risk of albuminuria in a study of type 2 diabetes from Australia.[9] The correlation of age with renal disease progression is yet unclear in type 1 diabetes, though those diagnosed before the age of 5 are typically at low risk for progression to ESRD.

Prevention

- To prevent progression to DN, individuals with diabetes are screened for the presence of microalbuminuria—a precursor to DN and an early indication of renal damage.
- Screening for DN consists of regular evaluations for microalbuminuria.
  - Microalbuminuria refers to a small quantity of albumin that can be detected in the urine during early DN.
    - **Microalbuminuria** is the excretion of between 30 and 300 mg of albumin in a 24-hour period.
    - **Albuminuria** (sometimes called macroalbuminuria) is the excretion of >300 mg of albumin in a 24-hour period. This degree of urinary albumin excretion characterizes the progression to DN.
  - **Tests for microalbuminuria:**
    - Microalbuminuria can be detected with a 24-hour urine collection. However, this can be cumbersome and often difficult to interpret because of improper sampling and the logistical difficulties of saving urine through 24 hours.

TABLE 19-1	CLASSIFICATION OF ALBUMINURIA	
	24-h Collection (mg per 24 h)	Adjusted for Urine Cr (mg per g creatinine)
Normal	<30	<30
Microalbuminuria	30–300	30–300
Albuminuria	>300	>300

- A ratio of albumin-to-creatinine excretion has sufficient correlation to 24-hour protein excretion and can be used instead.
- This study is often called a spot microalbumin test or a microalbumin/creatinine ratio. The ratio of albumin excreted per gram of creatinine correlates to the amount of albumin excreted in a 24-hour period (see Table 19-1).
- As a result, microalbuminuria is defined as 30 to 300 mg of albumin per g of creatinine, and albuminuria is defined as >300 mg of albumin per g of creatinine.
  ○ **Screening is conducted yearly in patients with type 2 diabetes,** but can be deferred for the first 5 years in those with type 1 diabetes.
    - As screening for microalbuminuria requires the detection of minute elevations in urine albumin, a routine urinalysis should not be used as screening of DN.
    - If a routine urine dipstick test result is negative for protein, a spot microalbumin screening test should still be checked, as microalbuminuria may not be detected by dipstick test alone.
    - If a routine urine dipstick test result is positive for protein, a spot microalbumin screening test remains necessary to quantify the extent of albumin excretion.

DIAGNOSIS

Clinical Presentation

- The natural history and progression of kidney disease is likely similar in both types of diabetes. However, the early course of the diabetic kidney disease is better studied in type 1 diabetes because of a more accurate correlation between the onset of disease and the time of diagnosis.
- In type 1 diabetes, the first 5 years are typically characterized by normal laboratory values for serum creatinine, electrolytes, and urine protein levels.
  ○ Despite the normal laboratory values, high glucose levels lead to glomerular hyperfiltration and the initiation of subtle histopathological changes.
- **Microalbuminuria typically develops between 5 and 10 years from diagnosis.**
  ○ This is one of the earliest markers for diabetic kidney involvement and forms the cornerstone of the screening process for DN.
- From 15 to 20 years, albuminuria and hypertension develop, with a fairly steep decline to ESRD occurring after 20 years.

- Diabetic patients are frequently referred to the nephrology clinic with albuminuria or elevations in serum creatinine levels. A complete evaluation of such patients requires a detailed evaluation for the presence of DN risk factors, manifestations of extra-renal microvascular disease, and a thorough review of long-term patterns in biochemical markers such as hemoglobin A1C, serum creatinine, and urine albumin levels. The goal of this detailed investigation is twofold.
  ○ First, it is necessary to establish whether the underlying renal condition is consistent with the pattern and progression of DN.
  ○ Second, it is crucial to identify the presence of modifiable risk factors and to establish appropriate goals of therapy.

History

- A detailed history should elicit the duration of diabetes, the level of glycemic control, and the presence of diagnoses, suggesting other end-organ microvascular disease associated with diabetes.
- As mentioned previously, patients typically develop microalbuminuria 5 to 10 years after the onset of disease. The risk of DN is further increased in those with poor glycemic control.
- During each visit, patients should be asked about adherence to the diabetic diet and their current level of glycemic control. A written log of recorded blood sugars is often helpful in tracking overall trends and daily variations in glucose levels.
- A **concurrent history of retinopathy or neuropathy** often supports the diagnosis of DN.
  ○ Type 1 diabetics with nephropathy almost always manifest evidence of retinopathy and/or neuropathy.[10]
  ○ The association is less established in type 2 diabetes. Although the absence of retinopathy should not exclude consideration of DN in these patients, physicians should consider alternative diagnoses as well.

Physical Examination

- **Blood pressure** recordings should be checked routinely at each office visit. Hypertension is a common comorbidity among diabetics and plays an important role in both the development and progression of DN.
- The patient's **volume status** should also be carefully assessed, as an expansion of the body's interstitial fluid compartment, manifesting as edema, may reflect avid sodium retention in hypertension or a loss in oncotic pressure due to nephrotic range urinary albumin excretion.
- Evidence of retinopathy and neuropathy may reflect concurrent microvascular disease and should be evaluated with a **fundoscopic and neurologic exam.**

Differential Diagnoses

- Although the term "diabetic nephropathy" specifically refers to the glomerular disease caused by the mechanisms discussed above, there are other forms of kidney injury that can occur in the diabetic patient.
- Of the other glomerular diseases, **membranous nephropathy** is associated with diabetes, and can occur in longstanding diabetics between the ages of 40 and 60 years.
- Diabetics are also susceptible to the development of **renal vascular disease**, which may be unmasked with the initiation of an angiotensin antagonist, and obstructive nephropathy, which is a particular concern among the 40% of diabetics who develop autonomic neuropathy of the bladder.

- Diabetics are more prone to developing certain infectious sequelae as well, such as renal papillary necrosis or renal tuberculosis.
  - ○ **Papillary necrosis** may present in individuals with frequent urinary tract infections (UTIs) who develop hematuria, pyuria, and mild kidney disease. A small degree of proteinuria is also common.
  - ○ **Renal tuberculosis** may also present with sterile pyuria, hematuria, and azotemia; the diagnosis is based on clinical suspicion and the growth of mycobacterial species in the urine.
- In a diabetic who develops proteinuria or renal insufficiency, **the following should raise suspicion of a diagnosis other than DN:**
  - ○ Development of albuminuria <5 years from diabetic disease onset
  - ○ Acute kidney injury
  - ○ Active urine sediment
  - ○ Thrombosis associated with nephrotic syndrome
  - ○ Absence of retinopathy or neuropathy, particularly in type 1 diabetes

Diagnostic Testing
Laboratories
- Recent laboratory data **should always be interpreted in the context of long-term trends and current clinical contexts.** A single elevation in serum creatinine or urine albumin should be confirmed with repeat testing, especially if there are clues to suggest a transient rise in such markers (dehydration, febrile illnesses, UTIs, and new medications).
- DN is confirmed by the persistence of albuminuria in two separate samples separated by 3 to 6 months.
- As the changes in renal function with DN typically follow a gradual but progressive course over time, serum creatinine would initially be expected to rise slowly, and small subtle increments are often noted when laboratory trends over the preceding months and years are scrutinized. Sudden fluctuations in laboratory data warrant confirmation with repeat values and consideration of alternative diagnoses (see below).

Diagnostic Procedures
- The **definitive diagnosis requires renal biopsy.**
- Biopsy should be pursued if alternative diagnoses are being considered due to an atypical presentation for DN.
  - ○ Glomerular hypertrophy can be seen early in DN, coinciding with mesangial expansion and thickening of the glomerular basement membrane.
    - ■ This typically progresses to a nodular pattern of glomerulosclerosis, known as Kimmelstiel–Wilson nodules. Although this is often considered the most pathognomonic lesion in DN, nodular glomerular lesions can also be seen in other conditions, such as light-chain nephropathy and amyloidosis.
  - ○ Structural lesions outside the glomerulus include changes in renal vasculature, tubular architecture, and the interstitium.
    - ■ Hyalinosis of both afferent and efferent arterioles can be seen, and may be particularly noticeable in patients with concurrent hypertension.
    - ■ Tubular changes include thickening of the tubular basement membrane and the Armanni–Ebstein lesion, a specific, although rarely appreciated, manifestation of tubular glycogen deposition and subsequent tubular vacuolization.

- Tubulointerstitial fibrosis can feature prominently in patients with longstanding DN and is suggestive of irreversible chronicity of the disease process.

TREATMENT

- **Modifiable risk factors of hyperglycemia and hypertension are the primary target of both preventive and treatment strategies.** Weight loss and smoking cessation are also thought to mediate some protective benefit from DN. Optimal care includes the reduction of hemoglobin A1C to levels under 7% and the reduction of blood pressure to levels under 130/80 mm Hg.
- **Glycemic control:**
  - Glycemic control remains the most important modifiable risk factor and should be pursued to a **goal of Hemoglobin A1C of under 7%.**
  - Some studies now propose a stricter goal of hemoglobin A1C <6.5%.[11]
  - Early and aggressive glycemic control results in a decreased incidence of microalbuminuria as well as a decrease in the prevalence of hypertension.
  - In type 1 diabetics, intensive insulin therapy has also been shown to reduce the rate of progression from microalbuminuria to overt albuminuria by 54%.[12]
  - Once patients develop overt nephropathy and marked albuminuria, the evidence that strict glycemic control slows progressive renal dysfunction is controversial. Some suggest that a lack of apparent benefit may be due to the significant contribution of concurrent hypertensive disease. This clearly emphasizes the importance of preventive interventions and early, comprehensive treatment in the diabetic population.
- **Hypertension:**
  - The current Kidney Disease Outcomes Quality Initiative (K/DOQI) and Joint National Committee on Prevention, Detection, Evaluation, and Treatment of High Blood Pressure (JNC 7) treatment guidelines support a **blood pressure target of <130/80 mm Hg** in patients with diabetes and patients with chronic kidney disease.[13]
  - In hypertensive diabetics without proteinuria, **angiotensin inhibitors** and **thiazide diuretics** are often prescribed as first-line agents.[14,15]
    - Inhibitors of the angiotensin system are known to decrease proteinuria and are the only agents associated with a significant reduction in the risk of developing microalbuminuria.
    - Some speculate that further benefit is conferred through anti-inflammatory effects of angiotensin inhibition, and not merely through blood pressure control and the reduction of intraglomerular pressure by efferent vasodilation.[16]
    - Often patients will require two agents to reduce blood pressure to target goal, and the combination of a diuretic with an ACE inhibitor or angiotensin receptor blocker (ARB) is usually necessary as well as optimally protective.
  - Once patients develop microalbuminuria, the control of hypertension becomes a crucial intervention to prevent progression of nephropathy and the incidence of additional diabetic complications.

- Data suggest that each 10 mm Hg reduction in systolic blood pressure is correlated with a 12% reduction in diabetic complications.[17]
- Additionally, a more aggressive goal of 125/75 mm Hg may be more beneficial in slowing the progression of renal disease in patients with over 1 g of proteinuria per day.
- In the context of increased urinary albumin excretion, angiotensin-inhibiting agents become a clear first choice among antihypertensives based on their ability to reduce both blood pressure and albuminuria.

- **Albuminuria:**
  - Albuminuria is often used as a surrogate marker for the extent of renal involvement, but there is expanding evidence to suggest that it is an independent risk factor associated with further disease progression.
    - Studies suggest that a reduction in albuminuria may confer improvements in both renal and cardiovascular outcomes.[18,19]
    - In trials using **ACE inhibitors and ARBs** in diabetic patients with proteinuria, the reduction of proteinuria was associated with reduced risk of progressive renal dysfunction.[20–23]
    - This beneficial effect is independent of blood pressure reduction, and has been demonstrated in trials comparing angiotensin-inhibiting agents to other antihypertensive medications titrated to equivalent blood pressure control.[22,23]
    - The question of whether ACE inhibitors and ARBs are equivalent has not yet been fully answered, though in clinical practice they are frequently used interchangeably.
    - One comparison of ACE inhibitors and ARBs in type 2 diabetics showed no significant differences in the primary end point (decline in glomerular filtration rate) or secondary end points (blood pressure control, albuminuria, serum creatinine, ESRD, cardiovascular end points, and death).[24]
    - Another area of controversy involves the combination of ACE inhibitors and ARBs for maximal reduction of proteinuria. Although this combination has been shown to reduce severe proteinuria in nondiabetic patients,[25] the concomitant use of ACE inhibitors and ARBs should generally be avoided due to the increased risk of adverse effects.
    - Direct renin inhibitors have also been used in conjunction with ARBs and have demonstrated a decrease in proteinuria among patients with DN. However, its utility as a single agent has not yet been demonstrated.[26]

COMPLICATIONS

- Clinical complications that may result from DN or the treatment of DN include hypoglycemia, acute renal failure, hyperkalemia, and metabolic acidosis.
- **Hypoglycemia:**
  - Pharmacological agents should be dosed with careful consideration of diminished renal clearances in patients who develop DN. Although glycemic control should be pursued by any means possible, the degree of renal insufficiency must be considered in the selection and titration of pharmacological agents.
  - The clearance of the biguanide metformin is notably decreased in the setting of impaired renal function, predisposing patients with renal disease to lactic acidosis. **Metformin is not recommended for patients with a creatinine clearance of <60 to 70 mL/min.**

○ Sulfonylureas are also not recommended in patients with a clearance of <50 mL/min because of the increased risk of severe hypoglycemia. Routine calculations of a patient's estimated renal function can be done using formulas described elsewhere in this book and may serve as a reminder to dose drugs appropriately in the clinical setting.

- **Acute renal failure:**
  ○ Acute renal failure is manifested by a sudden increase in creatinine that exceeds the predicted gradual decline of function seen with DN.
  ○ Both pre- and postrenal etiologies should be kept in mind, as diabetics are prone to both intravascular depletion and obstruction due to autonomic neuropathies.
  ○ An elevation in creatinine is often encountered in patients initiating on an angiotensin-inhibiting agent.
    ■ This usually reflects an expected physiological response to the change in glomerular filtration with efferent arterial vasodilation.
    ■ However, a rise in creatinine of >30% should prompt the cessation of the ACE inhibitor or ARB until renal function returns to baseline.
    ■ A slow retitration with gradual dose increments is warranted for most patients, given the known benefits of angiotensin inhibition in this population.
    ■ An evaluation for unmasked renal artery stenosis may be appropriate as well.
- **Hyperkalemia:**
  ○ Hyperkalemia is another complication often associated with the institution of angiotensin-inhibiting agents in diabetic patients.
    ■ Serum potassium levels under 5.5 mEq/L can be managed medically. Dietary potassium restriction and the titration of diuretics, particularly loop diuretics, are usually sufficient to lower potassium levels and promote kaliuresis.
    ■ For more severe cases of hyperkalemia, a decrease or cessation of dose may be necessary. After normalization of potassium levels and dietary education, a gradual retitration can be attempted.
  ○ Diabetic patients with chronic kidney disease may also develop a **type 4 renal tubular acidosis** that may manifest as hyperkalemia with a nonanion gap metabolic acidosis.
    ■ The hyperkalemia, which results from hyporeninemic hypoaldosteronism, impairs the generation of ammonia necessary for sufficient acid excretion, resulting in a metabolic acidosis.
    ■ Although type 4 renal tubular acidosis is often managed with mineralocorticoid replacement, the potential for exacerbation of fluid retention or hypertension often limits clinical application.
    ■ The institution of dietary potassium restriction and the stimulation of potassium excretion with diuretics can be used to control the hyperkalemia and restore normal ammoniagenesis.

MONITORING/FOLLOW-UP

- Patients with overt nephropathy should be followed regularly in the nephrology clinic. Achievement of glycemic goals, attainment of adequate blood pressure control, and maximal reduction of albuminuria should be checked at each visit. In those with progressive nephropathy, management of common complications of chronic kidney disease, including anemia and renal osteodystrophy, should be addressed as discussed elsewhere in this book.

REFERENCES

1. Wolf G, Ziyadeh FN. Molecular mechanisms of diabetic renal hypertrophy. *Kidney Int.* 1999;56(2):393–405.
2. Makita Z, Radoff S, Rayfield EJ, et al. Advanced glycosylation end products in patients with diabetic nephropathy. *N Engl J Med.* 1991;325:836.
3. Wolf G, Ziyadeh FN. Molecular mechanisms of diabetic renal hypertrophy. *Kidney Int.* 1999;56:393.
4. Fioretto P, Steffes MW, Brown DM, et al. An overview of renal pathology in insulin-dependent diabetes mellitus in relationship to altered glomerular hemodynamics. *Am J Kidney Dis.* 1992;20(6):549–558.
5. Adler AI, Stevens RJ, Manley SE, et al. Development and progression of nephropathy in type 2 diabetes: the United Kingdom Prospective Diabetes Study (UKPDS). *Kidney Int.* 2003;63(1):225–232.
6. The Diabetes Control and Complications Trial Research Group. The effect of intensive treatment of diabetes on the development and progression of long-term complications in insulin-dependent diabetes mellitus. *N Engl J Med.* 1993;329:977–986.
7. Jeffers BW, Estacio RO, Raynolds MV, et al. Angiotensin-converting enzyme gene polymorphism in non-insulin dependent diabetes mellitus and its relationship with diabetic nephropathy. *Kidney Int.* 1997;52:473.
8. Nelson RG, Knowler WC, Pettitt DJ, et al. Diabetic kidney disease in Pima Indians. *Diabetes Care.* 1993;16(1):335–341.
9. Tapp RJ, Shaw JE, Zimmet PZ, et al. Albuminuria is evident in the early stages of diabetes onset: results from the Australian Diabetes, Obesity, and Lifestyle Study. *Am J Kidney Dis.* 2004;44(5):792–798.
10. Chavers BM, Mauer SM, Ramsay RC, et al. Relationship between retinal and glomerular lesions in IDDM patients. *Diabetes* 1994;43:441.
11. Shichiri M, Kishikawa H, Ohkubo Y, Wake N. Long-term results of the Kumamoto Study on optimal diabetes control in type 2 diabetic patients. *Diabetes Care* 2000;23(suppl 2):B21–B29.
12. The Diabetes Control and Complications Trial Research Group. The effect of intensive treatment of diabetes on the development and progression of long-term complications in insulin-dependent diabetes mellitus. *N Engl J Med* 1993;329(14):977–986.
13. Chobanian AV, Bakris GL, Black HR, et al. The Seventh Report of the Joint National Committee on Prevention, Detection, Evaluation, and Treatment of High Blood Pressure: The JNC 7 Report. *JAMA* 2003;289:2560.
14. ALLHAT Officers and Coordinators for the ALLHAT Collaborative Research Group. The Antihypertensive and Lipid-Lowering Treatment to Prevent Heart Attack Trial. Major outcomes in high-risk hypertensive patients randomized to angiotensin-converting enzyme inhibitor or calcium channel blocker vs diuretic: ALLHAT. *JAMA* 2002;288:2981.
15. Strippoli G, Craig M, Schena FP, et al. Antihypertensive agents for primary prevention of diabetic nephropathy. *J Am Soc Nephrol* 2005;16:3081–3091.
16. Sharma K, Eltayeb B, McGowan TA, et al. Captopril-induced reduction of serum levels of transforming growth factor-beta 1 correlates with long-term renoprotection in insulin-dependent diabetic patients. *Am J Kidney Dis.* 1999;34:818.
17. Adler AI, Stratton IM, Neil HA, et al. Association of systolic blood pressure with macrovascular and microvascular complications of type 2 diabetes (UKPDS 36): prospective observational study. *BMJ* 2000;321:412–419.
18. Brenner BM, Cooper ME, de Zeeuw D, et al. Effects of Losartan on renal and cardiovascular outcomes in patients with type 2 diabetes and nephropathy. *N Engl J Med.* 2001; 345:861.
19. De Zeeuw D, Remuzzi G, Parving HH, et al. Albuminuria, a therapeutic target for cardiovascular protection in type 2 diabetic patients with nephropathy. *Circulation.* 2004;110: 921–927.

20. The Microalbuminuria Captopril Study Group. Captopril reduces the risk of nephropathy in IDDM patients with microalbuminuria. *Diabetologia*. 1996;39(5):587–593.

21. De Zeeuw D, Remuzzi G, Parving HH, et al. Proteinuria, a target for renoprotection in patients with type 2 diabetic nephropathy: Lessons from RENAAL. *Kidney Int*. 2004;65(6): 2309–2320.

22. Atkins RC, Briganti EM, Lewis JB, et al. Proteinuria reduction and progression to renal failure in patients with type 2 diabetes mellitus and overt nephropathy. *Am J Kidney Dis*. 2005;45(2):281–287.

23. Lewis EJ, Hunsicker LG, Clarke WR, et al. Renoprotective effect of the angiotensin-receptor antagonist irbesartan in patients with nephropathy due to type 2 diabetes. *N Engl J Med*. 2001;345:851.

24. Barnett AH, Bain SC, Bouter P, et al. Angiotensin-receptor blockade versus converting-enzyme inhibition in type 2 diabetes and nephropathy. *N Engl J Med*. 2004;351:1952–1961.

25. Nakao N, Yoshimura A, Morita H, et al. Combination treatment of angiotensin-II receptor blocker and angiotensin-converting enzyme inhibitor in non-diabetic renal disease (COOPERATE): a randomized controlled trial. *Lancet*. 2003;361(9364):1230.

26. Parving HH, Persson F, Lewis JB, et al. Aliskiren combined with losartan in type 2 diabetes and nephropathy. *N Engl J Med*. 2008;358(23):2433–2446.

Renal Artery Stenosis and Renovascular Hypertension

20

Ahsan Usman

GENERAL PRINCIPLES

- Renovascular hypertension (RVHTN) is a common cause of secondary hypertension in adults. The structural finding of a narrowed renal artery alone defines renal artery stenosis (RAS). RVHTN is the resultant increase in blood pressure produced from decreased renal perfusion because of a stenotic lesion in the renal artery(s).
- Injury to the renal parenchyma can occur from decreased renal perfusion as well, resulting in a decrease in kidney function known as *ischemic nephropathy*.
- It is often thought that hypertension in a patient with RAS is caused by the stenotic lesion and the physiologic response of the kidney. However, it is likely to be a more complex process.
- **RAS can be found incidentally in patients without hypertension** and with normal renal function. Moreover, correcting the lesion may or may not improve blood pressure control or renal function.
- Thus, the diagnosis and management of renal artery disease and hypertension requires experience, use of clinical and prognostic factors, and a good understanding of interventions and outcomes.

Causes of RAS

- **Atherosclerotic renal vascular disease** (ASRVD) is the most common cause of RAS (80% of cases).
- **Fibromuscular dysplasia** (FMD) is the second most common cause of RAS (~20%).
- **Other causes of** RAS include vasculitis (i.e., polyarteritis nodosa, Takayasu arteritis), aortic or arterial aneurysm (including dissection), embolic disease, trauma, radiation, or mass effect. These are extremely rare.

Epidemiology

Atherosclerotic Renovascular Disease

- The prevalence of RAS in the general population is unclear, as most data are from autopsy series or patients undergoing angiography for evaluation of other atherosclerotic disease (e.g., cardiac catheterization or lower extremity angiography). In addition, methods and criteria for defining a significant stenosis vary.
- The prevalence of RAS does not equal the prevalence of RVHTN, because a causal relationship is not always clear. A large autopsy study noted RAS in 4.3% of cases, and if there was a history of type 2 diabetes mellitus, the incidence was as high as 8.3%. A combined history of type 2 diabetes and hypertension was associated with a **10% risk** of RAS.[1,2]

- Population-based studies using Doppler techniques in persons aged >65 years found RAS in 6.8% (males, 9.1%; females, 5.5%). RAS was unilateral in 88% of cases and bilateral in 12%. Medicare claims from 1999 to 2001 showed an incidence of newly diagnosed ASRVD of 3.7 per 1000 patient years. Follow-up of this group for another 2 years showed that cardiovascular events from atherosclerotic heart disease in the incident ASRVD patients were higher than in the general population (304 vs. 73 per 1000 patient years).
- It stands to reason that patients with atherosclerotic disease of other vascular beds would be more likely to have ASRVD. For instance, RAS of >50% can be found incidentally in up to 20% of patients undergoing coronary angiography. **A finding of RAS of >75% in this setting is an independent predictor of all-cause mortality.** In patients undergoing angiography for atherosclerotic disease in the aorta or legs, RAS of >50% can be seen in up to 50% of the cases.[3,4]
- **Ischemic nephropathy** is defined as the diminution of renal function due to low blood flow caused by an obstructive lesion in the renal artery. According to the U.S. Renal Data System report from 2000 to 2004, the incidence of ESRD from RAS was 1.8%. Other studies suggest that ischemic nephropathy may be the **cause of ESRD in up to 11% to 15% of cases.** As the elderly population in the United States is steadily increasing, it is also expected that the incidence of RAS and ischemic nephropathy will rise.[5]

Fibromuscular Dysplasia

- FMD is most common in women with **onset of hypertension below 30 years of age** or in women **under the age of 50 years with refractory or suddenly worsening hypertension.** The most common form of FMD is medial fibroplasias, present with the classic **"string of beads"** appearance on the angiogram. Other arteries may also be affected in this disease.

Pathophysiology

- In 1934, Goldblatt experimentally produced hypertension in dogs by clamping their renal arteries, demonstrating that decreasing perfusion to the kidney(s) could cause systemic hypertension.
- For a lesion to cause significant hemodynamic impairment of blood flow through the renal artery, it must occlude the luminal diameter of the artery by 75% to 80%. When this critical level of stenosis is reached, numerous mechanisms are activated in an attempt to restore renal perfusion. Fundamental to this process is the production of renin in the juxtaglomerular apparatus, which then activates the renin–angiotensin–aldosterone system (RAAS).
- Subsequently, systemic arterial pressure increases until renal perfusion is restored or improved. By experimentally blocking the RAAS, medically or by genetic knockout in animal models for the angiotensin II 1A receptor, this rise in systemic arterial pressure can be prevented.[6]
- Other mechanisms may play a larger role in the long-term elevation of blood pressure such as chronic activation of the sympathetic nervous system, activation of oxidative stress pathways, impaired nitric oxide production, endothelin production, and hypertensive nephrosclerosis.

Maintenance of Hypertension

- Mechanisms of continued RVHTN depend on whether the RAS affects one or both kidneys. The terminology that has evolved from experimental animal models illustrates pathophysiologic concepts in human disease.

- The Goldblatt **2-kidney, 1-clip (2K1C) model** represents **unilateral RAS** in a patient with two functioning kidneys. Central to this concept is the fact that the kidney contralateral to the stenosis is normal and experiences increased perfusion pressure. This kidney adapts to the increased arterial pressure with local suppression of the RAAS and excretion of excess sodium and water. Because of normalization of volume status, poor perfusion to the stenotic kidney is maintained and persistent activation of the RAAS in this kidney occurs. This model is known as *angiotensin II-dependent* RVHTN.[7]
- The **1-kidney, 1-clip (1C1K) model** means that the entire renal mass is distal to a hemodynamically significant stenosis, whether this is bilateral RAS in a patient with two functioning kidneys or unilateral RAS in a patient with a single functioning kidney. In the 1C1K model, the entire renal mass is underperfused, leading to RAAS activation with **sodium retention and volume expansion** leading to increased renal perfusion pressure. Once this occurs, the RAAS is then suppressed and hypertension is thought to be more related to persistent volume expansion. This scenario is known as *angiotensin-independent* or *volume-dependent* RVHTN.[7]

DIAGNOSIS

Clinical Presentation

- There are no clinical characteristics that absolutely differentiate RVHTN from other causes of hypertension.
- Features that may be of use include **acute onset of moderate-to-severe hypertension early or late** in life, and hypertension **refractory to standard therapy.** A list of characteristics that raise clinical suspicion are given in Table 20-1.
- Improved and more aggressive medical treatments for hypertension make refractory hypertension less common; therefore, one should have a high index of suspicion when evaluating patients with hypertension. Early recognition of

TABLE 20-1	CLINICAL CHARACTERISTICS SUGGESTIVE OF RENOVASCULAR HYPERTENSION

Abrupt onset of HTN <30 females (FMD)
Abrupt onset of HTN >50 years of age (ASRVD)
Negative family history for HTN
Worsening of previously controlled HTN
HTN refractory to multiple medications
Recurrent flash pulmonary edema
Unexplained heart failure
Evidence of end-organ damage from malignant HTN
Abdominal bruit
Hypokalemia and metabolic alkalosis with HTN
Increase in serum creatinine after initiation of ACE inhibitor or angiotensin II receptor blocker
Renal asymmetry of >1.5 cm

ACE, angiotensin-converting enzyme; ASRVD, atherosclerotic renovascular disease; FMD, fibromuscular dysplasia; HTN, hypertension.

RVHTN is thought to be important, as success of revascularization appears to be inversely related to the duration of hypertension.

- Episodes of **recurrent flash pulmonary edema** with accelerated hypertension should raise the suspicion of RVHTN and are more commonly found in patients with bilateral disease. This is related to the pathophysiology of the 1C1K model and the resultant tendency toward volume overload and to left ventricular hypertrophy with diastolic dysfunction.
- One series showed that RVHTN was present in 30% of patients reporting to the emergency department with accelerated hypertension and severe hypertensive retinopathy (grade III/grade IV Keith–Wagner changes).[8]
- A **significant and persistent rise (at least 30% to 40%) in serum creatinine after initiation of an angiotensin-converting enzyme inhibitor (ACEI) or angiotensin II receptor blocker (ARB)** suggests the presence of bilateral RAS or RAS in a patient with a single functioning kidney.
- Other characteristics associated with RVHTN include smoking, elevated cholesterol, increased body mass index, and progressive renal failure.
- Reports suggest that RVHTN may rarely be associated with nephrotic range proteinuria.
- Patients may have polydipsia with hyponatremia secondary to the dipsogenic properties of angiotensin II and **may have hypokalemia** related to increased aldosterone activity.[9,10]

Diagnostic Testing

- Before embarking on an extensive diagnostic evaluation for renal artery disease, the clinician should consider whether further intervention will occur if disease is found. Renal artery disease is a relatively common unsuspected finding in certain high-risk groups, as discussed above.
- Most experts **only advocate looking for RAS if it is deemed that the patient would benefit from revascularization therapy.** Factors such as comorbid conditions, age, and risk of intervention should be considered in the decision process (see Table 20-2).
- Given that functional tests measuring renin activity in the blood lack statistical power for diagnosis, **radiographic imaging of the renal vasculature** has become the primary approach to RAS diagnosis. The test chosen depends on institutional expertise, but less-invasive tests are generally preferred initially.

Imaging

- **Renal ultrasound with Doppler:**
  - ○ Blood flow velocities in the renal arteries and aorta are measured using ultrasound with Doppler examination for RAS. Higher velocities indicate a narrowed luminal diameter.

TABLE 20-2	CHARACTERISTICS OF PATIENTS *NOT* LIKELY TO BENEFIT FROM REVASCULARIZATION

Preexisting longstanding hypertension (>3 years)
Kidney size <8 cm
Resistive index >0.8 on renal artery Doppler
Physiologically insignificant stenosis on captopril renogram
Advanced age

○ Doppler ultrasound is widely available, relatively inexpensive, and extends little, if any, risk to the patient. Peak **systolic velocities of >180 cm/s are consistent with RAS.**

○ Ultrasound also allows for assessment of kidney size, asymmetry, as well as other structural abnormalities such as cysts or obstruction.[11] Small kidneys suggest chronic damage, with very low likelihood of improvement in renal function after revascularization.

○ **Resistive index** (RI) can be measured by Doppler ultrasonography and is a measure of overall resistance to renal arterial blood flow. Evidence suggests that a **RI >0.8** is associated with a higher degree of irreversible intrarenal vascular or parenchymal disease, and the kidney may be less functional. Therefore, the RI may be helpful in **predicting the response to revascularization.** Larger studies are needed to further determine its predictive value.[12]

○ *Disadvantages* of renal Doppler ultrasonography are that it is highly dependent on patient body habitus, operator skill, interpreter expertise, and the type of equipment. For these reasons, the sensitivity and specificity vary in the literature, but can be as high as 98% when proficiency is great. Technology and expertise with Doppler ultrasound is growing and it is now often utilized as an initial test for RAS.

- **Spiral computed tomography (CT) scan and CT angiography:**
  ○ CT scanning with CT angiography is a highly sensitive and specific tool for the diagnosis of RAS. However, it is invasive and requires administration of iodinated contrast, which places the patient at high risk for contrast-induced nephropathy. Therefore, CT angiogram is not performed at most centers for diagnosis of RAS.

- **Magnetic resonance angiography (MRA):**
  ○ MRA is being increasingly used as the initial test for RAS. It is also highly sensitive and specific and is noninvasive. It is less operator dependent compared with Doppler ultrasound.
  ○ Iodinated contrast is not required, as in CT angiography. On the other hand, gadolinium has been associated with nephrogenic systemic fibrosis in patients with advanced chronic kidney disease (CKD) and should be used with caution.
  ○ MRA tends to slightly overestimate the severity of a stenotic lesion when compared with angiography because of issues related to maximum spatial resolution.
  ○ MRA is contraindicated in patients with pacemakers, cochlear implants, intracranial aneurysm clips, or other metallic implants.

- **Renal angiography:**
  ○ The **gold standard for the diagnosis of RAS is still renal angiography.** Problems with this procedure include its invasiveness and risk of catheter-induced injury, such as atheroemboli and arterial dissection.
  ○ Patients are also at risk for contrast-induced nephropathy, although digital imaging procedures and use of carbon dioxide as the contrast medium can minimize this complication.
  ○ Angiography is now usually performed only at the time of a percutaneous intervention after another less-invasive test has made the diagnosis of RAS very likely. If noninvasive testing is inconclusive, angiography should be performed.

Functional Testing

- Knowledge of the pathophysiology of RVHTN can be used to help determine the physiologic significance of a stenotic lesion and possibly whether or not it is contributing to or causing RVHTN. These tests are most helpful in patients with **unilateral disease** and with **normal renal function.**

- **Captopril plasma renin activity:**
  - Although increased renin production, measured as plasma renin activity (PRA), is fundamental to the initial rise in blood pressure, the chronic elevation of blood pressure in RVHTN is thought to be from other mechanisms, as noted in the pathophysiology section in this chapter. Renin levels can fall within a few weeks, despite persistently elevated blood pressure. Renin levels are also highly dependent on other factors such as sodium intake, posture, age, race, gender, and medications.
  - Consequently, the usefulness of PRA alone in the evaluation of RVHTN is extremely limited. On the other hand, the predictive value of PRA measurement can be increased by measuring it 1 hour after administration of 25 to 50 mg of captopril, a rapid-acting ACEI. This is called the *captopril PRA* or the *captopril stimulation test.*
  - If RVHTN is being maintained by high angiotensin II levels, renin will be suppressed by normal negative feedback mechanisms. **ACE inhibition will remove this suppression,** and renin production from the stenotic kidney should increase.
  - A major limitation of this test is that antihypertensive medications, including ACEIs, ARBs, diuretics, and β-blockers, must be **held for up to 2 weeks** prior to the test.
  - The test should not be performed in patients with congestive heart failure, edema, cardiovascular instability, or significant renal dysfunction.
  - Sensitivities and specificities in the literature, when done properly, have ranged from 75% to 100% and 60% to 95%, respectively. It may be lower in those with preexisting renal dysfunction.

- **Captopril radionuclide renogram:**
  - Radionuclide imaging of the kidneys can be helpful in evaluating the individual contribution of each kidney to the glomerular filtration rate (GFR).
  - However, its use in diagnosing RAS has a false-positive rate of up to 25%. When combined with the administration of captopril, similar to the captopril PRA, the predictive value can be improved. A rapid-acting intravenous ACEI, such as **enalaprilat,** is used at some institutions.
  - In the kidney distal to a stenosis, GFR is maintained by the efferent arteriolar constrictive effects of angiotensin II. When angiotensin II is blocked by captopril, efferent arteriolar dilatation occurs and GFR in the stenotic kidney often decreases, usually with a corresponding increase in GFR in the nonstenotic kidney. When a radioactive isotope such as Tc-99m diethylene-triamine-penta-acetic acid (DTPA) is given in this setting to measure GFR, the **stenotic kidney will exhibit decreased uptake** with a **delayed peak time and a slower washout time** compared with the nonstenotic kidney.
  - ACEIs or ARBs must be held prior to this test, but other antihypertensive agents can be continued and loop diuretics may even enhance the sensitivity.
  - A **positive captopril renogram indicates the presence of a physiologically significant stenosis that is likely causing RVHTN.** Furthermore, there is evidence to suggest that it can predict a good blood pressure response after percutaneous transluminal renal angioplasty (PTRA), with a sensitivity of 90%.
  - This test has a lower sensitivity in CKD and is generally not used in this setting.

TREATMENT

Natural History

- As with any disease, the approach to management must take into account the natural history of the disease.
- Recent prospective studies using Doppler ultrasound show that progression of ASRVD may not occur as frequently and rapidly as was once thought.
- Progression can occur in as many as 30% of higher-risk patients at 3 years, or as little as 4% in lower-risk patients followed up to 8 years.
- **Progression of disease is related to the initial degree of stenosis.** Progression to complete occlusion may develop in up to 3% to 7% of patients. Risk factors for progression are still poorly understood, but appear to be similar to risk factors for general atherosclerotic disease.[13]
- Complicating matters further, progression of a stenotic lesion may not translate clinically into worsening hypertension or renal function. In a group of patients with high-grade RAS (>70%) followed up for just over 3 years, only 8% eventually required revascularization for refractory hypertension. In the entire group, antihypertensive medication requirement increased, but blood pressure remained relatively unchanged and creatinine rose from 1.4 to 2 mg/dL. This increase in serum creatinine was more pronounced in patients with bilateral RAS. Mortality in this group was 30% and was primarily due to cardiovascular disease.[14]
- As described above, the finding of a high-grade stenosis has been shown to be an independent predictor for all-cause mortality, and patients with ASRVD have been shown to have a higher incidence of atherothrombotic cardiovascular events than the general population.
- It is possible that the **long-term neuroendocrine defects** caused by ASRVD could contribute to **worsening cardiovascular disease.** Therefore, end points of therapy should not only be targeted at blood pressure control and preservation of renal function but should also include reduction in cardiovascular events overall.[15,16]

Indications for Intervention

- Patients with **newly diagnosed, accelerated hypertension** and **rapidly progressive** kidney disease found to have RAS will most likely benefit from revascularization (see **Tables 20-2** and **20-3**). Other indications for revascularization include **recurrent episodes of congestive heart failure** or **flash pulmonary edema.**[17]
- The most common dilemma regarding intervention is the patient with ASRVD who has well-controlled hypertension and stable renal function. Even though

TABLE 20-3	CHARACTERISTICS OF PATIENTS LIKELY TO BENEFIT FROM REVASCULARIZATION

Recent onset or accelerated hypertension
Recent onset or progressive renal failure
Bilateral disease or stenosis in a single functioning kidney
Recurrent flash pulmonary edema
Possibly
Resistive index <0.8 on renal artery Doppler
Physiologically significant stenosis on captopril renogram

the presence of ASRVD portends a higher likelihood of a future cardiovascular event, intervening may or may not change that risk.[18,19]

- Present therapy available for RVHTN and ischemic nephropathy includes medical management, PTRA with or without stent placement, and surgical revascularization.[20]

Medical Management

- **Aggressive medical therapy** targeted at reducing atherosclerotic disease is recommended in all patients with ASRVD. This includes **smoking cessation,** control of dyslipidemia (usually with statins and **low-density lipoprotein goal of <70 mg/dL), glycemic control, aspirin,** and **blood pressure control** according to Joint National Committee (JNC) 7 goals.[21]

- ACEIs and ARBs are the preferred first-line agents, as they have proven benefit in RAS and cardiovascular disease. It is rare for patients to experience a clinically significant drop in their GFR after initiation of these agents, but **close monitoring of serum creatinine** and **optimization of volume status** after initiation of these drugs is recommended.[22,23]

- If GFR does decline, it is usually in a patient with bilateral disease or RAS in a single functioning kidney, and revascularization should be considered.

- Refractory hypertension is generally defined as **inadequate control with three medications,** and in this case revascularization may be considered, but it is unclear if it is beneficial. Even after successful revascularization is performed, medical management is usually necessary and the ability to discontinue all antihypertensive drugs is rare.[24]

Angioplasty and Stent Placement

- PTRA is the preferred revascularization procedure in most institutions. Owing to **high rates of restenosis with balloon angioplasty alone,** especially with ostial lesions, **stent** deployment has been increasingly utilized. This has improved technical success and is now the most widely used procedure for revascularization of RAS.

- Unfortunately, technical success does not guarantee "cure" of hypertension. In fact, three recent prospective randomized controlled trials comparing PTRA with medical therapy alone failed to show a blood pressure difference between the groups. In other analyses, the literature has concluded that there is evidence to support trends toward improvement (not cure) in blood pressure control and renal function with angioplasty compared with medical therapy alone.[25,26]

- The recently published, randomized controlled **ASTRAL trial** (Angioplasty and STenting for Renal Artery Lesions) is the largest study (860 patients) to date in this population and the first trial that analyzed hard end points—renal and cardiovascular events and mortality. It randomized patients with RAS to medical management versus percutaneous renal revascularization, and patients were followed for 34 months. Both groups had similar blood pressure control, but patients in the medical arm were taking slightly higher number of blood pressure medications at 1-year follow-up. However, there was no difference in renal function or the number of cardiovascular events in both groups. There were higher number of amputations in the intervention arm, due to cholesterol emboli after the procedure.[27]

- Given these new data, the decision for revascularization in a patient with RAS should be made after careful assessment of the clinical information and should be individualized. The potential benefits and risks should be explained to the

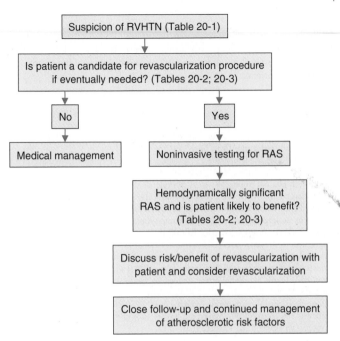

FIGURE 20-1. Approach to treatment.

patient in detail. Figure 20-1 outlines the treatment algorithm for atherosclerotic renal artery stenosis.

Risks of PTRA

- **Restenosis** is estimated to occur in 15% to 20% of cases. Contrast nephropathy complicates the procedure up to 13% of the time but is self-limited. Conversely, acute and progressive deterioration in renal function has been reported to have an incidence of up to 20% in some series.
- Atheroembolic disease is thought to be responsible for a majority of these cases. Studies using distal filter devices after stent placement show that atheroembolic debris can be recovered almost all the time and that by using these devices postprocedure renal function deterioration is less frequent.
- Other complications are **renal artery dissection, renal artery thrombosis, and segmental renal infarction.** Periprocedural death or cardiovascular events each occur with a reported incidence of up to 3%. In ASTRAL trial, 23 patients out of 403 patients in the revascularization arm experienced serious complications, including 2 deaths and 3 amputations.[27]

Surgery

- Before the era of interventional radiology, surgery was the definitive treatment for RAS. Now, it is reserved for situations in which revascularization is necessary but cannot be achieved by the percutaneous route.

Treatment of FMD

- The decision to perform revascularization with PTRA or surgery is less controversial with FMD than with atherosclerotic disease and is usually recommended. Intervention results in a cure or improvement of hypertension in 70% to 90% of patients.[28]

REFERENCES

1. Hansen KJ, Edwards MS, Craven TE, et al. Prevalence of renovascular disease in the elderly: a population based study. *J Vasc Surg.* 2002;36:443–451.
2. Sawicki PT, Kaiser S, Heinemann L. Prevalence of renal artery stenosis in diabetes mellitus—an autopsy study. *J Intern Med.* 1991;229:489–492.
3. Olin JW, Melia M, Young JR, et al. Prevalence of atherosclerotic RAS in patients with atherosclerosis elsewhere. *Am J Med.* 1990;88(1N):46N–51N.
4. Conlon PJ, Little MA, Pieper K, et al. Severity of renal vascular disease predicts mortality in patients undergoing coronary angiography. *Kidney Int.* 2001;60:1490–1497.
5. Caps MT, Perissinotto C, Zierler RE, et al. Prospective study of atherosclerotic disease progression in the renal artery. *Circulation.* 1998;98:2866.
6. Balk E, Raman G, Chung M, et al. Effectiveness of management strategies for renal artery stenosis: a systematic review. *Ann Intern Med.* 2006;145:901.
7. Safian RD, Textor SC. Renal-artery stenosis. *N Engl J Med.* 2001;344:431–442.
8. Davis BA, Crook JE, Vestal RE, et al. Prevalence of renovascular hypertension in patients with grade III or IV retinopathy. *N Engl J Med.* 1979;301:1273.
9. Krijnen P, van Jaarsveld BC, Steyerberg EW, et al. A clinical prediction rule for renal artery stenosis. *Ann Intern Med.* 1998;129:705–711.
10. Chen, R, Novick, AC, Pohl, M. Reversible renin mediated massive proteinuria successfully treated by nephrectomy. *J Urology.* 1995;153:133–134.
11. Olin JW, Piedmonte MR, Young JR, et al. The utility of duplex ultrasound scanning of the renal arteries for diagnosing significant renal artery stenosis. *Ann Intern Med.* 1995;122:833.
12. Radermacher J, Chavan A, Bleck J, et al. Use of Doppler ultrasonography to predict the outcome of therapy for renal-artery stenosis. *N Engl J Med.* 2001;344:410.
13. Pearce JD, Craven BL, Craven TE, et al. Progression of atherosclerotic renovascular disease: a prospective population-based study. *J Vasc Surg.* 2006;44:955.
14. Plouin P-F, Chatellier G, Darne B, et al. Essai Multicentrique Medicaments vs. Angioplastie (EMMA) Study Group. Blood pressure outcome of angioplasty in atherosclerotic renal artery stenosis: a randomized trial. *Hypertension.* 1998;31:823.
15. Mann SJ, Pickering TG. Detection of renovascular hypertension. State of the art: 1992. *Ann Intern Med.* 1992;117:845.
16. Maxwell MH. Cooperative study of renovascular hypertension: current status. *Kidney Int.* 1975;8(suppl):S153.
17. Pickering, TG, Devereux, RB, James, GD, et al. Recurrent pulmonary edema in hypertension due to bilateral renal artery stenosis: treatment by angioplasty or surgical revascularization. *Lancet.* 1988;2:551.
18. Kalra PA, Guo H, Kausz AT, et al. Atherosclerotic renovascular disease in United States patients aged 67 years or older: risk factors, revascularization, and prognosis. *Kidney Int.* 2005;68:293–301.
19. Textor SC. Renovascular hypertension update. *Curr Hypertens Rep.* 2006;8:521.
20. Cooper CJ, Murphy TP, Malsumoto A, et al. Stent revascularization for the prevention of cardiovascular and renal events among patients with renal artery stenosis and systolic hypertension: rationale and design of the CORAL trial. *Am Heart J.* 2006;152:59–66.
21. Plouin PF. Controversies in nephrology: stable patients with atherosclerotic renal artery stenosis should be treated first with medical management—pro. *Am J Kidney Dis.* 2003; 42(5):851.

22. Textor SC. Controversies in nephrology: stable patients with atherosclerotic renal artery stenosis should be treated first with medical management—con. *Am J Kidney Dis.* 2003; 42(5):858.
23. Chabova V, Schirger A, Stanson AW, et al. Outcomes of atherosclerotic renal artery stenosis managed without revascularization. *Mayo Clin Proc.* 2000;75:437.
24. Van Jaarsveld BC, Krijnen P, Pieterman H, et al. The effect of balloon angioplasty on hypertension in atherosclerotic renal-artery stenosis. Dutch Renal Artery Stenosis Intervention Cooperative Study Group. *N Engl J Med.* 2000;342:1007.
25. Webster J, Marshall F, Abdalla M, et al. Randomised comparison of percutaneous angioplasty vs. continued medical therapy for hypertensive patients with atheromatous renal artery stenosis. Scottish and Newcastle Renal Artery Stenosis Collaborative Group. *J Hum Hypertens.* 1998;12:329.
26. Rihal CS, Textor SC, Breen JF, et al. Incidental renal artery stenosis among a prospective cohort of hypertensive patients undergoing coronary angiography. *Mayo Clin Proc.* 2002; 77:309–316.
27. Wheatley K, Ives N, Gray R, et al. Angioplasty and STenting for Renal Artery Lesions (ASTRAL). Revascularization versus medical therapy for renal-artery stenosis, *N Engl J Med.* 2009;361:1953–1962.
28. Slovut DP, Olin JW. Fibromuscular dysplasia. *N Engl J Med.* 2004;350:1862.

Cystic Diseases
of the Kidney

21

Seth Goldberg

POLYCYSTIC KIDNEY DISEASE

GENERAL PRINCIPLES

Classification

- Polycystic kidney disease has two well-defined autosomal dominant forms (autosomal dominant polycystic kidney disease 1 [ADPKD1] and ADPKD2) as well as one with an autosomal recessive inheritance pattern (ARPKD).
- ARPKD leads to severe renal failure in infancy, while both ADPKD forms can remain asymptomatic for several decades before renal dysfunction is evident.

Epidemiology

- ADPKD has an incidence of 1 in 400 to 1000 live births, with no racial or gender predilection; ~85% have a defect in the *PKD1* gene (chromosome 16); whereas 15% have a defect at the *PKD2* locus (chromosome 4).
- ARPKD has an incidence of 1 in 10,000 to 40,000 live births.

Pathophysiology

- The gene products of *PKD1* (polycystin-1) and *PKD2* (polycystin-2) localize to the primary cilia of the nephron, the hepatic bile, and pancreatic ductal epithelium, and to various other tissues in the body.
- These gene products are thought to play a role in flow-mediated mechanosensation as well as cell–cell interactions, and defects lead to abnormal epithelial cell proliferation.
- In ADPKD, epithelial cells proliferate in response to a variety of signals; vasopressin signaling may be impaired and affected cells show an abnormal response to increases in cyclic adenosine monophosphate (cAMP).
- It is unclear why ADPKD has such a variable course even between related patients; only a small percentage of tubules develop cysts, suggesting that a "second-hit" somatic mutation to the normal allele is required to initiate cystogenesis.
- As the cysts enlarge, they become walled off from the rest of the collecting system, explaining why events occurring within the cyst (such as hemorrhage or infection) may not be evident in the urine.
- Enlarging cysts may impinge upon the blood flow to normal nephrons, leading to resistant hypertension and interstitial fibrosis.

DIAGNOSIS

Clinical Presentation

- Diagnosis is often delayed because the disease is **asymptomatic until late in the course.**

- It is frequently discovered on abdominal imaging performed for an alternate indication; ADPKD-specific reasons for ultrasonography include unexplained early-onset hypertension, elevated creatinine, or pain from an expanding cyst, cyst hemorrhage, or cyst infection.

History
- The history should include an in-depth **family history,** including relatives who may have required dialysis or a transplant and the age that they reached end-stage renal disease.
- Family history of **cerebral aneurysms or sudden death of unknown etiology** must be ascertained, as this would put the patient at risk for a similar event and necessitate screening.
- A personal history of headaches or neurological symptoms must be sought.
- Flank and abdominal pain may be suggestive of symptomatic renal or hepatic cysts.
- A history of hematuria, dysuria, and nephrolithiasis should be investigated.
- **Caffeine intake** should be quantified.[1]
- In women, the history of **estrogen exposure** (pregnancy, contraception, hormone replacement therapy) should be assessed.

Physical Examination
- The physical examination is **often normal in the early stages** of ADPKD.
- The first presenting sign of an underlying problem is frequently early-onset hypertension.
- As the kidneys progressively enlarge, the cysts may be palpable on abdominal examination.
- Hepatic cysts may also be palpable and elicit epigastric tenderness.
- Cardiac auscultation may reveal the mid-systolic click of mitral stenosis.

Diagnostic Criteria

- The diagnosis of ADPKD is made using the **combination of renal cysts, family history, and the constellation of extrarenal manifestations.**
- **Ultrasound diagnostic criteria** have been established for patients at risk for type 1 ADPKD (Table 21-1); however, the absence of cysts in a patient under the age of 30 does not rule out the disease.[2]
- As computed tomography (CT) scans or magnetic resonance imaging (MRI) can detect smaller cysts, the conventional diagnostic criteria do not apply to these modalities and no guidelines have been validated.
- The use of MRI technology is primarily limited to the research setting, where the growth rate of kidney and cyst volume can be measured as a surrogate marker for disease progression.[3,4]

TABLE 21-1	ULTRASOUND CRITERIA FOR DIAGNOSIS OF TYPE 1 ADPKD
Age	**Number of Cysts Required**
<30	At least two cysts in one or both kidneys
30–59	At least two cysts in each kidney
≥60	At least four cysts in each kidney

- Commercial **genetic testing** is available for ADPKD (types 1 and 2), with use primarily in young patients contemplating living kidney donation to an affected family member in order to rule out subclinical disease; the accuracy of the test depends on identifying the specific mutation (which differs between families) and so the utility of the genetic test is limited in patients with few or no affected relatives.
- Routine **screening of at-risk family members** (with ultrasonography or genetic testing) is **not currently recommended,** as there is no specific disease-modifying therapy available for the asymptomatic patient; early diagnosis may lead to emotional anguish and possible difficulties in obtaining health insurance.
- It is, however, prudent for at-risk relatives to obtain regular blood pressure checks, and to pursue further evaluation if indicated.

Differential Diagnosis

- The diagnosis of ADPKD is not difficult when there is an established family history of disease; when absent, the possibility of an alternative renal cystic disease must be excluded.
- Acquired cystic disease in the presence of renal dysfunction typically exhibits small, shrunken kidneys.
- The cysts in medullary cystic kidney disease (MCKD) are often a late manifestation, with small-to-normal–sized smooth-contoured kidneys and cysts confined to the corticomedullary junction or renal medulla.
- Medullary sponge kidney (MSK) can also be distinguished from ADPKD by the medullary location of the cysts and collecting duct dilation.
- Solid renal nodules are uncommon in ADPKD, but may be seen in tuberous sclerosis and von Hippel–Lindau (VHL) syndrome.
- The presence of extrarenal manifestations, such as hepatic cysts, can be a helpful clue to make the diagnosis of ADPKD.

TREATMENT

- There is **no specific therapy currently available** for ADPKD, although numerous medications are being studied for efficacy and safety (vasopressin antagonists, water therapy, inhibitors of the mammalian target of rapamycin, somatostatin analogues, growth factor receptor blockers).[5,6]
- Management is primarily centered on **strict blood pressure control** and addressing the complications of chronic kidney disease as they develop.
- Angiotensin-converting enzyme inhibitors and angiotensin receptor blockers are considered first-line antihypertensive agents.
- Anemia is not often an early problem for these patients, as compared to other causes of chronic kidney disease, because of the production of erythropoietin by cells surrounding the cysts.
- **Caffeine intake should be reduced or avoided,** as animal models have implicated caffeine as a promoter of cyst growth; however, evidence in human studies is not available.
- Large-volume surgical cyst reduction does not affect long-term renal outcomes, although selected aspiration and sclerosis of severely symptomatic renal or hepatic cysts can provide relief.

COMPLICATIONS

Renal Manifestations

- **Hematuria** is a common finding in patients with ADPKD and may represent a ruptured cyst, nephrolithiasis, or infection.
- **Cyst hemorrhage** is self-limited, lasting for several days to 1 to 2 weeks and can be very painful; as cysts may have become walled off from the rest of the urinary tract, hematuria is not always present. Cyst hemorrhage is treated conservatively with oral hydration, bed rest, and analgesia.
- **Cyst infection** may present with fever, dysuria, pyuria, and flank pain; however, as with cyst hemorrhage, there may not be direct communication with the rest of the collecting system and so lower urinary findings may be minimal and the urine culture may be negative. Treatment of cyst infection should include an antibiotic with good cyst penetration (ciprofloxacin, sulfamethoxazole–trimethoprim, or chloramphenicol) for at least 3 to 4 weeks.
- **Nephrolithiasis** can occur in patients with ADPKD, with an increased frequency of uric acid stones as compared to the general population; calcium-based stones are also common in this group.
- A full metabolic stone workup should be performed in ADPKD patients with nephrolithiasis to look for hypocitraturia, hypercalciuria, hyperuricosuria, and low urine volume.
- **Hypertension** in this population is thought to be mediated, at least partially, through activation of the renin–angiotensin–aldosterone axis through local ischemia from external compression by enlarging cysts; the onset of hypertension is often early, with preserved renal filtration.
- A concentrating defect is generally mild and may be seen early in the disease course; this may be accounted for by vasopressin receptor (V_2) signaling abnormalities.

Extrarenal Manifestations

- **Liver cysts** are common and are present in up to 80% of patients with ADPKD; progression to liver dysfunction, however, is very uncommon.
  - Liver enlargement may lead to abdominal fullness, discomfort, or early satiety; in unusual circumstances, the pain may be severe enough as to prompt cyst drainage with sclerosis or surgical unroofing.
  - Liver cysts are more common in women with increased estrogen exposure.
- **Cerebral aneurysms** constitute the most serious extrarenal manifestation and are found to cluster within families with certain mutations.
  - When there is a family history of a cerebral aneurysm or sudden death of unknown cause, the incidence is increased to 20%; in the absence of such a family history, the risk is no greater than in the general population (1% to 2%).
  - The risk of aneurysm rupture is greater in patients with uncontrolled hypertension.
  - Patients with neurological symptoms or those with a family history of cerebral aneurysms should undergo magnetic resonance angiography testing; others who should be screened include patients with high-risk occupations in which loss of consciousness would put others at risk (such as commercial pilots), patients needing anticoagulation, or those undergoing surgery with potential hemodynamic instability.

○ Smaller cysts (<5 to 7 mm) may be followed serially by a neurosurgeon, while those that are at higher risk of rupture should undergo repair.

○ For patients at increased risk for cerebral aneurysms but with negative scans, reimaging at 10 years can be performed to detect new lesions.

• **Colonic diverticulosis** occurs with greater frequency in patients with ADPKD with a higher risk of perforation compared to the general population.

• **Cardiac valvular disease,** particularly mitral valve prolapsed, is common in ADPKD patients; most are asymptomatic, although antibiotic prophylaxis for invasive procedures is recommended in these patients.

• **Abdominal wall hernias** occur with increased frequency, and may worsen if peritoneal dialysis is pursued in these patients without surgical correction.

PATIENT EDUCATION

• All patients with ADPKD should be counseled regarding the mode of inheritance and the 50% risk to each offspring.

• Other relatives may also be at risk (depending on whether the patient's disease is familial or sporadic); however, routine screening is not currently recommended as there is yet no disease-modifying therapy available.

• Monitoring of blood pressure and for neurological symptoms suggestive of cerebral aneurysm should be undertaken in at-risk family members, and ultrasonography should be performed only if the results would significantly alter management.

• Although the exact nature of the risk has not been defined, patients should be counseled in restricting caffeine intake and avoiding estrogen-based therapies.

PROGNOSIS

• At the present time, without proven therapies to slow cyst growth, the **typical outcome is progression toward end-stage renal disease.**

• In ADPKD1, ~50% of patients require renal replacement therapy by the age of 60; this is delayed by 15 years in ADPKD2.

• Appropriate candidates for renal transplantation should be identified and evaluated early, anticipating their need for renal replacement therapy to minimize or entirely avoid time spent on dialysis.

SIMPLE RENAL CYSTS

GENERAL PRINCIPLES

Epidemiology

• Simple renal cysts are very common in the general population (5%) and can be found in healthy kidneys.

• Prevalence increases with age, with roughly one-quarter of the general population having a simple cyst on ultrasound by the age of 50.

Pathophysiology

• Simple cysts are typically solitary, but the finding of multiple cysts is not uncommon.

• They can be unilocular or multilocular.

- They are lined with a single layer of flattened epithelial cells and are confined to the renal cortex.
- The etiology of simple cyst formation is not fully understood.

DIAGNOSIS

Clinical Presentation

- Simple cysts are **almost always asymptomatic,** usually found incidentally on imaging for an alternate purpose.
- In rare circumstances, large cysts (>10 cm in diameter) can cause local symptoms such as a palpable abdominal mass or abdominal pain.
- Cyst infection, hemorrhage, or urinary obstruction (if near the renal pelvis) rarely complicate simple cysts.
- Renal function is typically preserved, although hypertension may be noted if the cyst compresses a large vessel.

Diagnostic Criteria

- Size is quite variable, and can range from <1 cm to >10 cm in diameter.
- **Ultrasonography** is the best initial modality to evaluate simple cysts.
- Typically, on ultrasound, simple cysts are (a) anechoic, (b) round in shape with smooth walls, and (c) exhibit sharp definition of the posterior wall with a strong acoustic enhancement.
- Scanning under CT can further characterize renal cysts, should the diagnosis be in question.[7]

Differential Diagnosis

- Simple cysts can be differentiated from polycystic disease by their fewer numbers, lack of extrarenal manifestations, normal kidney size and function, and lack of family history.
- Unlike acquired cystic disease, simple cysts are generally associated with a normal creatinine level (unless a separate disease has caused renal dysfunction).
- The primary differential is to distinguish simple cysts from malignant masses.
- If the appearance is typical for a simple cyst on ultrasonography, no further evaluation is indicated; the Bosniak classification system on CT scanning (Table 21-2) can help characterize the lesion if there is still concern, with categories III and IV needing surgical evaluation as the risk of malignancy is high.

TREATMENT

- Almost all simple cysts are asymptomatic and require **no specific therapy.**
- Pain from a large cyst is managed conservatively.
- If clinically warranted, a painful cyst resistant to therapy can be aspirated and sclerosed by either a percutaneous or surgical route.

PROGNOSIS

- Simple cysts do not cause progressive renal dysfunction.
- If there is a decline in renal function, obstruction should be ruled out and an alternative explanation sought.

TABLE 21-2	BOSNIAK RENAL CYST CLASSIFICATION SYSTEM

Category	Description
I	**Simple benign cyst** Hairline-thin wall Measures water density No enhancement No septa, calcifications, or solid components
II	**Benign cyst with additional features** Fine calcifications Few hairline-thin septa "Perceived" enhancement Mass <3 cm with high attenuation but no enhancement
IIF	**Cysts with minimally complicated features** Multiple hairline-thin septa or smooth thickening of wall or septa Calcifications may be thick and nodular No measurable enhancement Generally well marginated Lesions >3 cm with high attenuation
III	**"Indeterminate" cystic mass** Thickened irregular or smooth walls or septa with enhancement
IV	**Mass with high likelihood of malignancy** All criteria of category III Adjacent enhancing soft-tissue components

ACQUIRED RENAL CYSTS

GENERAL PRINCIPLES

Epidemiology

- Acquired cystic disease occurs in patients with advanced chronic kidney disease or end-stage renal disease.
- The incidence increases with time on dialysis, with up to 90% of patients affected after 10 years or more.
- African-American men tend to develop the disease earlier in the course.

Pathophysiology

- Chronic uremia with compensatory hyperplasia of the nephron is believed to underlie the development of acquired cystic disease, with bilateral involvement in most cases.
- Cysts form primarily from the proximal tubules with epithelial hyperplasia.
- The overall size of the kidney tends to be small to normal, as opposed to the massive enlargement frequently seen in ADPKD.
- Transformation into renal cell carcinoma occurs more frequently than in the absence of acquired cystic disease; the papillary subtype predominates as opposed to otherwise more common clear cell or granular subtypes.

DIAGNOSIS

Clinical Presentation
- Most often, acquired cystic disease is **asymptomatic.**
- Cyst hemorrhage can occur, presenting with flank or back pain as well as hematuria.
- Pain may arise from an enlarging cyst itself, although this is uncommon.

Diagnostic Criteria
- Ultrasonography can easily identify cysts; however, **CT/MRI is recommended for evaluating symptomatic patients or those with suspicious cysts.**
- Screening for transformation into renal cell carcinoma remains controversial, given the typically reduced life expectancy in patients on dialysis; patients who have extended life expectancies, have survived on dialysis for more than 3 years, or who are being evaluated for transplantation may benefit from screening, although formalized guidelines are not available.[8]

Differential Diagnosis
- Acquired cystic disease can be distinguished from ADPKD, as the kidneys remain small to normal in size, with a smooth contour.
- Simple cysts typically appear in fewer numbers than acquired cysts.

TREATMENT

- Acquired cysts are **generally asymptomatic and require no specific treatment.**
- Cyst hemorrhage is typically a self-limited process and can be managed with bed rest, hydration, and analgesia, as well as avoiding heparin on dialysis.
- Severe bleeding episodes are unusual, but may require embolization or nephrectomy.
- Patients with a suspicious lesion on CT/MRI that is >3 cm in diameter should undergo nephrectomy.

PROGNOSIS

- Approximately 2% to 7% of patients with acquired cystic disease will have transformation to renal cell carcinoma.
- Screening may be useful for patients with an anticipated life expectancy longer than the average patient on dialysis.

MEDULLARY CYSTIC KIDNEY DISEASE

GENERAL PRINCIPLES

Classification
- MCKD is a complex of disorders manifesting as cyst development at the corticomedullary junction; progression with interstitial fibrosis typically leads to end-stage renal disease.

- Nephronophthisis is a childhood disorder usually diagnosed by age 15; it is an autosomal recessive disorder.
- The adult forms of MCKD have an autosomal dominant inheritance, with MCKD1 (chromosome 1) and MCKD2 (chromosome 16) from two distinct genetic loci.

Epidemiology

- All forms of MCKD are rare.
- Although juvenile nephronophthisis has an incidence of 1 in 1,000,000, it is the most common genetic cause of end-stage renal disease under the age of 20.
- There is no racial or gender predilection for MCKD.

Pathophysiology

- The gene products of MCKD appear to localize to the primary cilia in the nephron.
- As in ADPKD, there may be a defect in flow-mediated sensation or cell–cell interaction that results in cell proliferation and cyst formation.[9]
- Cysts form at the corticomedullary junction and arise late in the course of disease; they are not absolutely necessary for diagnosis.

DIAGNOSIS

Clinical Presentation

- Patients with the adult forms typically present in the third and fourth decades of life.
- A family history is common given the autosomal dominant inheritance pattern, but sporadic mutation can occur.
- A **concentrating defect** in the kidney may be pronounced, with **severe sodium wasting.**
- Other defects of the distal nephron are common, such as impaired H^+ excretion leading to a distal renal tubular acidosis (type 1 RTA).

Diagnostic Criteria

- **CT scans** may detect numerous small cysts at the corticomedullary junction, with sizes ranging from <0.5 to 2 cm in diameter.
- **Ultrasonography** can also be used to detect the larger cysts, showing small-to-normal–sized kidneys with smooth outlines.

Differential Diagnosis

- Unlike ADPKD, the kidneys in MCKD are smooth and not enlarged, whereas the cysts, when present, are confined to the corticomedullary junction or renal medulla.
- Also, extrarenal cysts are not common in MCKD.

TREATMENT

- As no specific therapy is available for MCKD, **treatment is generally supportive.**
- **Maintenance of an adequate fluid volume** is important to replace urinary salt and water losses.

PROGNOSIS

- **Progression to end-stage renal disease** is the typical pattern for MCKD.
- MCKD1 has a more rapid progression, with a median age of 62 years for end-stage renal disease versus 32 years for MCKD2.

MEDULLARY SPONGE KIDNEY

GENERAL PRINCIPLES

Epidemiology
- MSK is a developmental disorder with cystic dilation of the distal nephron (collecting ducts within the medullary pyramids).
- It is not believed to be a genetically inherited disorder.
- Incidence is 1 in 5000 live births with no racial or gender predilection, although many more cases are probably undiagnosed.

Pathophysiology
- The pathogenesis is unknown.
- Only the inner papillary portions of the medulla are affected with cystic dilation, ranging from 1 to 7 mm in size.
- Most cysts communicate directly with the collecting system.
- Abnormalities of distal tubular function are common and account for the typical complications of MSK.
- Defects in urinary concentration may result from impaired vasopressin response (nephrogenic diabetes insipidus).
- Impaired H^+ excretion results in a distal renal tubular acidosis (type I RTA), and the accompanying hypocitraturia and increased calcium filtration can lead to nephrolithiasis.
- Urinary stasis within the cysts predisposes to infection, pyelonephritis, and abscess formation.

DIAGNOSIS

Clinical Presentation
- Patients are **typically asymptomatic** and the abnormality is frequently picked up on imaging for another cause.
- Complications of the disease, such as nephrolithiasis or recurrent urinary tract infections, can bring these patients to medical attention.
- **Gross hematuria** can occur in up to 20% of patients, either in isolation or in association with a renal stone or infection.
- Renal function is typically normal, and deterioration is not seen as long as the stone and infectious complications are appropriately managed.

Diagnostic Criteria
- The gold standard for making the diagnosis of MSK is **intravenous excretory pyelography.**
  - Dilated collecting ducts appear as linear striations, causing a classic "paintbrush" effect.

○ Ectatic areas appear as "bouquets of flowers" or as "bunches of grapes."
- Ultrasonography is generally unable to identify the small cysts.

Differential Diagnosis
- Like with MSK, MCKD also involves the deeper portions of the kidney; however, renal dysfunction and a family history are typically absent in MSK.
- MSK can usually be distinguished from ADPKD by the smaller size of the cysts, normal renal function, and absence of a family history.

TREATMENT

- Patients with MSK should be encouraged to **maintain adequate fluid intake** to avoid urinary stasis and reduce stone formation.
- Close vigilance and early eradication of urinary tract infections can reduce infectious complications.
- Persistent hematuria, particularly in patients >50 years of age, should prompt an evaluation for malignancy or other causes.
- **Acid–base balance should be monitored** and **persistent metabolic acidosis treated** in order to protect long-term bone health.

PROGNOSIS

- As MSK is a developmental disorder and not a progressive one, **long-term prognosis is excellent.**
- Overall patient health is determined by correction of disease complications and not the renal malformations themselves.

TUBEROUS SCLEROSIS

GENERAL PRINCIPLES

Epidemiology
- Tuberous sclerosis is an inherited disease complex, involving benign growths in the kidneys (angiomyolipomas), brain, retina, lungs, and soft tissues.
- Two distinct types are defined genetically: TSC1 on chromosome 9 (hamartin) and TSC2 on chromosome 16 (tuberin), with autosomal dominant transmission.
- Incidence is estimated at 1 in 6000 to 10,000 live births, affecting all races and ethnicities.
- The genetic locus for TSC2 is adjacent to the locus for PKD1, and thus ~2% of patients with TSC2 will also have PKD1 (with a more severe renal phenotype and earlier progression).

Pathophysiology
- The gene products of TSC1 and TSC2 are tumor suppressors acting on the mTOR (Mammalian target of rapamycin) complex.
- Hamartomas, angiomyolipomas, and renal cysts develop from unopposed cell proliferation.

DIAGNOSIS

Clinical Presentation

- Extrarenal manifestations are most characteristic, with **hamartomas** in the brain, retina, soft tissue, and lungs; a history of **epilepsy** is common.
- The kidneys typically develop angiomyolipomas, which can lead to **hematuria**.
- Although cyst formation occurs in only 20% to 30% of patients, they can be quite large in size.
- Renal dysfunction is uncommon and development of renal cell carcinoma is rare, but the risk is elevated as compared to the general population.
- Symptoms tend to be more severe with mutations in TSC2 as compared to TSC1.

Diagnostic Criteria

- Diagnosis rests on the typically clinical extrarenal manifestations; major and minor criteria have been defined (Table 21-3).[10]
- **Renal angiomyolipomas** constitute a major criterion; whereas **renal cysts** make up a minor criterion.

TABLE 21-3	CRITERIA FOR DIAGNOSIS OF TUBEROUS SCLEROSIS
Major features	Facial angiofibromas or forehead plaque
	Nontraumatic ungula or periungual fibromas
	Three or more hypomelanotic macules
	Connective tissue nevus (Shagreen patch)
	Multiple renal nodular hamartomas
	Cortical tuber
	Subependymal nodule
	Subependymal giant cell astrocytoma
	Cardiac rhabdomyoma
	Lymphangiomyomatosis
	Renal angiomyolipoma
Minor features	Multiple random pits in dental enamel
	Hamartomatous rectal polyps
	Bone cysts
	Cerebral white matter radial migration lines
	Gingival fibromas
	Nonrenal hamartomas
	Retinal achromatic patch
	"Confetti" skin lesions
	Multiple renal cysts

Definite TSC: Two major features or one major feature plus two minor features

Probable TSC: One major feature plus one minor feature

Possible TSC: One major feature OR two or more minor features

TSC, tuberous sclerosis.

- Ultrasonography can define the cystic structures, but angiomyolipomas may be better evaluated with CT scanning or MRI.
- Genetic tests for TSC1 and TSC2 have been available since 2002, although they have a significant false-negative rate.

Differential Diagnosis

- The presence of fat in the renal lesions, as detected on imaging, can help identify them as angiomyolipomas.
- Yearly CT/MRI follow-up of known lesions should be undertaken to determine if suspicious growth patterns develop.

TREATMENT

- Management is primarily **centered on the neurological manifestations**, with **antiepileptic medications** to treat seizures.
- Given the implication of an overactive mTOR pathway, studies using the mTOR inhibitors, sirolimus and everolimus, have shown promise, particularly for neurological manifestations.[11]
- **Renal disease is not typically progressive** and thus requires no specific treatment.
- **Yearly imaging** can identify suspicious changes for renal cell carcinoma.

VON HIPPEL–LINDAU SYNDROME

GENERAL PRINCIPLES

Epidemiology

- The VHL syndrome is an inherited disease complex of cerebellar and retinal hemangioblastomas, adrenal pheochromocytomas (up to 20%), renal/pancreatic cysts and carcinomas (40% incidence).
- Inheritance is autosomal dominant with the genetic abnormality on chromosome 3.
- The incidence of this disease is ~1 in 35,000.

Pathophysiology

- The precise nature of the underlying tumor and cyst development has not been fully elucidated.
- Studies have implicated uncontrolled angiogenesis, through abnormal regulation of hypoxia-inducible factors, mTOR overactivity, and microtubular abnormalities during cell division.

DIAGNOSIS

Clinical Presentation

- The VHL syndrome can present with **malignancies of the kidney, pancreas, adrenal glands (pheochromocytoma), or brain and retina (hemangioblastoma)**.

- **Neurologic symptoms** depend on the local expansion of the nonmetastatic cerebellar hemangioblastomas.
- **Renal cysts** may be large and plentiful, simulating ADPKD with renal dysfunction.
- **Malignant tumors** generally arise separately from the cysts, although renal cysts can show evidence of epithelial dysplasia and progress to solid malignant lesions.
- Not all mutations confer the same risk for developing renal cell carcinoma; mutations that result in the production of truncated proteins are associated with a higher risk of developing this malignancy, and thus tends to cluster within families.[12]

Diagnostic Criteria

- **CT scans** are preferred over ultrasonography, given their ability to identify smaller lesions.
- However, ultrasonography can be helpful in distinguishing cystic lesions from solid masses.
- **Genetic testing** is available for VHL and can determine the need for cancer screening in at-risk relatives.

Differential Diagnosis

- VHL may be difficult to distinguish from ADPKD when a family history is absent and the cysts are large and numerous; extrarenal manifestations can be helpful in separating these diseases.
- A high index of suspicion is necessary when evaluating a patient with cysts but without a family history of a cystic syndrome.

TREATMENT

- **Imaging of renal lesions with CT scanning** every 6 months to 1 year is recommended.
- Suspicious enlarging solid lesions should undergo nephron-sparing surgical removal.

REFERENCES

1. Belibi FA, Wallace DP, Yamaguchi T, et al. The effect of caffeine on renal epithelial cells from patients with autosomal dominant polycystic kidney disease. *J Am Soc Nephrol.* 2002; 13:2723–2729.
2. Ravine D, Gibson RN, Walker RG, et al. Evaluation of ultrasonographic diagnostic criteria for autosomal dominant polycystic kidney disease 1. *Lancet.* 1994;343:824–827.
3. Chapman AB, Guay-Woodford LM, Grantham JJ, et al. Renal structure in early autosomal-dominant polycystic kidney disease (ADPKD): the consortium for radiologic imaging studies of polycystic kidney disease (CRISP) cohort. *Kidney Int.* 2003;64:1035–1045.
4. Grantham JJ, Torres VE, Chapman AB, et al. Volume progression in polycystic kidney disease. *New Engl J Med.* 2006;354:2122–2130.
5. Serra AL, Poster D, Kistler AD, et al. Sirolimus and kidney growth in autosomal dominant polycystic kidney disease. *N Engl J Med.* 2010;363:820–829.
6. Walz G, Budde K, Mannaa M, et al. Everolimus in patients with autosomal dominant polycystic kidney disease. *N Engl J Med.* 2010;363:830–840.

7. Israel GM, Bosniak MA. An update of the Bosniak renal cyst classification system. *Urology.* 2005;66:484–488.

8. Choyke PL. Acquired cystic kidney disease. *Eur Radiol.* 2000;10:1716–1721.

9. Kiser RL, Wolf MTF, Martin JL, et al. Medullary cystic kidney disease type 1 in a large Native-American kindred. *Am J Kidney Dis.* 2004;44:611–617.

10. Roach ES, DiMario FJ, Kandt RS, Northrup H. Tuberous sclerosis consensus conference: recommendations for diagnostic evaluation. National Tuberous Sclerosis Association. *J Child Neurol.* 1999;14:401–407.

11. Krueger DA, Care MM, Holland K, et al. Everolimus for subependymal giant-cell astrocytomas in tuberous sclerosis. *N Engl J Med.* 2010;363:1801–1811.

12. Gallou C, Joly D, Mejean A, et al. Mutations of the VHL gene in sporadic renal cell carcinoma: definition of a risk factor for VHL patients to develop an RCC. *Hum Mutat.* 1999; 13:464–475.

Renal Diseases in Pregnancy

Sindhu Garg and Tingting Li

GENERAL PRINCIPLES

- Pregnancy is associated with predictable anatomic changes of the kidney and is characterized by physiologic changes of systemic and renal hemodynamics.
- Hypertension and proteinuria should be considered pathologic, and the presence of these findings must lead to consideration of preeclampsia as well as other conditions.
- Women with mild kidney disease have a slightly higher risk of maternal and fetal complications, but their pregnancies are generally successful.
- More advanced kidney disease is associated with lower fertility rates and worse maternal and fetal outcomes.

Normal Anatomic Renal Changes in Pregnancy

- **Kidney size increases** by 1.0 to 1.5 cm in pregnancy. Kidney volume increases by 30% due to increased renal blood flow and increased interstitial volume.[1]
- Renal histology and nephron numbers are unchanged.[1]
- **Dilation of the ureters** (hydroureter) and renal pelvis/calyces (hydronephrosis) occurs due to the smooth muscle relaxing effect of progesterone, causing reduced ureteral tone and peristalsis. These are physiologic findings and occur in ~80% of pregnant women, more prominent on the right side.[2]
- Extrinsic compression of the ureters by the gravid uterus may cause **mechanical obstruction** as the pregnancy progresses, but this is usually of no clinical significance.
- The dilated collecting system can result in urinary stasis, leading to an **increased risk for ascending infection** of the urinary tract.

Normal Hemodynamic Changes in Pregnancy

- Systemic hemodynamics[3]:
  - There is **reduction in systemic vascular resistance** in early pregnancy, leading to a drop in mean arterial blood pressure by 10 mm Hg by the second trimester.
  - The reduced systemic vascular resistance leads to increased sympathetic activity, resulting in 15% to 20% **increase in heart rate.**
  - Cardiac output increased by 30% to 50% due to increased heart rate and stroke volume, and reduced after load.
  - Renin–angiotensin–aldosterone system is activated, leading to **increased sodium and water reabsorption,** resulting in retention of up to 900 mEq of extra sodium during the entire pregnancy and increase of total body water by 6 to 8 L. As a result, **physiologic anemia and edema** are common during normal pregnancy.

TABLE 22-1	EXPECTED LABORATORY VALUES IN PREGNANCY	
	Nonpregnant	Pregnant
Hematocrit (vol/dL)	41	33
Plasma creatinine (mg/dL)	0.7–0.8	0.4–0.5
Plasma osmolality (mOsm/kg)	285	275
Plasma sodium (mmol/L)	140	135
Arterial PCO2 (mm Hg)	40	30
pH	7.40	7.44
Bicarbonate (mmol/L)	25	22
Uric acid (mg/dL)	4.0	3.0
Plasma protein (g/dL)	7.0	6.0

- Renal hemodynamics:
  - Renal vascular resistance decreases during early pregnancy due to incompletely understood mechanisms, leading to a significant **increase in renal blood flow.**
  - Glomerular filtration rate (**GFR**) **increases** during early pregnancy by 50% because of both increased renal blood flow and increased cardiac output.[4]
  - The increase in GFR results in a decrease in serum creatinine (from 0.8 mg/dL to 0.4 to 0.5 mg/dL), serum blood urea nitrogen (from 13 mg/dL to 8 to 10 mg/dL), and serum uric acid levels (from 4 mg/dL to 2 to 3 mg/dL) (see Table 22-1).
  - It is important to remember that **serum creatinine that is considered normal in a non-pregnant female might actually signify significant renal impairment in a pregnant patient.**

Changes in Water Homeostasis

- Mild, asymptomatic **hyponatremia** is due to downward resetting of osmotic threshold for antidiuretic hormone (ADH) secretion and thirst (frequently known as the "**reset osmostat**"). This leads to a new steady-state plasma osmolality of 270 to 275 mOsm/kg and fall in serum sodium level by 5 mEq/L.[5] Reset osmostat is thought to be mediated by human chorionic gonadotropin (hCG).
- During the second half of pregnancy, high levels of placental vasopressinase can lead to increased ADH catabolism. Rarely, **diabetes insipidus** (DI) can ensue but is usually transient.[6]
- DI in pregnancy can be treated with desmopressin, a vasopressin analog that is resistant to the actions of vasopressinase.

Acid–Base Regulation

- In pregnancy, there is increase in minute ventilation and **mild chronic respiratory alkalosis** (PCO_2 falls to 30 mm Hg, pH increases to 7.44, and serum bicarbonate level decreases to 20 to 22 mEq/L because of compensatory increase in renal bicarbonate excretion). This can occur even in the first trimester, as progesterone directly stimulates central respiratory receptors.[7]

Other Renal Changes

- Urinary **protein excretion increases** during pregnancy, **up to 200 mg per 24 hours.** Proteinuria of >300 mg per 24 hours is pathologic.
- Owing to increased filtered load of glucose and amino acids, as well as less efficient tubular reabsorption, pregnant women may have mild glycosuria and aminoaciduria.[3]

HYPERTENSIVE DISORDERS IN PREGNANCY

Definition

- Absolute blood pressure ≥140/90 mm Hg, taken on two separate occasions 6 hours apart, is considered abnormal.

Classification

- **Chronic hypertension** (or preexisting hypertension)[8]:
  - Hypertension diagnosed **prior to 20th week** of gestation, or persisting longer than 12 weeks postpartum
- **Gestational hypertension:**
  - *De novo* hypertension occurring **after 20th week** of gestation and resolving within 12 weeks postpartum
- **Preeclampsia:**
  - **New onset hypertension and proteinuria** (>300 mg per 24 hours) occurring after 20th week of gestation
  - Diagnosis is changed to eclampsia with development of seizures
- **Preeclampsia superimposed on chronic hypertension**

Chronic Hypertension in Pregnancy

- Chronic hypertension occurs in 3% to 5% of all pregnancies[3] and contributes significantly to maternal and fetal morbidity and mortality.
- Pregnancies complicated by hypertension have an increased risk of preeclampsia, intrauterine growth retardation, placental abruption, preterm delivery, and fetal loss.
- Chronic hypertension can be masked in early pregnancy because of the physiologic decrease in blood pressure.
- **Tight blood pressure control does not improve neonatal outcome or prevent superimposed preeclampsia** and **can compromise fetal growth** because of decreased placental perfusion.[9]
- Target blood pressure is ill-defined. Most experts recommend a **goal of 140 to 150/90 mm Hg.**
- Management (see Table 22-2):
  - Pharmacological treatment is recommended when blood pressure is >150/100 mm Hg to prevent maternal end-organ damage.[10]
  - Severe hypertension (≥170/110 mm Hg) can be managed using intravenous labetalol, hydralazine, or nicardipine, as these have been extensively used during pregnancy.
  - Oral agents that are used to treat elevated blood pressure in pregnancy include methyldopa, labetalol, long-acting nifedipine, and hydralazine.
  - Diuretics are generally not recommended during pregnancy because of risk of volume depletion in the fetus.

TABLE 22-2	DRUG OPTIONS FOR HYPERTENSION IN PREGNANCY
Subacute Antihypertensive Therapy	**Acute Antihypertensive Therapy**
Methyldopa: 250 mg PO bid or tid; usual dose, 1.0–1.5 g/d; maximum dose, 3 g/d	Labetalol: 20 mg IV; can be repeated at 10–15-min intervals (with escalating doses, i.e., 40 mg, 60 mg, and so forth) to a total cumulative dose of 300 mg
Nifedipine, long acting: 30 mg/d PO; maximum dose 120 mg/d	Hydralazine: 5–10 mg IV; can be repeated at 15-min intervals to a maximum cumulative dose of 30 mg
Labetalol: 100 mg PO bid or tid; maximum dose, 1200 mg/d	—

○ **Angiotensin-converting enzyme (ACE) inhibitors and angiotensin receptor blockers (ARBs) are CONTRAINDICATED** because of extremely high risk of teratogenicity. Other inhibitors of the renin–angiotensin–aldosterone axis also fall into this category.

Preeclampsia

Epidemiology
- Preeclampsia affects ~5% of all pregnancies and remains the leading cause of maternal and fetal mortality in the world.[11]
- Risk factors for preeclampsia are listed in Table 22-3.

Pathophysiology
- Initiating events in preeclampsia are poorly understood, but the origin appears to be the placenta and the target is the maternal endothelium.
- In normal pregnancy, cytotrophoblasts invade the uterine spiral arterioles, converting them from small-caliber vessels to large-caliber capacitance vessels capable of carrying larger amount of blood flow through the placenta.
- In preeclampsia, this process of cytotrophoblast invasion is defective and there is deficient transformation of the spiral arterioles, leading to reduced placental perfusion.[12]

TABLE 22-3	RISK FACTORS FOR PREECLAMPSIA
Maternal age ≥40	Multiple gestation
Nulliparity	Diabetes mellitus
Preeclampsia in previous pregnancy	Chronic hypertension
Family history of preeclampsia	Chronic kidney disease
Time between pregnancy >10 years	Connective tissue disorder
Obesity	Antiphospholipid syndrome

- The diseased placenta secretes an increased amount of antiangiogenic factor (soluble fms-like tyrosine kinase-1), which antagonizes the proangiogenic effects of vascular endothelial growth factor and placental growth factor, resulting in systemic vascular endothelial dysfunction characteristic of preeclampsia.[13]
- Maternal endothelial dysfunction causes increased production of reactive oxygen species, thromboxane, and endothelin-1. Also, there is increased vascular sensitivity to angiotensin II and decreased nitric oxide and prostacyclin bioavailability.[13]
- The end result is potent vasoconstriction and end-organ damage.

Clinical Presentation

- Symptom onset is usually in the latter part of the third trimester, but can happen anytime after 20th week of gestation, or can be delayed until after delivery.
- Clinical features of preeclampsia are detailed in Table 22-4.
- **Signs and laboratory findings in severe preeclampsia are**[8,14]:
  ○ Blood pressure ≥160/110 mm Hg
  ○ Proteinuria ≥5g per 24 hours or 3+ protein on urine dipstick results
  ○ Oliguria <500 mL urine in 24 hours or elevated serum creatinine
  ○ Hemolysis, elevated liver enzymes, and low platelets (HELLP) syndrome
  ○ Pulmonary edema, impaired liver function
  ○ Headaches, visual disturbances, epigastric or right upper quadrant pain
  ○ Fetal growth restriction

Treatment

- **Definitive treatment is delivery.** Gestational age, severity of preeclampsia, and maternal and fetal condition are all important factors when deciding the appropriate course of action.

TABLE 22-4	CLINICAL FINDINGS IN PREECLAMPSIA
Neurologic	Headache, blurred vision, visual scotomata, hyperreflexia, clonus, and seizures. Cerebral edema and intracerebral hemorrhage can be seen.
Renal	Proteinuria (>300 mg/d), azotemia (decreased renal blood flow and average GFR decreases by 30%–40%), and acute kidney injury—rare and often secondary to acute tubular necrosis. Increased urate reabsorption results in hyperuricemia.
Hematologic	Microangiopathic hemolytic anemia, thrombocytopenia, disseminated intravascular coagulation
Hepatic	Elevated liver enzymes (HELLP syndrome)
Cardiovascular	Hypertension, decreased cardiac output
Gastrointestinal	Elevated liver enzymes, epigastric/right upper quadrant pain, subcapsular hemorrhage, liver rupture
Other	Pulmonary edema, peripheral edema—often facial and lower extremity

GFR, glomerular filtration rate: HELLP, hemolysis, elevated liver enzymes, and low platelets.

- **Indications for urgent delivery**[8]:
  - Greater than or equal to 37 weeks of gestation
  - Refractory hypertension despite adequate therapy
  - Progressive organ system failure (kidney, liver, hematologic parameters, neurological dysfunction)
  - Eclampsia
  - HELLP syndrome
  - Fetal compromise
  - Abruptio placentae
- Management of hypertension:
  - The **goal of treatment is prevention of cerebrovascular and cardiovascular events.**
  - Treatment **does not change the course of preeclampsia and does not prevent progression to eclampsia.**
  - Aggressive lowering of blood pressure in patients with preeclampsia is NOT recommended, as it can further decrease placental perfusion and compromise fetal growth.
  - The blood pressure level at which treatment should begin is undefined. In general, most experts initiate therapy with blood pressure at ≥150 to 160/100 to 110 mm Hg. **Target blood pressure is usually 140 to 150/90 mm Hg.**
  - Please refer to Chronic Hypertension in Pregnancy for recommendations on antihypertensive therapy.
- **Mild preeclampsia management:**
  - Supportive therapy until delivery
  - Complete or partial bed rest
  - Frequent fetal monitoring
  - Blood pressure check twice weekly
  - Laboratory tests: hemoglobin and hematocrit, platelet count, creatinine, hepatic enzymes (aspartate aminotransferase, alanine transaminase, lactate dehydrogenase), uric acid, urine dipstick test.
- **Severe preeclampsia management** includes:
  - Immediate hospitalization
  - **Seizure prophylaxis with magnesium sulfate**
  - **Corticosteroids between 25 and 34 weeks** to decrease the risk of respiratory distress syndrome in infants
  - Acute **management of severe hypertension** with intravenous labetalol, hydralazine, or nicardipine to a target blood pressure of 140 to 150/90 mm Hg
  - **Delivery of fetus**

ACUTE KIDNEY INJURY IN PREGNANCY

- Pregnant patients are susceptible to a variety of causes of acute kidney injury (AKI), including disorders that are pregnancy specific.

Causes of AKI in Pregnancy

Prerenal Azotemia

- Hyperemesis gravidarum
- Other prerenal causes

Acute Tubular Necrosis
- Hyperemesis gravidarum
- Hemorrhage
- Shock/sepsis (e.g., septic abortion, pyelonephritis)

Obstructive Uropathy
- Gravid uterus (rare)
- Large uterine fibroids
- Stones:
  - These are **usually calcium containing** as urinary calcium excretion increases in pregnancy.
  - They are often located in the distal ureter.
  - Most stones tend to **pass spontaneously.**
  - Ureteral stents can be placed in patients unable to pass the stone; percutaneous nephrostomy may be required to decompress the urinary system.
  - Extracorporeal shock wave lithotripsy is not recommended during pregnancy.
  - Obstructive stones with hydronephrosis/pyonephrosis may require cystoscopic or ureteroscopic stone removal.[15]
  - **Risk of infection is increased.**

Acute Pyelonephritis
- Risk factors[16]:
  - **Urinary stasis** due to physiologic hydroureter and hydronephrosis increases risk for upper tract infection.
  - **Anatomic displacement** of ureters by the gravid uterus can also lead to stasis and obstruction, thus increasing risk for pyelonephritis.
  - **Untreated asymptomatic bacteriuria** is a well-known risk factor for urinary tract infections. This is defined by the presence of positive urine culture in an asymptomatic person: $\geq 10^5$ colony-forming units per mL in voided urine on two separate collections or $\geq 10^2$ colony-forming units per mL in a catheterized specimen. It increases risk for adverse fetal outcomes, and routine screen at 12 to 16 weeks is recommended. Treatment is always warranted for asymptomatic bacteriuria.
- Clinical presentation:
  - Fever, dysuria, flank pain
  - Can lead to sepsis and shock
  - AKI can result from focal microabscesses and sepsis/shock
- Treatment:
  - Aggressive treatment with intravenous antibiotics and supportive measures

Renal Cortical Necrosis
- Renal cortical necrosis is secondary to rare catastrophic events resulting in prolonged hypotension and profound renal ischemia, especially to the renal cortex.[17,18] The **damage is irreversible in most cases,** with survivors often requiring long-term dialysis. The well-described causes for renal cortical necrosis are listed below.
- **Causes:**
  - Septic abortion
  - Amniotic fluid embolism
  - Fetal demise with retained fetus
  - Abruptio placentae

- The precipitating event usually leads to disseminated intravascular coagulation and severe renal ischemia.
- **Clinical presentation** includes:
  - ○ Abrupt onset of oliguria/anuria
  - ○ Flank pain
  - ○ Gross hematuria
  - ○ Hypotension (±)
- **Diagnosis:**
  - ○ Ultrasound or computed tomography scan shows hypoechoic or hypodense areas in the renal cortex.
  - ○ Renal biopsy is not routinely done.
- **Treatment:**
  - ○ Supportive measures only as there is no effective therapy.
  - ○ A total of 20% to 40% patients initially require renal replacement therapy.
  - ○ Partial renal recovery can occur, but may take months.

Preeclampsia/HELLP Syndrome
- This is a rare cause of AKI, and has been explained in detailed under preeclampsia.

Acute Fatty Liver of Pregnancy
- This is extremely rare but can be fatal.[18]
- Fatty liver of pregnancy **typically presents in the third trimester.**
- It is extremely important to distinguish from HELLP syndrome and hemolytic uremic syndrome (HUS) (Table 22-5).
- **Clinical features** include:
  - ○ Anorexia
  - ○ Jaundice

TABLE 22-5 DIFFERENTIAL DIGNOSIS OF AKI IN LATE PREGNANCY

Features	HUS	HELLP	Acute Fatty Liver of Pregnancy
Time of onset	Usually postpartum	After 20 weeks	Third trimester
Hepatic involvement	None	Yes	Yes
Thrombocytopenia	Severe	Moderate	Maybe
Coagulopathy	None	Maybe	Often
Hemolytic anemia	Yes	Yes	No
Hypertension	Maybe	Yes	Maybe
Proteinuria	Maybe	Yes	Maybe
Renal dysfunction	Severe	Mild	Severe
Therapy	Plasmapheresis	Delivery	Delivery

AKI, acute kidney injury; HELLP, hemolysis, elevated liver enzymes, and low platelets; HUS, hemolytic uremic syndrome.

○ Nausea and vomiting
○ Abdominal pain
○ AKI: the mechanism is unclear and renal pathology is usually unremarkable.
- Etiology:
  ○ There is extensive microvesicular fatty infiltration of hepatocytes due to defective mitochondrial fatty acid oxidation. The trigger for this is unknown.
- **Laboratory data:**
  ○ Elevated transaminases
  ○ Increased bilirubin/ammonia level
  ○ Prolongation of PTT and PT
  ○ Thrombocytopenia (not prominent)
  ○ Hypoglycemia
- **Treatment:**
  ○ Prompt delivery and supportive care
  ○ Most patients fully recover, but some may require liver transplantation

Hemolytic Uremic Syndrome

- HUS usually presents in the near term or in the immediate postpartum period, but can occur at any stage of pregnancy.
- **Clinical features:**
  ○ Microangiopathic hemolytic anemia
  ○ Thrombocytopenia
  ○ AKI: thrombotic microangiopathy is noted on renal pathology
  ○ Hypertension
- **Treatment:**
  ○ Plasma exchange is the primary treatment.
  ○ Delivery does not appear to change the course of the disease.

CHRONIC KIDNEY DISEASE AND PREGNANCY

- **Fertility is diminished in women with chronic kidney disease (CKD),** especially in those with serum creatinine >3.0 mg/dL or who are dialysis dependent. CKD leads to impairment in the hypothalamic–pituitary–gonadal axis, causing decreased fertility.[19]
- If patients with CKD (regardless of underlying etiology) become pregnant, they are at increased risk for adverse maternal and fetal outcomes.[19]
  ○ **Maternal complications:**
    ■ Increased proteinuria
    ■ Worsening hypertension
    ■ Increased risk for preeclampsia
    ■ Permanently diminished renal function
  ○ **Fetal complications:**
    ■ Prematurity
    ■ Intrauterine growth retardation
    ■ Increased risk for fetal loss
- This risk depends on the severity of baseline renal dysfunction, presence of uncontrolled hypertension, and degree of proteinuria.[20,21]
- Women with preexisting mild CKD (creatinine <1.4 mg/dL), normal blood pressure, and no proteinuria generally have good maternal and fetal outcomes.

- Patients with moderate (creatinine 1.4 to 2.5 mg/dL) or severe (creatinine >2.5 mg/dL) CKD have significantly increased risk of developing worsening renal function, proteinuria, hypertension, as well as increased rates of fetal complications.[22,23]
- In one study, the combined presence of **GFR <40 mL/min/1.73 m²** (CKD stage 3) and **proteinuria >1 g/d** before conception **predicted faster GFR loss after delivery, shorter time to dialysis, and low birth weight.**[24]
- Necessary discontinuation of certain medications (ACE inhibitor, ARB, or certain immunosuppressants) may lead to renal exacerbation or disease flare.
- Women of reproductive age with CKD should be advised of the potential adverse maternal and fetal effects related to pregnancy.

Pregnancy in the Dialysis Patient

- Conception in dialysis patients is very rare (only 0.3% to 1.5% of all women of childbearing age).[20]
- Early pregnancy is **difficult to diagnose as β-HCG is not reliable.**[20]
- **Outcomes** are similar in patients treated with hemodialysis and peritoneal dialysis.[25]
  - **Fetal:**
    - High spontaneous fetal loss (50%)
    - Premature labor (86%)
    - Fetal growth retardation (30%)
  - **Maternal:**
    - Severe hypertension (85%)
    - Increased mortality rate
- Management[26,27]:
  - Hemodialysis:
    - **Longer and more frequent dialysis sessions** can improve fetal outcome (>20 h/wk).
    - It is important to avoid hypotension, hypocalcemia, and metabolic acidosis.
  - Peritoneal dialysis:
    - Decreased fill volume and frequent exchanges might be beneficial.
  - Anemia:
    - Hemoglobin should be maintained above 10 g/dL.
    - Iron and folic acid supplementation should be administered.
    - Erythropoietin should be prescribed cautiously given risk of hypertension, but there does not appear to be a risk for teratogenicity.
  - Nutrition:
    - Protein intake should be ~1.8 g/kg/d and supplemented with vitamins.
  - Blood pressure control:
    - Diuretics do not have a significant role in a dialysis patient and should be used with caution in a non-dialysis CKD patient.
    - ACE inhibitors and ARBs are CONTRAINDICATED in pregnancy.
  - Obstetric care:
    - High-risk obstetric care and serial fetal monitoring during hemodialysis is recommended.

Pregnancy after Renal Transplant

- Return of fertility is the rule in female transplant patients of childbearing age, occurring as early as 1 month following renal transplantation.[28]

- Patients are advised to **wait for at least 1 year and preferably 2 years following renal transplantation before conception.**
- Prior to conception:
  - The pregnancy should be planned and the patient should discuss with treating nephrologist prior to conception.
  - Renal function should be stable with serum creatinine <1.5 mg/dL.
  - Proteinuria should be <500 mg/d.
  - Blood pressure should be controlled with minimal number of medications.
  - There should be no recent episodes of rejection or other transplant-related complications.
  - **Mycophenolate, sirolimus, statins, ACE inhibitor, and ARB should be discontinued prior to pregnancy.**
  - It is important to change these medications to others that are considered "safe" in pregnancy ahead of time and to ensure that the serum creatinine and blood pressure are stable, before conception.
  - Azathioprine, calcineurin inhibitors, and calcium channel blockers may be continued during pregnancy.

Systemic Lupus Erythematosus and Pregnancy

- **Best pregnancy outcomes** occur in women with **quiescent lupus for at least 6 months prior to conception.**[29]
- Pregnancy in women with **active lupus nephritis** is associated with an **increased risk of fetal loss** (up to 75%) and **worsening of both renal and extrarenal manifestations.**[30]
- Women with severe active disease or a high degree of irreversible organ damage, such as symptomatic pulmonary hypertension, heart failure, severe restrictive pulmonary disease, or advanced chronic kidney disease/lupus nephritis, should avoid pregnancy.[31]
- Maintenance therapy for systemic lupus erythematosus or lupus nephritis should be continued during pregnancy to prevent flares, although the choice of therapy is frequently limited by teratogenicity.
- When renal function or proteinuria worsens, low complement levels, rising double stranded DNA antibody levels, and active urine sediment could help differentiate lupus nephritis from preeclampsia.[32]
- There is an **increased risk of thrombosis and fetal loss in the presence of antiphospholipid antibody.**
- The presence of **SSA/SSB antibodies is a risk factor for neonatal heart block.**

REFERENCES

1. Bailey RR, Rolleston GL. Kidney length and ureteric dilatation in the puerperium. *J Obstet Gynaecol Br Commonw.* 1971;78(1):55–61.
2. Rasmussen PE, Nielsen FR. Hydronephrosis during pregnancy: a literature survey. *Eur J Obstet Gynecol Reprod Biol.* 1988;27(3):249–259.
3. Maynard SE, Karumanchi SA, Thadhani R. Hypertension and kidney disease in pregnancy. In: Brenner BM, ed. *Brenner & Rector's The Kidney.* 8th ed. Philadelphia, PA: Saunders Elsevier; 2008:1567–1595.
4. Baylis C. The determinants of renal hemodynamics in pregnancy. *Am J Kidney Dis.* 1987; 9(4):260–264.
5. Lindheimer MD, Barron WM, Davison JM. Osmoregulation of thirst and vasopressin release in pregnancy. *Am J Physiol.* 1989;257(2 Pt 2):F159–F169.

6. Durr JA, Hoggard JG, Hunt JM, et al. Diabetes insipidus in pregnancy associated with abnormally high circulating vasopressinase activity. *N Engl J Med.* 1987;316(17):1070–1074.

7. Lim VS, Katz AI, Lindheimer MD. Acid-base regulation in pregnancy. *Am J Physiol.* 1976; 231(6):1764–1769.

8. National Institutes of Health. *Working Group Report on High Blood Pressure in Pregnancy.* Washington, DC: National Institutes of Health; 2000.

9. Von Dadelszen P, Magee LA. Fall in mean arterial pressure and fetal growth restriction in pregnancy hypertension: an updated metaregression analysis. *J Obstet Gynaecol Can.* 2002; 24(12):941–945.

10. Lindheimer MD, Taler SJ, Cunningham FG. Hypertension in pregnancy. *J Am Soc Hypertens.* 2008;2(6):484–494.

11. Karumanchi SA, Maynard SE, Stillman IE, et al. Preeclampsia: a renal perspective. *Kidney Int.* 2005;67:2101–2113.

12. Meekins JW, Pijnenborg R, Hanssens M, et al. A study of placental bed spiral arteries and trophoblast invasion in normal and severe pre-eclamptic pregnancies. *Br J Obstet Gynaecol.* 1994;101(8):669–674.

13. Gilbert JS, Ryan MJ, LaMarca BB, et al. Pathophysiology of hypertension during pre-eclampsia: linking placental ischemia with endothelial dysfunction. *Am J Physiol Heart Circ Physiol.* 2008;294;H541–H550.

14. ACOG Committee on Practice Bulletins–Obstetrics. ACOG Practice Bulletin. Diagnosis and Management of Preeclampsia and Eclampsia Number 33, January 2002. *Obstet Gynecol.* 2002;99(1):159–167.

15. Stothers L, Lee LM. Renal colic in pregnancy. *J Urol.* 1992;148(5):1383–1387.

16. Thompson C, Verani R, Evanoff G, et al. Suppurative bacterial pyelonephritis as a cause of acute renal failure. *Am J Kidney Dis.* 1986;8(4):271–273.

17. Matlin RA, Gary NE. Acute cortical necrosis. Case report and review of the literature. *Am J Med.* 1974;56(1):110–118.

18. Grunfeld JP, Pertuiset N. Acute renal failure in pregnancy. *Am J Kidney Dis.* 1987;9(4):359–362.

19. Hou S. Pregnancy in women with chronic renal disease. *N Engl J Med.* 1985;312(13):836–839.

20. Hou S. Pregnancy in chronic renal insufficiency and end-stage renal disease. *Am J Kidney Dis.* 1999;33(2):235–252.

21. Fischer MJ, Lehnerz SD, Hebert JR, et al. Kidney disease is an independent risk factor for adverse fetal and maternal outcomes in pregnancy. *Am J Kidney Dis.* 2004;43(3):415–423.

22. Bar J, Ben-Rafael Z, Padoa A, et al. Prediction of pregnancy outcome in subgroups of women with renal disease. *Clin Nephrol.* 2000;53(6):437–444.

23. Jones DC, Hayslett JP. Outcome of pregnancy in women with moderate or severe renal insufficiency. *N Engl J Med.* 1996;335(4):226–232.

24. Imbasciati E, Gregorini G, Cabiddu G, et al. Pregnancy in CKD stages 3 to 5: fetal and maternal outcomes. *Am J Kidney Dis.* 2007;49(6):753–762.

25. Okundaye I, Abrinko P, Hou S. Registry of pregnancy in dialysis patients. *Am J Kidney Dis.* 1998;31(5):766–773.

26. Hou S. Modification of dialysis regimens for pregnancy. *Int J Artif Organs.* 2002;25(9):823–826.

27. Giatras I, Levy DP, Malone FD, et al. Pregnancy during dialysis: case report and management guidelines. *Nephrol Dial Transplant.* 1998;13(12):3266–3272.

28. McKay DB, Josephson MA. Pregnancy in recipients of solid organs–effects on mother and child. *N Engl J Med.* 2006;354(12):1281–1293.

29. Day CJ, Lipkin GW, Savage CO. Lupus nephritis and pregnancy in the 21st century. *Nephrol Dial Transplant.* 2009;24:344–347.

30. Bobrie G, Liote F, Houillier P, et al. Pregnancy in lupus nephritis and related disorders. *Am J Kidney Dis.* 1987;9(4):339–343.

31. Ruiz-Irastorza G, Khamashta MA. Lupus and pregnancy: ten questions and some answers. *Lupus.* 2008;17(5):416–420.

32. Buyon JP, Cronstein BN, Morris M, et al. Serum complement values (C3 and C4) to differentiate between systemic lupus activity and pre-eclampsia. *Am J Med.* 1986;81(2):194–200.

Nephrolithiasis

23

Raghavender Boothpur

GENERAL PRINCIPLES

- Kidney stones are crystalline structures in the urinary tract that have achieved sufficient size to cause symptoms or be visible by radiographic imaging techniques.
- Most kidney stones in Western countries are composed of calcium salts and occur in the upper urinary tract. Conversely, in developing countries, the majority of stones are composed of uric acid and occur in the urinary bladder.
- It is believed that a protein-rich Western diet and lifestyle is responsible for this difference. The economic impact of kidney stones relates to surgical extraction or fragmentation of stones, loss of productivity, and need for preventive treatment.
- Stone formation is associated with increased risk of chronic kidney disease.[1]

Classification

- Chemical composition of stones can be determined in specialized laboratories. On the basis of chemical composition, urinary stones can be classified in the following manner:
- **Stones composed of calcium salts:** In Western societies, 80% of all kidney stones are composed of calcium salts. Of these, 35% are composed exclusively of calcium oxalate; 40% are mixed (i.e., composed of calcium oxalate and calcium phosphate), whereas 5% of stones are composed exclusively of calcium phosphate (hydroxyapatite or brushite).
- **Uric acid stones and struvite stones:** These form roughly 10% to 20% of all stones in the urinary tract. Uric acid stones are radiolucent.
- **Cystine stones:** The hereditary disorder *cystinuria* (not to be confused with *cystinosis*) accounts for ~1% of all cases. Cystinuria is characterized by an amino acid transport defect in the proximal renal tubule, resulting in a urinary loss of dibasic amino acids (Fig. 23-1).
- **Other:** Rarely, stones can be formed by poorly soluble drugs (e.g., triamterene, indinavir), xanthine, hypoxanthine, or ammonium urate.

Epidemiology

- Nephrolithiasis is one of the most common diseases in Western countries. In the United States, the prevalence of nephrolithiasis has increased over the years. Whites are affected more frequently than blacks, Hispanics, or Asian Americans. Prevalence is influenced by age, sex, race, body size, and geographic distribution.[2]
- The peak age of onset is the third decade, with increasing prevalence until the age of 70 years. In women, there is a second peak at the age of 55 years.[2,3]

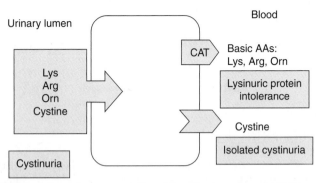

FIGURE 23-1. Schematic representation of the dibasic amino acid (AA) transport in the proximal renal tubule. Cystinuria results from a defect in the dibasic AA transporter on the apical side of the membrane. Hence, cystinuria is also attended by elevated urinary excretion of lysine (Lys), arginine (Arg), and ornithine (Orn). CAT, cationic amino acid transporter. (Data obtained from Lopez-Nieto CE, Brenner BM. Molecular basis of inherited disorders of renal solute transport. *Curr Opin Nephrol Hypertens*. 1997;6:411–421.)

- Historically, men have had a two to three times greater risk than women. More recently, an increasing rate of nephrolithiasis in females has been attributed to more obesity. Larger body mass index (BMI) is associated with an increased risk of nephrolithiasis.[4]
- Lifetime risk of developing a kidney stone is ~12% for men and 6% for women.
- The southeastern states have the highest incidence of nephrolithiasis, which is attributed to higher average temperatures and greater sun exposure, resulting in oversaturation of stone-forming salts in the urine.

Pathophysiology

One can infer from the variety of stones observed that several pathophysiologic mechanisms are responsible for stone formation. Nevertheless, a common pathway leading to stone formation is urinary supersaturation. Crystals form when the amount of solute in the urine exceeds its solubility limits.

Stone Formation

Three steps are necessary to form a stone:

1. Formation of a small initial crystal, or *nidus.*
2. Retention of a nidus in the urinary tract. If washed away by urine flow, crystal formation would remain a mere physiologic curiosity.
3. Growth of a nidus to a size at which it either becomes symptomatic or visible by imaging techniques.

Solubility Product, Formation Product, and Nucleation

- **Solubility product:** Solubility product describes the **level of a solution's saturation with solute at which solid-phase material exists in equilibrium with liquid-phase material.** For a calcium oxalate crystal immersed in a calcium oxalate solution, the solubility product describes a concentration of calcium and oxalate that does not allow the crystal to dissolve. At the same time, the product is too low to permit crystal growth; the size of the calcium oxalate crystal remains unchanged. Concentrations lower than solubility products are **undersaturated.** Concentrations higher than the solubility product are **supersaturated.**

- **Formation product:**
  ○ **Formation product** is the **level of supersaturation at which a solute can no longer remain in a solution and precipitates out spontaneously (homogeneous nucleation).**
  ○ **Nucleation** can take place at a lower level of supersaturation if a solid phase is already present (**heterogeneous nucleation**). Even normal urine is often supersaturated with calcium oxalate. Urinary calcium oxalate product can exceed its solubility by three to four times. Calcium oxalate crystalluria occurs in both stone formers and nonstone formers. Studies suggest that calcium oxalate crystal formation occurs by heterogeneous nucleation. Potential nucleating agents are calcium phosphate crystals, uric acid crystals, and cellular debris. Indeed, calcium phosphate is commonly present in stones composed primarily of calcium oxalate. By a similar mechanism of heterogeneous nucleation, hyperuricosuria contributes to calcium oxalate stone formation.
- **Urinary saturation:** Urinary saturation levels are influenced by the amount of solute and urine volume. The importance of the absolute amount of solute and urine volume is obvious: The more the solute is excreted in a lower volume, the higher the levels of saturation achieved.
- **Urine pH:** Urinary pH has a variable effect depending on the solutes involved.
  ○ **Low urine pH** significantly **lowers the solubility of uric acid.** This effect is a result of different solubilities of the protonated and dissociated forms of uric acid. Solubility of the undissociated form in acidic urine is very poor. Low urine pH makes uric acid supersaturation easy to achieve, even at normal uric acid excretion rates of 600 to 800 mg/d (3.6 to 4.8 mM/d). Uric acid crystals not only form into uric acid stones but also can nucleate out calcium oxalate (heterogeneous nucleation). Hence, low urine pH is a risk factor for uric acid and calcium oxalate stones.
  ○ **Alkaline urine pH predisposes to the formation of crystals containing phosphates:** calcium phosphate and struvite (ammonium magnesium phosphate) stones.
    ■ **Calcium phosphate** nephrolithiasis is most commonly observed in patients with distal renal tubular acidosis (RTA), a condition leading to a persistently high urine pH.
    ■ **Struvite** stones form in the presence of a urinary tract infection (UTI) caused by urease-producing bacteria. Urease-producing bacteria split abundant urinary urea into ammonia and carbon dioxide. Ammonia alkalinizes the urine and, together with magnesium, combines with phosphate to form struvite crystals.
- **Amount of inhibitors of crystallization:**
  ○ **Citrate,** the main inhibitor of crystallization of calcium salts, complexes with calcium to form a soluble calcium citrate compound. By doing so, it makes calcium unavailable to precipitate out as calcium oxalate or calcium phosphate. Hypocitraturia is a common finding among calcium stone formers.
  ○ **Magnesium** also inhibits crystallization of calcium salts, although its effect is not as important as that of citrate.

Risk Factors

Risk Factors for Calcium Oxalate and Calcium Phosphate Nephrolithiasis

- **Hypercalciuria:** Hypercalciuria is the **most common metabolic derangement among stone formers.** The amount of calcium excreted in the urine varies with body size and dietary calcium intake. The upper limit of normal calcium excretion in the urine is 4 mg/kg/d (approximately 280 mg/d for men, 240 mg/d for women) for patients consuming 1000 mg of elemental calcium. For patients consuming only 400 mg, the upper value becomes approximately 200 mg/d. Hypercalciuria can be classified as either idiopathic or secondary to hypercalcemia (Table 23-1).
  - ○ **Hypercalciuria due to hypercalcemia:** Hypercalcemia imposes an increased filtered load of calcium and results in an overflow hypercalciuria. The causes and approach to hypercalcemia are discussed in Chapter 8.
  - ○ **Idiopathic hypercalciuria:**
    - ■ Idiopathic hypercalciuria, by definition, is **not a consequence of hypercalcemia.** It is currently believed that most cases of idiopathic hypercalciuria are caused by excessive calcium absorption from the gastrointestinal (GI) tract (absorptive hypercalciuria). This disorder has a strong familial component. The pathophysiology of this disorder is not clear, but vitamin D receptor polymorphisms have been implicated.
    - ■ The degree of hypercalciuria can also be influenced by dietary sodium intake. Excessive sodium intake causes extracellular fluid volume expansion and diminished sodium resorption along the nephron. Volume expansion results not only in natriuresis but in calciuresis as well. Hence, dietary salt restriction can be an effective method of lowering hypercalciuria.
    - ■ **Thiazide diuretics reduce hypercalciuria** predominantly through reduction in extracellular fluid volume, leading to enhanced proximal and distal reabsorption of calcium.[5]
- **Hyperoxaluria:** Hyperoxaluria is divided into dietary, enteric, or primary forms (Table 23-2).
  - ○ **Dietary hyperoxaluria:** Normal daily urinary excretion of oxalate is <40 mg/d. Excessive dietary intake of oxalate-rich foods can result in a mild form of dietary hyperoxaluria (urinary oxalate excretion of 50 to 60 mg/d).

TABLE 23-1 DIFFERENTIAL DIAGNOSIS OF HYPERCALCIURIA

Normal serum calcium
Idiopathic hypercalciuria

PTH-dependent elevated serum calcium
Primary hyperparathyroidism: adenoma or hyperplasia

PTH-independent elevated serum calcium
Malignancy: squamous cell carcinoma, breast cancer, bladder cancer, multiple myeloma, lymphoma
Granulomatous disease: sarcoidosis, tuberculosis, berylliosis
Hypervitaminosis D
Hyperthyroidism

PTH, parathyroid hormone.

TABLE 23-2 CAUSES OF HYPEROXALURIA

Dietary Hyperoxaluria	Enteric Hyperoxaluria	Primary Hyperoxaluria
Cause: excessive dietary oxalate intake	*Cause:* small bowel malabsorption, Crohn's disease, jejunoileal bypass, celiac sprue, short bowel syndrome, chronic pancreatitis, biliary obstruction	*Type I:* deficiency of alanine glyoxylate aminotransferase
Foods rich in oxalate: cocoa, chocolate, black tea, green beans, beets, celery, green onions, leafy greens (spinach, rhubarb), Swiss chard, mustard greens, berries, dried figs, orange and lemon peel, summer squash, nuts, peanut butter	Moderate-to-severe elevation of urinary oxalate excretion; may result in nephrocalcinosis and renal failure	*Type II:* D-glycerate dehydrogenase or glyoxylate reductase deficiency
Mild elevation in urinary oxalate excretion		Severe hyperoxaluria, resulting in nephrocalcinosis and renal failure

Oxalate-rich foods include nuts, sunflower seeds, spinach, rhubarb, chocolate, Swiss chard, lime peel, star fruit, peppers, and tea. Intake of vitamin C exceeding 100 mg/d can cause hyperoxaluria.[6]

○ **Enteric hyperoxaluria:** Fat malabsorption and saponification of calcium in the gut by free fatty acids result in increased colonic absorption of oxalate. Detergent bile acids nonselectively increase the permeability of colonic mucosa to a number of substances, including oxalate. The resultant hyperoxaluria is more severe than the dietary form. Urinary oxalate excretion often exceeds 100 mg/d. Thus, small bowel resection, jejunal bypass surgery, and inflammatory bowel disorders can lead to hyperoxaluria, calcium oxalate nephrolithiasis, and even chronic renal failure due to nephrocalcinosis. In addition to hyperoxaluria, malabsorption has several other consequences that predispose to stone formation, including:
  ▪ Low urine volumes due to diarrheal loss of water
  ▪ Low urine pH due to colonic loss of bicarbonate
  ▪ Hypocitraturia due to chronic metabolic acidosis and hypokalemia
  ▪ Hypomagnesemia due to magnesium malabsorption

○ **Primary hyperoxaluria:** Primary forms of hyperoxaluria result from well-described metabolic defects. These are characterized by excessive endogenous production of oxalate, resulting in profound hyperoxaluria (135 to 270 mg/d). Stone formation often begins in childhood. Deposition of calcium oxalate in the tubulointerstitial compartment of the kidneys (renal oxalosis) often leads to progressive loss of renal function. Deposition of calcium oxalate also occurs in the heart, bone, joints, eyes, and other tissues. Two major defects are worth mentioning:
  ▪ **Type I primary hyperoxaluria** is an autosomal-recessive disorder that results from reduced activity of hepatic peroxisomal alanine glyoxylate aminotransferase. This increases the availability of glyoxylate, which is irreversibly converted to oxalic acid.

- **Type II primary hyperoxaluria** is a much rarer form of the disease due to D-glycerate dehydrogenase or glyoxylate reductase deficiency.[5]
- **Hypocitraturia:**
  - Hypocitraturia is defined as a **urinary citrate excretion <250 mg/d.** It is observed in ~40% of patients with nephrolithiasis.
  - The presence of hypocitraturia should arouse suspicions of a disorder associated with chronic metabolic acidosis, such as distal RTA or a GI disorder. The eubicarbonatemic form of distal RTA should be suspected in patients with persistently high urine pH but normal or near-normal plasma bicarbonate concentrations. Such patients may develop overt metabolic acidosis only when challenged with an acid load. Patients with complete or incomplete distal RTA make stones composed predominantly of calcium phosphate (apatite).
  - Hypocitraturia can also be seen in the setting of hypokalemia or with the use of carbonic anhydrase inhibitors such as topiramate.[7]
- **Hyperuricosuria:** Hyperuricosuria is a common finding noted in 10% to 26% of calcium stone formers. The amount of uric acid in the urine is determined by daily production of uric acid and is not necessarily associated with hyperuricemia. Studies have demonstrated that allopurinol, a xanthine oxidase inhibitor, significantly reduces the rate of calcium oxalate stone recurrences. The benefits are attributed to a decreased urinary excretion of uric acid.
- **Urinary proteins:** Although a number of urinary proteins have been implicated in the pathogenesis of calcium nephrolithiasis, their role remains to be further elucidated. Uropontin and nephrocalcin both inhibit crystal growth. Their role in nephrolithiasis is still not fully established.

Risk Factors for Uric Acid Nephrolithiasis

Uric acid is a product of purine metabolism and is primarily derived from endogenous sources, with dietary purines generally providing little substrate. **Four abnormalities have been strongly associated with uric acid stones:** persistently low urine pH, hyperuricemia, hyperuricosuria, and low urine volume.

- **Persistently low urine pH:** The pK_a of uric acid is 5.35. Hence, low urine pH makes urinary saturation with uric acid easy to achieve even at normal excretion rates of 600 to 800 mg/d (3.6 to 4.8 mM/d). Patients with gout, obesity, diabetes, or metabolic syndrome are at greater risk of forming uric acid stones, presumably secondary to excretion of abnormally acidic urine. A linear drop in urine pH with increase in BMI has been demonstrated, which is thought to be the link between obesity and risk of forming uric acid stones.
- **Hyperuricemia and hyperuricosuria:**
  - **Hyperuricosuria** can be secondary to an increased production of uric acid with an increased burden of excretion; alternatively, it can result from enhanced renal excretion of uric acid in the absence of hyperuricemia.
  - **Increased uric acid production** can be either congenital or acquired.
    - **Congenital causes of uric acid overproduction** are typically diseases of single-gene defects such as hypoxanthine guanine phosphoribosyltransferase deficiency and other similarly rare diseases.
    - **Acquired uric acid overproduction** is common in myeloproliferative disorders, such as polycythemia vera, or after chemotherapy for certain cancers resulting in large-scale cell death (tumor lysis syndrome).
  - **Hyperuricosuria with normal uric acid levels** can occur due to uricosuric agents such as probenecid and high-dose salicylates. Other commonly

used medications have uricosuric effects. Several examples include losartan (increases uric acid excretion by approximately 10%), fenofibrate (increases uric acid excretion by 20% to 30%), and atorvastatin.

- **Low urine volume:** Low urine volume is not a specific risk factor for uric acid nephrolithiasis, but increases the risk of all stone types by increasing the urinary supersaturation, as mentioned above.

Risk Factors for Struvite Nephrolithiasis

Struvite stones are also referred to as magnesium ammonium phosphate, triple phosphate, urease, or infection stones.

- **UTI:** Struvite stones form only during a UTI caused by urease-producing bacteria, such as *Proteus* species, *Providencia* species, *Pseudomonas,* and *Enterococcus.* These bacteria cleave ammonia from urea, causing an elevation of urinary pH >7.0. Abundant ammonium and magnesium combine with phosphates to give rise to struvite stones. Sometimes, calcium phosphate (apatite) may become incorporated into stones.[8]
- **Primary calcium stones:** Mixed struvite and calcium stones can occur in cases in which primary calcium stones cause a UTI by one of the urea-splitting organisms. Mixed struvite and calcium stones occur more often in men with idiopathic hypercalciuria, in which calcium stones become secondarily infected or when alkaline urine becomes supersaturated for calcium phosphate.
- **Factors that predispose one to recurrent UTIs,** such as urinary retention, increase the likelihood of struvite stone formation (neurogenic bladder, indwelling bladder catheters, ileal conduit, urethral stricture, benign prostatic hyperplasia, bladder and caliceal diverticuli, cystocele). Patients with **history of diabetes mellitus** or **laxative or analgesic abuse** are at increased risk for struvite stones.

Prevention

- The first tenet of prevention of nephrolithiasis is **maintenance of high urine volume.** Nephrolithiasis patients should achieve a **daily urine volume of ≥2.5 L.**
  - High urine volumes lower urine saturation with all salts.[9,10]
  - There are several helpful hints to assist patients in increasing urine volume.
    - They can be instructed to drink sufficient amounts of fluids to a point that the urine appears clear. Patients may take metered quantities of water throughout the day, including in the evenings, to avoid excessive urinary concentration during the night. This is particularly important for those patients who suffer from chronic diarrheal disorders resulting in excessive fluid loss from the GI tract.
    - Adequate fluid intake is also very important for patients who demonstrate significant hyperuricosuria, as urine can become easily saturated with uric acid even at normal levels of uric acid excretion.
- Having a low sodium, low protein, and normal calcium diet decreases the formation of calcium stones. Low protein diet also decreases the formation of uric acid stones, as meat is the major contributor for purines. Additional therapies to prevent the recurrence of specific types of stones are discussed under Treatment (Table 23-3).

TABLE 23-3	NONSPECIFIC AND SPECIFIC TREATMENT OPTIONS FOR CALCIUM STONE FORMERS

Nonspecific treatment options:
Adequate oral liquid intake to maintain UOP of 2 L/d
Restrict salt intake to <100 mEq/d
Restrict protein consumption to <12 oz of beef/poultry/fish per day or <0.8–1 g/kg/d

Specific treatment options:

Hypercalciuria	**Hypocitraturia**
Eliminate dietary excess	K citrate
Thiazides	Neutral phosphates
No added-salt diet	
Hyperoxaluria	**Hyperuricosuria**
Low-oxalate diet	Dietary purine restriction
Oral calcium	Allopurinol
Cholestyramine	K citrate if pH is low
Pyridoxine	

Associated Conditions

- **Cystinuria** is a hereditary disorder of dibasic amino acid transport in the proximal renal tubule.
  - The defect rests in a common dibasic amino acid transporter located on the apical membrane of the proximal tubular cell (Fig. 3-1). A genetic defect of this transporter results in urinary wasting of the dibasic amino acids cysteine, ornithine, arginine, and lysine.
  - Cystine is a poorly soluble disulfide of the amino acid cysteine. The solubility of cystine is ~300 mg/L (1.25 mmol/L).
  - Normal urinary cystine excretion is only 30 to 50 mg/d (0.12 to 0.21 mmol/d). Patients with cystinuria often excrete as much as 480 to 3600 mg/d (2 to 15 mmol/d), easily achieving urinary supersaturation status. The other three dibasic amino acids are soluble, and their loss in the urine is inconsequential.
- **Structural abnormalities in the kidney** such as polycystic kidney disease, horseshoe kidney, and ureteropelvic junction obstruction cause more stasis of the urine and predispose to stone formation.[11]
  - Medullary sponge kidney, a radiologic diagnosis of dilated distal collecting ducts seen on intravenous (IV) pyelogram, may reflect damage to the collecting ducts by hypercalciuria, which also predisposes to the formation of calcium oxalate nephrolithiasis.

DIAGNOSIS

Clinical Presentation

The clinical presentation of nephrolithiasis ranges from incidental diagnosis of otherwise asymptomatic disease to presentation with severe symptoms, such as abdominal or flank pain (renal colic), macroscopic or microscopic hematuria, UTIs, or even renal failure resulting from bilateral urinary tract obstruction.

- **Asymptomatic disease:** Patients with nephrolithiasis may remain asymptomatic for years. They usually become symptomatic if a calculus or its fragments begin to move along the urinary tract or cause obstruction. However, even chronic obstruction can be asymptomatic, but may eventually result in a permanent loss of renal function.

- **Renal colic:** In renal colic, the pain is usually abrupt in onset, colicky in nature, and located in the flank area. It often loops around and radiates down along the path of the affected ureter; sometimes, it migrates anteriorly and inferiorly into the groin and testicles or labia majora. Usually, hematuria, urinary frequency, urgency, nausea, and vomiting accompany the pain.
- **Hematuria:** Trauma to the urinary tract incited by passage of gravel or a stone leads to hematuria. It may be gross or microscopic and can occur even in completely asymptomatic patients.

History

When interviewing a patient with kidney stone, history of prior stones and dietary history, occupational history, and family history of stones and medicinal use, including supplements such as calcium and vitamin C, should be asked. Clinicians should also **identify various risk factors such as inflammatory bowel diseases, bowel surgeries, recurrent UTIs, conditions that predispose toward hypercalcemia, and so forth.**

Physical Examination

On physical examination, patient with renal colic may have costovertebral tenderness over the affected area.

Differential Diagnosis

In its classic form, the clinical presentation of renal colic is quite suggestive of the diagnosis. However, it is imperative to consider other serious conditions that can masquerade as renal colic in the differential diagnosis: Ectopic pregnancy, intestinal obstruction, acute appendicitis, diverticulitis, and many other abdominal catastrophes have been confused with renal colic. The presence of hematuria is suggestive of the diagnosis but not conclusive proof; an imaging study is required to make a positive diagnosis.

Diagnostic Testing

Laboratories

- **Urinalysis:** The presence of hematuria is suggestive of nephrolithiasis, but its presence is insufficient to make the diagnosis.
- **Urine microscopy:** The appreciation of specific types of crystals in the urine identifies the type of stone being formed and can guide subsequent therapy. A review of the appearance of various crystals can be found in Chapter 1, Art and Science of Urinalysis.
- **Serum chemistries:** A basic chemistry panel should be checked to assess renal function, as well as any disturbances in electrolyte or mineral balance. Serum levels of calcium, magnesium, and uric acid can be helpful in determining the underlying processes leading to stone formation. An intact parathyroid hormone level and 1,25 $(OH)2$ D_3 levels should be assessed in patients with hypercalcemia.

Imaging

- **Plain abdominal radiograph:**
  - **Approximately 90% of renal stones are radiopaque** and can be seen on plain radiographs of the abdomen. However, the plain x-ray provides no information

concerning presence or absence of urinary obstruction, and it may not add significant insight to the differential diagnosis of acute abdominal pain. Thus, plain abdominal x-rays have limited use in the evaluation of acute renal colic.

○ **Radiographic appearance of stones:** The radiographic appearance of stones on a plain abdominal radiograph may help identify stone type and guide further evaluation.

■ **Calcium phosphate and calcium oxalate stones** are radiodense.

■ **Struvite stones** (magnesium ammonium phosphate), when complexed with calcium carbonate or phosphate, are also visible as large, irregular stones. They sometimes take the shape of the calyces and are referred to as staghorn calculi.

■ A plain x-ray of the abdomen (kidneys, ureter, and bladder) may miss radiolucent **uric acid or** poorly visible **cystine stones.**

■ Xanthine and hypoxanthine stones are also radiolucent, but occur very rarely.

• **IV urography and CT scan:** IV urography used to be the preferred test of choice for evaluation of these patients. The application of helical noncontrast CT has largely replaced it as the initial step in evaluation of suspected renal colic. It allows nephrolithiasis to be excluded or confirmed expeditiously and without administration of potentially nephrotoxic radiocontrast material. The sensitivity and specificity of CT scan is superior to IV urography.[12,13]

• **Renal ultrasound:** Ultrasound is useful to rule out significant hydronephrosis or hydroureter; however, it may not detect stones until they are relatively large. At times, the exact site of obstruction may also not be clearly delineated. Although the sensitivity of ultrasound for stones is low compared to CT scan, it remains very useful for evaluation of patients who cannot receive radiation, such as pregnant women.[14]

TREATMENT

Treatment of Renal Colic

• The treatment of acute renal colic consists of pain management, relief of obstruction, and control of infection, if present.

• The bigger the size of the stone, it is less likely to pass spontaneously.[12,15,16]

○ If the stone is <5 mm, conservative management is adequate, as 80% to 90% of these stones pass spontaneously. The urine must be strained to retrieve the stone for analysis.

○ Stones 5 to 7 mm only pass spontaneously 50% of the time, and stones >7 mm rarely pass spontaneously.

○ If the stone is <7 mm, there is no obstruction, the urine is sterile, and the pain is controlled; conservative management is warranted.

• Fluid replacement should be designed to obtain a urine output of 2.5 L/d to assist with the passage of the stone.

• If the stone is passed but the patient had evidence of hydronephrosis or evidence of multiple stones, a follow-up imaging study, such as helical CT, within 2 weeks, is warranted. For the acute treatment of renal colic narcotics or nonsteroidal anti-inflammatory drugs can be used.[15]

Treatment of Calcium-Containing Nephrolithiasis

- **Thiazide diuretics:**
  - ○ Thiazide diuretics have long been the mainstay in treatment of idiopathic hypercalciuria, with metabolic abnormality noted with more than half of calcium oxalate nephrolithiasis.
  - ○ They lower urinary excretion of calcium by at least two mechanisms.
    - ▪ The main mechanism is contraction of the extracellular fluid volume. By reducing the extracellular volume, thiazide diuretics increase proximal reabsorption of calcium.
    - ▪ Thiazides also directly increase calcium reabsorption in the distal nephron.
  - ○ The effects of thiazide diuretics can be completely negated by high dietary salt intake. Urinary sodium excretion of ≥ 120 mEq/d suggests nonadherence to a low-sodium diet. If calcium excretion is not reduced, compliance with thiazide treatment and sodium intake should be questioned.
  - ○ **Hypokalemia and hypocitraturia** may complicate long-term therapy with thiazide diuretics and can be prevented by adding oral potassium citrate. Sometimes, to enhance the effect of thiazides and conserve potassium, amiloride may be added.
  - ○ The optional treatment regimens that have been studied include: **chlorthalidone** 12.5 to 25 mg every day to a maximum of 100 mg every day; **hydrochlorothiazide 25 to 50 mg bid; hydrochlorothiazide 50 mg with amiloride** (Moduretic) half tablet bid.
- **Oral phosphate:**
  - ○ Patients with urinary phosphate wasting and hypophosphatemia may benefit from phosphate replacement therapy.
  - ○ **Neutral potassium phosphate** (Neutraphos) divided into three to four doses (total daily dose 1500 mg) can lower urinary calcium excretion in some patients and as one study has shown, may be as effective as thiazide diuretics. However, compliance is difficult to achieve due to the frequent doses and side effects, such as diarrhea and bloating.
- **Citrate:**
  - ○ Citrate therapy is the principal intervention for a large number of calcium stone formers. In particular, hypocitraturia often occurs in patients with small bowel malabsorption syndromes and distal RTA. As an added advantage, in these patients with chronic acidosis, citrate serves as a source of alkali (citrate is metabolized in the liver to bicarbonate).
  - ○ Citrate is administered in divided doses throughout the day; the **starting dose is usually 10 mEq PO two or three times daily.**
  - ○ Administration of an excessive amount of citrate can result in a persistently alkaline urinary pH, which may increase the risk of calcium phosphate stone formation in some patients.
- **Dietary modifications:**
  - ○ Dietary hyperoxaluria is treated by dietary restriction of oxalate-rich foods.
  - ○ Treatment of the enteric form of hyperoxaluria should be directed toward correction of metabolic derangements resulting in stone formation and nephrocalcinosis. Thiazide diuretics are usually ineffective because patients with small bowel malabsorption demonstrate hypocalciuria.
  - ○ Absorptive hyperoxaluria is most often treated with a dietary restriction of oxalate-rich foods and administration of intestinal oxalate binders, such as

calcium carbonate, which form nonreabsorbable compounds in the GI tract. If calcium carbonate is ineffective, bile sequestrants, such as cholestyramine, could be added.

- **Management of type I primary hyperoxaluria:**
  - ○ Type I primary hyperoxaluria occasionally can respond to pyridoxine supplements. However, no good medical treatment short of liver transplantation exists.
  - ○ Increasing urinary volume to 3 L/d is beneficial.
  - ○ Liver transplantation restores the enzymatic defects responsible for the disease.
  - ○ Renal transplantation in patients who have developed end-stage renal disease due to primary hyperoxaluria requires a special protocol to avoid accelerated renal oxalosis in the allograft; the ideal approach is combined liver and kidney transplantation.

Treatment of Uric Acid Nephrolithiasis

Treatment of uric acid nephrolithiasis is based on attempts to increase the solubility of uric acid and to decrease its excretion.

- All patients should maintain urine volume >2.5 L/d.
- **Dietary counseling** about low purine and low protein intake is paramount. Alkalinization of urine to a pH >6.5 markedly increases the solubility of uric acid.[17]
- **Potassium citrate** (10 to 20 mEq PO tid; maximum, 100 mEq/d) is the preferred alkalinizing agent because, unlike sodium salts, it does not augment urinary calcium excretion. However, urinary alkalinization alone is rarely sufficient. It is very difficult to avoid temporary episodes of urinary acidification throughout the entire day (e.g., during the night).
- **Allopurinol,** a xanthine oxidase inhibitor that blocks the conversion of xanthine to uric acid, is well tolerated and very effective in reducing urinary uric acid excretion. The benefits of allopurinol are attributed to its ability to treat hyperuricosuria and reduce uric acid crystal-induced nucleation of calcium oxalate. The dose of allopurinol should be adjusted to achieve a target excretion of uric acid of <600 mg/d. The success of the treatment should be monitored by repeated 24-hour urinary collections for stone risk assessment.

Treatment of Struvite Stones

- **Surgical intervention is usually needed** to remove struvite stones. Referral to Urology is advised for an evaluation and stone removal.
- A variety of procedures are available, including percutaneous nephrolithotomy and/or shockwave lithotripsy. Open surgical removal (kidney-splitting surgery) is no longer the treatment of choice for staghorn struvite calculi, unless the patient's body habitus or stone burden precludes less-invasive techniques.
- Once patients are free of stones, they benefit from antibiotic therapy directed against the predominant urinary organism. Most patients with residual stone fragments progress despite treatment with antibiotics. Reducing the bacterial population with antibiotics often slows stone growth, but stone resolution with antibiotics is unlikely.

Treatment of Cystine Stones

- Preventive medical therapy is directed toward reducing urinary cystine concentration below its solubility limits.

- High fluid intake can prevent stones only in some patients with low levels of cystine excretion.
- Most patients require treatment with penicillamine, tiopronin, or captopril. These drugs reduce urinary saturation with cystine by forming soluble disulfides. However, side effects may limit their use.
- Dietary restriction of the essential amino acid methionine, a cystine precursor, is impractical.
- Urinary alkalinization to a pH >7.5 increases cystine solubility. However, persistently alkaline urine is difficult to attain.
- Once formed, cystine stones often require surgical removal.

Surgical Management

- **Indications for expedient stone removal** are complete obstruction, UTI, urosepsis, worsening renal failure, or uncontrollable colic with severe nausea and vomiting.[15]
- Symptomatic stones for more than 4 weeks can cause complications such as ureteral stricture.
- **Treatment modalities** include extracorporeal shockwave lithotripsy (ESWL), percutaneous nephrostolithotomy (PCN), ureteroscopic removal, surgery, and chemolysis. The **selection of treatment modality** is determined by the size, composition, and anatomic location of the stone, anatomy of the collecting system, health status, and patient preference.
  - Stones that are lodged in the proximal ureter above the iliac vessels, which are less than 1 cm, are treated with ESWL.
  - For proximal ureteral stones greater than 1 cm, ureteroscopy with YAG laser is superior to ESWL.
  - For distal ureteral stones, both ESWL and ureteroscopy have similar stone-free rates.[18]
  - Brushite and cystine stones are less responsive to ESWL.
  - Stones that are >2 cm are usually treated with PCN.
  - Surgical intervention is preferred for large staghorn calculi.

Diet

- Dietary intervention plays a cardinal role in the preventive treatment of calcium nephrolithiasis.
- Studies have shown that a **low-protein, low-salt diet** significantly reduces nephrolithiasis recurrence rates in patients with idiopathic hypercalciuria.[19] Long-term dietary compliance with a low-protein, low-salt diet has been shown to be superior to a low-calcium diet in prevention of nephrolithiasis.
- A low-calcium diet may increase the intestinal absorption of oxalate, reducing the effectiveness of this therapy. Therefore, **low-calcium diets are not recommended.** Diets containing 700 to 800 mg of calcium are adequate for patients with idiopathic hypercalciuria.
- Low-protein diets reduce purine intake, resulting in reduced systemic acid and uric acid loads. Low-sodium diets reduce the amount of calcium in the urine by the mechanisms described previously.

MONITORING/FOLLOW UP

- **Follow-up imaging:** Subsequent imaging studies are recommended at 1 year for evaluation of recurrence. The study may be a kidneys/ureter/bladder x-ray, ultrasound, or helical CT. If there is no evidence of new stones, then imaging studies may be repeated every 5 years. Recurrent nephrolithiasis may mandate more frequent imaging. All patients with nephrolithiasis deserve a screening evaluation for common problems that can lead to stone formation, although there is no consensus of how extensive evaluation should be after the first episode. Patients with recurrent nephrolithiasis deserve a thorough metabolic evaluation, which should be done once the acute episode has resolved and the patient has returned to his or her daily routine.

- A **24-hour urine** sample should be collected on at least two occasions, and ~4 weeks after the acute event has resolved and the patient has returned to his or her usual lifestyle. The drugs prescribed for stone disease, as well as vitamin supplements, should be stopped 5 days before urine collection.[20]
  - The following **urinary parameters** are routinely determined when performing **stone risk evaluation:**
    - Total urine volume: It is desirable to achieve urinary volume >2.5 L/d
    - Urine pH
    - Creatinine: Urinary excretion of creatinine is determined to assure adequacy of the collection. It is expected that in a 24-hour period, men excrete ~20 mg/kg and women 15 mg/kg of creatinine.
    - Calcium: normal 50 to 250 mg/d
    - Uric acid: normal <750 mg/d
    - Citrate: normal >250 mg/d
    - Oxalate: normal <40 mg/d
    - Sodium: <100 mmol/d is consistent with low dietary sodium intake
    - Phosphorus: normal <1100 mg/d
    - Magnesium: normal 18 to 130 mg/d
    - Ammonia: normal 25 to 50 mmol/d
    - Sulfate: normal 4 to 35 mmol/d
    - Urine culture and sensitivity for struvite stones
  - A number of commercial urine collection kits, quantitating urinary salt composition and saturations, are widely available. To account for day-to-day variability in urinary salt excretion, several 24-hour urinary collections may be necessary.

OUTCOME/PROGNOSIS

The incidence of kidney stones has increased over the years and if untreated stones have high recurrence rate. Fortunately, most kidney stones can be prevented by modifying the dietary habits and lifestyle such as increased fluid intake and decreasing the sodium and animal protein content in the diet.

REFERENCES

1. Rule AD, Bergstralh EJ, Melton LJ III, et al. Kidney stones and the risk for chronic kidney disease. *Clin J Am Soc Nephrol.* 2009;4:804–811.
2. Stamatelou KK, Francis ME, Jones CA, et al. Time trends in reported prevalence of kidney stones in the United States: 1976–1994. *Kidney Int.* 2003;63:1817–1823.
3. Soucie JM, Thun MJ, Coates RJ, et al. Demographic and geographic variability of kidney stones in the United States. *Kidney Int.* 1994;46:893–899.

4. Semins MJ, Shore AD, Makary MA, Johns R, Matlaga BR. The association of increasing body mass index and kidney stone disease. *J Urol.* 2010;183(2):571–575.
5. Coe FL, Parks JH, Asplin JR. The pathogenesis and treatment of kidney stones. *N Engl J Med.* 1992;327(16):1141–1152.
6. Taylor EN, Curhan GC. Determinants of 24-hour urinary oxalate excretion. *Clin J Am Soc Nephrol.* 2008;3:1453–1460.
7. Worcester EM, Coe FL. Calcium Kidney stones. *N Engl J Med.* 2010;363:954–963.
8. Rodman JS. Struvite stones. *Nephron.* 1999;81(suppl 1):50–59.
9. Borghi L, Meschi T, Amato F, et al. Urinary volume, water and recurrences of idiopathic calcium nephrolithiasis. A 5-year randomized prospective study. *J Urol.* 1996;155:839–843.
10. Curhan GC, Willett WC, Rimm EB, et al. A prospective study of dietary calcium and other nutrients and the risk of symptomatic kidney stones. *N Engl J Med.* 1993;328:833–838.
11. Gambaro G, Fabris A, Puliatta D, et al. Lithiasis in cystic disease and malformations of the urinary tract. *Urol Res.* 2006;34:102–107.
12. Portis AJ, Sundaram CP. Diagnosis and initial management of kidney stones. *Am Fam Physician.* 2001;63(7):1329–1338.
13. Vieweg J, Teh C, Freed K, et al. Unenhanced helical computerized tomography for the evaluation of patients with acute flank pain. *J Urol.* 1998;160:679–684.
14. Shokeir AA, Mahran MR, Abdulmaaboud M. Renal colic in pregnant women: role of resistive index. *Urology.* 2000;55:344–347.
15. Teichman JMH. Acute renal colic from ureteral calculus. *N Engl J Med.* 2004;350:684–693.
16. Ueno A, Kawamura T, Ogawa A, et al. Relation of spontaneous passage of ureteral calculi to size. *Urology.* 1977;10:544–546.
17. Liebman SE, Taylor JG, Bushinsky DA. Uric acid nephrolithiasis. *Curr Rheum Rep.* 2007: 9(3):251–257.
18. Lam JS, Greene TD, Gupta M. Treatment of proximal ureteral calculi: holmium:YAG laser ureterolithotripsy versus extracorporeal shock wave lithotripsy. *J Urol.* 2002;167:1972–1976.
19. Borghi L, Schianchi T, Meschi T, et al. Comparison of two diets for the prevention of recurrent stones in idiopathic hypercalciuria. *N Engl J Med.* 2002;346(2):77–84.
20. Lifshitz DA, Shalhav AL, Lingeman JE, et al. Metabolic evaluation of stone disease patients: a practical approach. *J Endourol.* 1999;13(9):669–678.

Management of Chronic Kidney Disease

24

Nicholas Taraska and Anitha Vijayan

GENERAL PRINCIPLES

Definition

- Chronic kidney disease (CKD) is a term used to describe a gradual reduction in renal function over the span of weeks to years.
- CKD can also be described as a renal injury manifested by proteinuria or hematuria of glomerular or interstitial origin in the setting of a normal or higher than normal glomerular filtration rate (GFR)[1] (e.g., diabetic nephropathy in early stages manifested by proteinuria or IgA nephropathy with hematuria).
- However, the term is more commonly applied to describe patients with a **GFR <60 mL/min.**
- The staging of CKD depends on the level of GFR, and the ensuing complications increase in severity with worsening renal function (Fig. 24-1).
- Majority of patients may require renal replacement therapy (RRT) or renal transplantation at GFR below 15 mL/min. The discussion in this chapter will focus on management of predialysis CKD.
- It must be kept in mind that management of CKD patients is complicated and involves close collaboration with their primary care physicians as well as other specialists (endocrinologists, cardiologists, vascular surgeons, and so forth).

Classification

- In 2002, a National Kidney Foundation (NKF) work group released guidelines for classifying CKD[1] (Table 24-1).
- This classification has helped to streamline the management of CKD, as the terminology helps the healthcare professional as well as the patients to clearly understand the severity of the illness and decide on treatment strategies appropriate for the stage of CKD.

Associated Conditions

- Figure 24-1 depicts the presentation of some of the comorbid conditions in relation to the GFR and stage of CKD.
- **Hypertension:** The pathophysiology of hypertension is multifactorial, but sodium and water retention as well as inappropriate renin secretion play key parts. A net positive sodium balance results in volume expansion and resultant hypertension.
  - The Seventh Report of the Joint National Committee on Prevention, Detection, Evaluation, and Treatment of High Blood Pressure (JNC 7) noted that hypertension was present in the majority of patients with GFR <60 mL/min.
  - The committee recommended a **goal of systolic blood pressure of <130** mm Hg and a **diastolic blood pressure** of **<80 mm Hg** in patients with diabetes and/or CKD.[2,3]

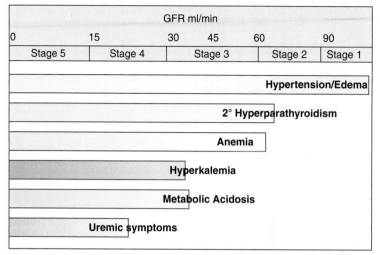

FIGURE 24-1. Onset of complications related to decreased GFR. This figure shows the complications of renal dysfunction in relation to GFR and stage of CKD. CKD, chronic kidney disease; GFR, glomerular filtration rate.

TABLE 24-1	NATIONAL KIDNEY FOUNDATION STAGES OF CHRONIC KIDNEY DISEASE		
Stage	Description	GFR (mL/min/1.73 m²)	Action
1	Kidney damage with normal or increased GFR	≥90	Diagnosis and treatment; slow progression
2	Kidney damage with mildly decreased GFR	60–89	Estimate progression
3	Moderately decreased GFR	30–59	Evaluate and treat complications
4	Severely decreased GFR	15–29	Prepare for kidney replacement therapy
5	Kidney failure	<15 or dialysis	Kidney replacement (if uremia present)

GFR, glomerular filtration rate.

Adapted from Levey AS, Coresh J, Balk E, et al. National Kidney Foundation practice guidelines for chronic kidney disease: evaluation, classification, and stratification. *Ann Intern Med.* 2003; 139(2):137–147.

- **Anemia:** The oxygen demand and use by the kidneys far exceeds the 20% to 25% of cardiac output that they receive, making them an excellent oxygen sensor for the body.
  - The kidneys produce and secrete **erythropoietin,** a hormone that stimulates red blood cell production by the bone marrow.
  - With advancing kidney damage, the kidneys are less able to produce adequate amounts of erythropoietin necessary to maintain normal hemoglobin levels.[4]
  - Resistance to the action of erythropoietin also plays a role in the development and maintenance of anemia.
- **Renal osteodystrophy:** Owing to the complex nature of this disease and its effects on other organs and tissues besides bone, this condition is also referred to as mineral and bone disorder or metabolic bone disease. Dysregulation of calcium and phosphorus metabolism can lead to cardiac, vascular and other tissue calcification.
  - Decreased GFR results in phosphorus retention, leading to increased production of parathyroid hormone (PTH).
  - Decreased 1-alpha hydroxylation of 25-OH vitamin D and decreased serum levels of active vitamin D lead to hypocalcemia and elevation of PTH levels.
  - Secondary hyperparathyroidism (SHPT) can lead to a state of high bone turnover called "osteitis fibrosa," placing CKD patients at high risk for bone fractures.[5,6]
- **Metabolic acidosis and hyperkalemia:**
  - With advancing CKD and decreasing GFR, the ability of the kidney to effectively eliminate the total acid load and potassium is reduced.
  - An individual typically generates 1 mEq H^+ (acid) per kg body weight daily, and as renal function deteriorates, the kidney in unable to excrete this acid load.
  - **Acidosis typically develops with GFR below 40 mL/min,** unless there is renal tubular acidosis associated with conditions such as diabetic nephropathy, obstructive nephropathy, sickle-cell anemia, and so forth, in which case acidosis is seen in earlier stages of CKD.
  - These patients are also at higher risk for developing hyperkalemia.
- **Hyperlipidemia and cardiovascular disease:**
  - CKD is associated with increased rates of cardiovascular events, deaths, and hospitalizations.[7]
  - It must be noted that a **significantly higher number of patients with stage 3 or 4 CKD die of cardiovascular causes before reaching the need for dialysis or transplantation.**
  - Modification of risk factors such as hyperlipidemia, hypertension, and bone and mineral disorders is critical in reducing mortality and morbidity from cardiovascular disease.

DIAGNOSIS

Diagnostic Testing
Laboratory Data
- The Modification of Diet in Renal Disease GFR (**MDRD GFR**) **calculation** is a creatinine-based equation used to estimate a patient's GFR.
  - It requires that the patient have a stable creatinine level.[8]
  - The equation depends on its ability to predict a patient's normal creatinine production level.

○ It has been validated in patients with CKD, African-Americans, Caucasians, and females.

○ It may be inaccurate in patients with unusual diets, extremes of age or weight, or unusual levels of skeletal muscle mass. A 24-hour urine collection may be more accurate in these patients.

• The Chronic Kidney Disease Epidemiology Collaboration (**CKD-EPI**) is an alternative equation used to estimate GFR in patients with stable creatinine levels.[9]

○ It may underestimate the incidence of CKD as compared with the MDRD equation in some patients, but it may be more accurate in patients with a higher GFR.[10]

○ Table 24-1 shows the correlation of the GFR with the different stages of CKD and highlights the clinical actions appropriate to each stage.

• Table 24-2 outlines the relevant laboratory and diagnostic studies that are useful in the evaluation of a patient with CKD.

• **Urine protein excretion:**

○ Heavy proteinuria is associated with progression of renal disease, and the amount of proteinuria serves as an indicator of the severity of disease in certain glomerulonephritis.

○ It can be assessed in a 24-hour urine collection or by calculating the urine protein to creatinine ratio in a spot collection (see chapter on proteinuria).

• **Evaluation of anemia:**

○ Complete blood cell count is required at initial and subsequent office visits.

○ Ferritin and transferrin saturation levels are required to help guide the treatment of anemia.

○ The Kidney Disease Outcomes Quality Initiative (KDOQI) work group recommends a **ferritin level >100 ng/mL** and a **transferrin saturation >20%** in predialysis CKD patients.[4]

○ However, these measures are not necessarily sufficient to determine which patients will or will not respond to iron supplementation, and so some clinicians may opt to administer iron and monitor for response even in patients whose markers are at recommended goal values.[11]

• **PTH, calcium, phosphorus, and 25-OH vitamin D levels** should be measured to assist in directing the management of renal osteodystrophy.

○ For stages 3 and 4 CKD, the KDOQI work group recommends maintaining corrected calcium in the "normal" range for the laboratory used and a phosphorus value between 2.7 and 4.6 mg/dL.

○ Measurement of intact PTH is recommended at least every 6 to 12 months.

▪ For patients with stage 3 CKD, the KDOQI clinical guidelines for bone metabolism recommend an opinion-based target of an intact PTH level between 35 and 70 pg/mL.

▪ For patients with stage 4 CKD, the recommended target range is 70 to 110 pg/mL and measurement should occur at least every 3 months.

• The KDOQI bone metabolism work group guidelines recommend maintaining a total CO_2 levels of $\geq$ **22 mEq/L** for patients with a GFR <60 mL/min.

• A **lipid panel** should be checked in all CKD patients at initial office visit and annually.

○ Patients with nephrotic syndrome are particularly susceptible to dyslipidemia.

○ The optimal low-density lipoprotein cholesterol target has not been defined for the CKD population, but given the risk for cardiovascular disease, it is generally recommended to be <100 mg/dL.

○ It is generally recommended that triglyceride level is kept below 200 mg/dL.

TABLE 24-2 DIAGNOSTIC WORKUP OF A CKD PATIENT

Tests and Diagnostics	Significance and/or Goal
• Serum creatinine	• Used to estimate GFR using equations • Historical values assist in determining chronicity and progression of disease
• Urinalysis with microscopy	• Presence of RBCs, RBC casts, and/or proteinuria suggests glomerular process • Additional workup is necessary to diagnose underlying disease
• Assessment of proteinuria	• A 24-h urine collection or spot urine protein to creatinine ratio is recommended on initial visit • If heavily proteinuric, then proteinuria should be assessed on follow-up visits to determine response to therapy
• Electrolyte panel	• Electrolyte values necessary to guide antihypertensive treatment (e.g., hyponatremia, hypokalemia with diuretics) • Potassium and bicarbonate values necessary to rule out hyperkalemia and acidosis • Usually performed at each office visit
• Calcium, phosphorus, intact PTH, 25-OH vitamin D	• Assist in management of metabolic bone disease • Usually done at initial office visit and every 3–6 mo
• Complete blood cell count	• Evaluation and treatment of anemia • Usually performed at each office visit
• Ferritin and iron panel	• Useful in the evaluation and treatment of iron deficiency • Iron deficient individuals require additional workup to find underlying etiology • Usually performed every 3–6 mo
• Fasting lipid panel	• CKD patients are at high risk for cardiovascular disease • Dyslipidemia seen often in nephrotic syndrome • Usually performed at initial visit and at every 6–12 mo
• Hepatitis B and C serologies	• Negative hepatitis B testing mandates vaccination • Positive hepatitis B surface antigen or core antibody may be a clue to underlying renal disease • Hepatitis C is associated with cryoglobulinemia and glomerulonephritis
• Serum and urine electrophoresis and immune fixation	• Strongly recommended for patients presenting with elevated creatinine and anemia, especially in elderly • Electrophoresis alone has low sensitivity, so immunofixation is required • Serum free light chains are more sensitive to diagnose monoclonal gammopathies

TABLE 24-2 DIAGNOSTIC WORKUP OF A CKD PATIENT (Continued)

Tests and Diagnostics	Significance and/or Goal
• HIV antibody	• Warranted for select populations with risk factors to rule out HIV-associated nephropathy
• Antinuclear antibody	• Warranted for adults with proteinuria to rule out lupus nephritis or other renal disease secondary to autoimmune disorders
• Renal ultrasound with or without arterial Dopplers	• Characterizes kidney number, size, echogenicity • Rules out obstruction • Evaluate for renovascular disease • Evaluate for presence of cysts/malignancy/stones
• Kidney biopsy	• Indicated for individuals with unexplained hematuria and/or proteinuria or elevated creatinine. Also useful in diagnosing and treating suspected glomerular disease (e.g., lupus nephritis, vasculitis)

CKD, Chronic kidney disease; GFR, glomerular filtration rate; RBC, red blood cell; PTH, parathyroid hormone; HIV, human immunodeficiency virus.

- The current KDOQI Nutrition guidelines recommend checking **serum albumin** every 1 to 3 months in patients with a GFR <20 mL/min as an assessment of nutritional status because albumin is a strong prognostic indicator in end-stage renal disease (ESRD) patients.
- **Hepatitis B and C and HIV serologies** may help diagnose the underlying cause of the patient's CKD (e.g., membranoproliferative glomerulonephritis secondary to Hepatitis C-induced cryoglobulinemia or HIV nephropathy). Hepatitis B titers are also useful to determine which patients need to be immunized against the disease as CKD progresses.
- An **antinuclear antibody** can suggest the presence of autoimmune disease as the cause of the patient's CKD, and high titers may warrant additional workup such as complement levels and extractable nuclear antibody screen.
- A patient with unexplained rise in serum creatinine and anemia (especially the elderly) needs to be ruled out for monoclonal gammopathies.
  - Serum and urine protein electrophoresis, along with immunofixation, are useful diagnostic tools to evaluate for paraproteinemia and related renal disorders such light chain deposition disease, cast nephropathy, and amyloidosis.
  - Serum-free light chains are more sensitive in picking up monoclonal gammopathies and should be considered in patients with high index of suspicion.

Imaging
- A **renal ultrasound** is usually performed after the initial visit for several reasons.
  - It helps to delineate renal anatomy and verify the presence of two normal sized kidneys.
  - It is useful to rule out obstruction.
  - It may detect abnormalities such as nephrocalcinosis/nephrolithiasis.

○ It aids in the detection of cysts or renal cell cancers. Renal cell malignancies are more common in patients with CKD.

○ Abnormally large kidneys (>13 cm) may suggest the presence of certain disease such as diabetic nephropathy, HIV-associated nephropathy, infiltrative disorders, interstitial nephritis, and so forth.

○ A follow-up renal ultrasound may be required if there is unexplained changes in renal function, presence of hematuria, back pain, or other changes on clinical evaluation.

• A **Doppler study of the renal arteries** can help rule out renal artery disease in a patient with resistant or difficult-to-control hypertension.

• Computed tomographic scan of the abdomen may be necessary to further evaluate for stones or to rule out malignancy.

Diagnostic Procedures

• **Urine microscopy:**

○ Any patient with hematuria on urine dipstick examination should have the urine microscopy examined by a nephrologist for the presence of casts or abnormal cells.

• A **kidney biopsy** is indicated in the setting of proteinuria and hematuria or unexplained rise in serum creatinine.

○ Risks of biopsy (especially risk for life-threatening bleeding) must be weighed against the benefit of diagnosing underlying disease. If the diagnosis will not significantly alter treatment of prognosis, then biopsy may not be necessary.

○ Kidney biopsy may be necessary in certain conditions (suspected lupus nephritis, vasculitis) to help guide therapy.

TREATMENT

Nephrology Consultation

• Referral to a nephrologist is **almost always indicated once the GFR has fallen to <30 mL/min.**

○ However, it is **highly recommended to refer at earlier stages of CKD (i.e., GFR <60 mL/min)** when the progression of renal disease is anticipated or when further evaluation is necessary (e.g., diabetic nephropathy, lupus nephritis, vasculitis).

○ The nephrology clinic is often better prepared to coordinate the care of the CKD patient with anemia, difficult-to-control hypertension, significant proteinuria, or primary renal disease.

○ Late nephrology referral is associated with poorer outcomes and increased cost.[12]

• Management of stage 3 CKD focuses primarily on complications that occur with this level of renal function.

• Management of stage 4 CKD involves both addressing complications of the disease in addition to preparation for RRT and transplantation.

• Management of stage 5 CKD involves continued management of the complications of CKD, optimal transition to dialysis, and, if appropriate, end-of-life discussions.

Hypertension

• As stated previously, the blood pressure **goal is <130/80 mm Hg.**

• Diuretics, beta-blockers, angiotensin-converting enzyme (ACE) inhibitors and/or angiotensin-receptor blockers (ARB), calcium channel blockers, alpha-blockers, alpha-2 agonists, aldosterone receptor antagonists, and vasodilators are all used to achieve blood pressure goals.[3,13]

- **ACE inhibitors and/or ARBs** are useful in patients with proteinuria.
  - ○ ACE inhibitors and ARBs classically lower intraglomerular pressure, thus protecting the kidneys from disease progression.
  - ○ A renal function panel should be checked 1 to 2 weeks after starting treatment with ACE inhibitors or ARBs.
  - ○ A 30% increase in creatinine is considered acceptable, although often hyperkalemia can limit the use of these medications.[14]
  - ○ The recent ONTARGET study that examined dual renin-angiotensin-aldosterone system blockade with both telmisartan and ramipril showed that in patients with high vascular risk, dual therapy reduced proteinuria better than ramipril alone but led to a higher incidence of doubling of the creatinine, dialysis, or death.[15]
  - ○ The patients in the ONTARGET study generally had nonnephrotic range proteinuria.
  - ○ The utility and safety of "dual therapy" in patients with heavy proteinuria remain under clinical investigation.
- A new medication, **aliskiren,** functions through direct inhibition of renin and may have more potent effects if combined with ACE inhibition.
- Recently, there has been interest in adding aldosterone receptor blockade to ACE inhibitor therapy as an antifibrotic strategy to lower blood pressure, reduce proteinuria, and abrogate the progression of renal disease. However, additional long-term studies are necessary before endorsing this additional promising therapy. Furthermore, hyperkalemia is a possible side effect to the use of this medication.[16]

Edema and Volume Overload

- Edema and volume overload are frequently seen in CKD, especially in the setting of nephrotic range proteinuria, congestive heart failure, pulmonary dysfunction, sleep apnea, and GFR <40 mL/min.
- **Diuretics** are an effective therapy in the management of hypertension and edema in CKD.
  - ○ The effectiveness of thiazide diuretics is reduced in patients with GFR <40 mL/min.
  - ○ Loop diuretics are useful in patients with low GFRs, but their effectiveness may be more limited in patients with a low serum albumin.
  - ○ A reasonable starting dose for a loop diuretic in a patient with CKD is **furosemide 40 mg PO bid or bumetanide 1 mg PO bid.** A new steady state will be reached within 1 to 2 weeks.
- **Sodium restriction** is also an essential component of management of edema.
- It is also important to **rule out concomitant etiologies** such as sleep apnea, diastolic or systolic hear failure, and so forth.

Anemia and Iron Deficiency

- If iron deficiency is diagnosed, appropriate gastrointestinal workup should be considered.
- Iron deficiency, even in the absence of anemia, is associated with neurological dysfunction, restless legs syndrome, fatigue, hair loss, and even worsening of cardiac dysfunction.

- If no contraindications exist, **iron replacement should begin via the oral route,** which is the preferred first line of treatment.
  - We recommend **ferrous sulfate 325 mg PO bid–tid.**
  - Iron is best absorbed on an empty stomach and in an acid environment.
  - Patients treated with antireflux medications will not absorb iron as efficiently as patients not taking these drugs.
- If patient has suboptimal response to oral iron or if the patient is unable to tolerate the treatment, then **intravenous iron** should be considered.
  - There are several options for intravenous iron—iron dextran, iron sucrose, ferric gluconate, or ferumoxytol.
  - The least expensive option is **iron dextran.** Because of risk of anaphylactic reactions, a 25-mg test dose should be administered and the patient monitored for any adverse events. If the patient tolerates the test dose without difficulty, a 500- to 1000-mg dose of iron dextran can be administered over 3 to 4 hours.
  - **Iron sucrose and ferric gluconate** preparations require multiple infusions of small doses (125 mg and 200 mg, respectively) since higher doses can be associated with hemodynamic changes and hypotension from sudden iron release into the circulation. These preparations are useful in patients with history of medication allergies.[17]
  - Ferumoxytol has been associated with anaphylactic reactions.
  - The lowest number of adverse events has been associated with iron sucrose.[17]
  - Not all CKD patients with anemia will have a renal-related pathophysiologic mechanism for their reduced hemoglobin level.
  - An iron-deficient stage 3 CKD patient requires a standard anemia workup, including age-appropriate cancer screening measures to rule out malignancies.
- **Erythropoiesis-stimulating agents** (ESAs):
  - Erythropoietin replacement or ESA is necessary once hemoglobin levels fall to <10 g/dL.
  - The current Food and Drug Administration guidelines recommend that ESA should be used only to prevent blood transfusion and not to treat symptoms such as fatigue and decreased energy.
  - Currently approved ESAs include **epoetin alfa** and **darbepoetin alfa.**
  - There is no well-defined critical threshold for initiating an ESA in CKD patients. In the opinion of the KDOQI anemia management work group, initial starting doses for the above-approved ESAs are not defined and should be determined according to clinical circumstances and the patient's starting hemoglobin levels.
  - A **typical starting dose** of epoetin alfa is 50 to 100 units/kg subcutaneously every week or darbepoetin alfa 40 mcg subcutaneously every 2 weeks.
  - The subcutaneous route is preferred in stages 3 and 4 CKD patients.
  - The 2006 NKF KDOQI guidelines recommend keeping the hemoglobin levels >11 g/dL; however, the Food and Drug Administration also recommends an upper target hemoglobin limit of 12 g/dL.[22]
  - Higher hemoglobin levels are not necessarily beneficial to patients (normal hematocrit and CHOIR trials).[18,19]
  - The TREAT study recently evaluated CKD patients given darbepoetin, targeting a hemoglobin level of 13 g/dL. Treated patients required significantly fewer transfusions but had a statistically significant higher incidence of stroke. There was no significant difference in cardiovascular event, progression to ESRD, or death.[20]

○ As hemoglobin levels >13 g/dL during ESA therapy have been associated with increased rates of blood clots, heart attacks, strokes, and death, the **complete blood cell count should be monitored at least monthly** while administering an ESA to avoid exceeding that level.[21]

Renal Osteodystrophy/Secondary Hyperparathyroidism

- The management of ROD is complex and involves reduction of phosphorus in diet, use of phosphate binders, and appropriate use of vitamin D analogs.
- **Dietary restriction:**
  ○ It is generally recommended to restrict phosphorus intake to 800 to 1200 mg/d.
  ○ See Table 24-3 for a list of commonly used high-phosphorus foods.
  ○ The list is not comprehensive and so patients should be counseled on reading food labels.
- **Phosphorus binders:**
  ○ Phosphorus binders are **primarily calcium compounds** (calcium carbonate or acetate). Aluminum compounds are rarely used because of risk of toxicity.
  ○ Other binders, such as **sevelamer hydrochloride or carbonate, are not approved for use in predialysis CKD.**
  ○ Similarly, **lanthanum carbonate** is a an effective phosphorus binder but **not approved for use in predialysis patients.**

TABLE 24-3	COMMON HIGH-PHOSPHORUS FOODS	
Beverages	Ale Chocolate drinks Drinks made with milk, canned, iced teas	Beer Cocoa Dark colas
Dairy products	Cheese Custard Milk Cream soups	Cottage cheese Ice cream Pudding Yogurt
Protein	Carp Beef liver Fish roe Oysters	Crayfish Chicken liver Organ meats Sardines

Vegetables	**Dried beans and peas:**
	    Baked beans
	    Chick peas
	    Kidney beans
	    Limas
	    Pork and beans
	    Soy beans
		
		Black beans
		Garbanzo beans
		Lentils
		Northern beans
		Split peas
		—

Other foods	Bran cereals Caramels Whole-grain products	Brewer's yeast Nuts/seeds Wheat germ

Reprinted with permission from the National Kidney Foundation.

○ Because of concern of excessive calcium loading and vascular calcification, it is generally recommended to **limit the amount of elemental calcium no more than 2000 mg/d.** As an example, a 500-mg tablet of calcium carbonate provides 200 mg of elemental calcium.

- **Vitamin D analogs:**
  ○ Active vitamin D (**1,25-dihydroxycholecalciferol** also known as "**calcitriol**") provides a feedback mechanism to the parathyroid gland to reduce PTH production and secretion.
  ○ Active vitamin D therapy can lead to unacceptable increases in calcium and phosphorus levels via its action on the small intestine. Therefore, it is primarily used in patients whose calcium and phosphorus are already controlled with the interventions listed above.
  ○ Some active vitamin D analogs, such as paricalcitol, retain the PTH-lowering effect of calcitriol with less hypercalcemia and hyperphosphatemia.[22]
  ○ Another analog that is available for use in the United States is doxercalciferol.[23]
  ○ The **typical starting dose** for calcitriol is 0.25 mcg PO daily, for paricalcitol it is 1 mcg PO daily or 2 mcg PO three times a week, and for doxercalciferol it is 1 mcg/d.
  ○ **Serum calcium and phosphorus should be evaluated within 2 to 4 weeks of therapy initiation** to check for hypercalcemia and hyperphosphatemia. Whether therapy is instituted with calcitriol or an analog such as paricalcitol, the calcium, phosphorus, and intact PTH should be checked in about 2 weeks.[23]
- **Vitamin D repletion:**
  ○ The KDOQI bone metabolism work group recommends replacement of 25-hydroxy vitamin D, the storage form, once levels fall to <30 ng/mL.
  ○ In stages 3 and 4 CKD patients with levels <5 ng/mL, **ergocalciferol** (50,000 IU, orally) should be given weekly for 12 weeks and then monthly thereafter.
  ○ For patients with milder deficiency (5 to 15 ng/mL), the same dose of ergocalciferol is given weekly for 4 weeks and then monthly thereafter.
  ○ For patients with insufficiency (16 to 30 ng/mL), the work group recommends monthly ergocalciferol (50,000 units).
  ○ For patients with deficiency (levels <30 ng/mL), the work group recommends repeating the blood measurement of 25-hydroxy vitamin D after 6 months of treatment.[6]

Metabolic Acidosis

- Metabolic acidosis can lead to decreased albumin production, increased calcium resorption from bone, and worsening of SHPT.
  ○ The best available option to treat acidosis is **sodium bicarbonate 650 to 1300 mg PO bid–tid.** A 650-mg tablet contains 7.6 mEq of bicarbonate.
- **Maintaining bicarbonate levels above 22 mEq/L** will help preserve bone histology and lessen the impact of acidosis on protein catabolism.
- Correction of acidosis will also help in the management of hyperkalemia.
- A recent randomized controlled study also noted that treatment with sodium bicarbonate **decelerated the rate of progression to ESRD,** while improving nutritional parameters in CKD patients.[24]

Hyperlipidemia

- CKD patients should be considered to be in the highest risk group for coronary artery disease.

- The updated National Cholesterol Education Program Adult Treatment Program (NCEP ATP) III guidelines for cholesterol management recommend a low-density lipoprotein cholesterol **goal of <100 mg/dL** for high-risk patients defined as those with established CHD or coronary heart disease risk equivalents.[25]
  - Lifestyle modifications are recommended for LDL 100 to 130 mg/dL as initial line of therapy.
  - Medications are recommended for those with LDL above 130 mg/dL or those failing lifestyle modifications.
  - Statins are first-line agents in CKD.
- Hypertriglyceridemia is treated using lifestyle and dietary modifications as well as medications with **goal of triglycerides of <200 mg/dL.**
  - Fibrates such as gemfibrozil are appropriate for use in CKD but the combination of fibrates and statins in the setting of CKD can result in **rhabdomyolysis.**
  - Appropriate **dose adjustments are necessary** for the levels of renal function.
- A recent review has concisely summarized the role, safety, initial dosing, and potential benefits of statins in patients with CKD and ESRD. In brief, statins are safe in the CKD population and, although they demonstrate similar relative risk reductions for cardiovascular events as compared with non-CKD patients, the absolute risk reductions are greater in the CKD population, given the high rates of underlying cardiovascular disease.[26]

Hyperkalemia

- Hyperkalemia is a potentially life-threatening complication of CKD.
- The acute management of this electrolyte imbalance is discussed elsewhere.
- **Dietary restriction:**
  - Patients should be counseled regarding the restriction of high-potassium foods in their diet.
  - High potassium content is seen in all types of foods, but the common ones are citrus fruits/juices; bananas; watermelons; dried foods such as raisins, prunes, and dates; vegetables such as tomatoes, potatoes, and broccoli; and other food products such as milk.
  - See Table 24-4 for a more comprehensive list of high-potassium foods. However, this does NOT include all possible food items that may contain high potassium content.
  - Patients should be offered medical nutritional therapy (MNT) by a licensed dietician and should be taught to **read food labels** regarding potassium concentration.
- **Medications:**
  - Patients should be counseled on avoiding medications such as nonsteroidal anti-inflammatory agents and cox-2 inhibitors.
  - Inhibitors of the renin–angiotensin–aldosterone system should be used with caution, as renal function deteriorates and electrolytes should be checked routinely.
- **Corrections of acidosis:**
  - Treatment of metabolic acidosis will help correct hyperkalemia.
- **Loop diuretics:**
  - Treatment with loop diuretics will also aid in potassium excretion.

Hyperuricemia

- Hyperuricemia is associated with metabolic syndrome and increased risk for cardiovascular disease and all-cause mortality.[27]

TABLE 24-4	COMMON HIGH-POTASSIUM FOODS (>200 mg per portion)[a]

Fruits	Vegetables	Other Foods
Apricot, raw (two medium)	Acorn squash	Bran/bran products
Avocado (one-fourth whole)	Artichoke	Chocolate (1.5–2 oz)
Banana (half whole)	Bamboo shoots	Granola
Cantaloupe	Baked/refried beans	Milk, all types (one cup)
Dates (five whole)	Butternut squash	Molasses (one tablespoon)
Dried fruits	Tomatoes/tomato products	Peanut butter (two tablespoons)
Figs, dried	Beets, fresh then boiled	Yogurt
Grapefruit juice	Black beans	Nuts and seeds (1 oz)
Honeydew	Broccoli, cooked	Salt-free broth
Kiwi (one medium)	Brussels sprouts	Salt substitutes/lite salt
Mango (one medium)	Chinese cabbage	Snuff/chewing tobacco
Nectarine (one medium)	Carrots, raw	Nutritional supplements
Orange (one medium)	Dried beans and peas	—
Orange juice	Greens, except kale/spinach	—
Papaya (half whole)	Hubbard squash	—
Pomegranate (one whole)	Kohlrabi	—
Pomegranate juice	Lentils/legumes	—
Prunes	Vegetable juices	—
Prune juice	Mushrooms, canned	—
Raisins	Parsnips	—
—	Potatoes, white and sweet	—
—	Pumpkin	—
—	Rutabagas	—

[a]The portion is half cup unless otherwise stated.

Reprinted with permission from the National Kidney Foundation.

- Hyperuricemia is prevalent in CKD due to decreased uric acid excretion as well as the use of diuretics, which further decrease uric acid excretion.[28]
- Hyperuricemia in CKD can manifest as painful gout flares or chronic tophaceous gout.[28]
- Treatment of hyperuricemia and gout involves use of **steroids or colchicine to treat acute flares.** Nonsteroidal anti-inflammatory medications, which are very effective, have to be used with extreme caution (if not at all) due to risk of worsening renal function, blood pressure control, and hyperkalemia.
- Once acute flare has been treated, it is recommended that a xanthine oxidase inhibitor such as **allopurinol** or febuxostat be used to lower uric acid levels.

- A recent small study suggested that treatment of hyperuricemia with allopurinol in CKD patients may slow down progression to ESRD.[29]

Prevention of Acute Kidney Injury and Monitoring of Concomitant Medications

- Prevention of additional renal insults is essential in decreasing progression to ESRD.
- Intravenous contrast is a frequent cause of acute kidney injury (AKI) in high-risk patients, and they should be aware of this risk. Please refer to the chapter on contrast-induced nephropathy.
- Likewise, surgeries or other procedures in the hospital associated with hypotension will increase the risk of AKI.
- Studies have shown that CKD patients who develop AKI and recover renal function, still progress faster to ESRD than those patients who do not develop AKI.[30]
- Concomitant medications should be addressed at every visit.
  - Medications should be dose-adjusted to prevent side effects from accumulation in the setting of decreased renal function.
  - Medications should be discontinued or dose-adjusted to decrease further renal injury.
  - Patients should be asked and counseled regarding use of over-the-counter medications, supplements, herbal products, and vitamins, since all of these agents can interact with other medications, exacerbate renal dysfunction, or cause electrolyte imbalances.

PREPARATION FOR DIALYSIS AND RENAL TRANSPLANT

Patient Education

- Lifestyle modifications are essential in decreasing cardiovascular risk and include, but are not restricted to, weight loss, reduction of dietary sodium intake, regular exercise, and smoking cessation.
- Smoking is associated with increased progression to ESRD.
- A **comprehensive education program** is usually offered to all CKD patients, typically when GFR falls below 30 mL/min, in order to prepare them for RRT.
  - The program should encompass educating patients regarding different modalities of RRT—hemodialysis (HD), peritoneal dialysis (PD), and renal transplantation.
  - The dieticians should be available to give nutritional counseling.
  - Patients should be encouraged to tour a HD facility and meet HD and PD patients.
  - Patients should also be given information regarding different types of HD options (nocturnal, in-center, home HD, etc.) as well as chance to be evaluated for kidney transplantation.
  - Social work staff should be available to address concerns such as insurance, cost, transportation to dialysis, and so forth.
- It is the **responsibility of the treating nephrologist to address the suitability of dialysis** initiation with his/her patients, and often their family members, and plan accordingly.
- Dialysis initiation **may not be appropriate** at extremely advanced age (in patients with multiple comorbid conditions) or patients in nursing home, since dialysis has not been shown to improve quality of life or significantly prolong it.[31]

Nutritional Counseling

- The 2004 KDOQI recommendations were made from modifications from the Dietary Approaches to Stop Hypertension (DASH) diet to apply to patients with CKD.
- Individualizing the dietetic therapy may ultimately prove to be the most appropriate strategy for CKD patients.
- It is essential that CKD patients receive **MNT counseling.** This is offered by licensed renal dieticians and covered under some insurance plans.
- Patients should be counseled about the **consequences of a high-protein diet,** including the generation of extra solute (i.e., urea) that will need to be eliminated and the enhanced production of an acid load that will also need to be excreted.
- Although current recommendations suggest reducing dietary protein intake to minimize the need for urea and acid excretion, a risk of malnutrition does exist.
- Malnutrition in the setting of a GFR higher than that normally recommended for initiating RRT maybe an indication to start dialysis.
- Appropriate counseling regarding **low-potassium or low-phosphorus diet** is also a part of nutritional management.
- MNT also involves counseling regarding food choices appropriate for those with diabetes mellitus and hyperlipidemia.

Immunizations

- The Center for Disease Control and Prevention's January 2010 adult vaccination schedule can be found online at http://www.cdc.gov/mmwr/PDF/wk/mm5901-Immunization.pdf.[32]
- The most commonly administered vaccines to CKD patients are listed below
- **Hepatitis B:**
  - ○ Although hepatitis B immunization is not required for all patients with CKD, it is generally recommended for those expected to start dialysis, given the risk of transmission in dialysis units.
  - ○ There is a three-dose regimen, with the second dose given at least 1 month later and the third given at least 2 months later but >4 months from the first dose.
  - ○ An alternative schedule is necessary if the combined hepatitis A and B vaccine is used.
  - ○ Surface antibody immunity can be checked 1 to 6 months after the vaccination has been completed. Levels of hepatitis B surface antibody should exceed >10 mIU/mL.
  - ○ Booster doses are recommended for dialysis patients if levels fall below this value.
- **Pneumococcal vaccination:**
  - ○ The CDC recommends pneumococcal polysaccharide vaccination for all patients with CKD.
  - ○ Current guidelines recommend a one-time revaccination 5 years after the initial vaccination for patients older than 65 years, if the initial vaccination was given when they were younger than 65 years.
- **Influenza vaccination:**
  - ○ Influenza vaccination is recommended annually for all individuals aged 50 years and older.
  - ○ The CDC also recommends annual influenza vaccination (inactivated vaccine) for all younger patients with CKD.

Referral for Dialysis Access and Transplantation

- Patients with GFR <30 mL/min (stage 4 CKD) should be referred for vascular access if **HD** is the preferred RRT of choice.
- The NKF also has KDOQI practice guidelines detailing recommendations for vascular access.
  - An **arteriovenous fistula (AVF)** is the most preferred access for HD patients; however, these take longer time to mature and may not be feasible in patients with extensive vascular disease.
  - The next preferred access is **arteriovenous graft (AVG)**, where a synthetic material is used to connect the artery to the vein. AVG has a higher tendency to thrombose compared with AVF but is preferred over tunneled HD catheters.
- Although it is difficult to anticipate exactly when a patient will need to initiate RRT, an **AVF should ideally be placed 6 months prior** to the start of HD and an **AVG placed at least 3 to 6 weeks prior** to the start of HD.
- **Early referral to a vascular surgeon** is extremely vital for several reasons:
  - Preoperative studies (e.g., vein mapping) can be completed and access placed in a timely manner.[33]
  - Further, the nondominant upper extremity is the preferred site for AVF placement. This arm should be protected from IV access, including peripheral IVs, peripherally inserted central catheter (PICC) lines, and subclavian lines. It may also be useful to avoid measuring blood pressures on the arm preferred for AVF placement.[33]
- If **PD** is the initial preferred modality of choice, then patients should be referred to the specific PD nurses for further assessment. Several issues need to be addressed before the patient is considered as an appropriate candidate.
  - Does the patient have adequate support at home?
  - Is the patient capable of understanding and performing the procedure at home?
  - Does the patient have a clean home environment?
- Early surgical evaluation is useful to rule out potential problems such as ventral/umbilical hernias.
- Ideally, the **PD catheter** should be placed **at least 2 weeks prior** to the anticipated start of PD.
- **Transplantation:**
  - Suitable candidates with stage 4 CKD should be referred for evaluation by a multidisciplinary kidney transplant clinic.
  - Typically, patients cannot be listed for transplantation until the GFR has fallen to <20 mL/min.
  - Not all patients are eligible for a kidney transplant, and it is responsibility of the treating nephrologist to advise the patient regarding the appropriateness of transplantation, which involves major surgery and complications of immunosuppression.

Initiation of Renal Replacement Therapy

- Timing of initiation of RRT is a very difficult problem in the management of CKD patients.
- In practical terms, it is advisable to initiate dialysis in patients with **CKD secondary to diabetic nephropathy** once the **GFR is <15 mL/min.**
- In patients with **CKD from other causes,** dialysis may be delayed until **GFR declines below 10 mL/min.**

- Although the values presented here are convenient, they are not absolute.
- In cases of severe malnutrition, diuretic resistant volume overload, or profound, resistant metabolic acidosis, RRT may need to be initiated at higher levels of GFR.
- However, **starting dialysis based on GFR levels alone is no longer recommended** on the basis of recent data.
- The Initiating Dialysis Early and Late trial examined starting dialysis with a GFR between 10 and 14 cc/min versus 5 to 7 cc/min and found no benefit in early initiation with respect to dialysis complications, infections, or cardiovascular events.[34]
- Signs and symptoms of uremia such as poor appetite, nausea, vomiting, restless legs, severe itching, headaches, shortness of breath, volume overload refractory to diuretics, and laboratory manifestations such persistent hyperkalemia, metabolic acidosis, and SHPT despite adequate treatment are good indicators to guide the timing of initiation of RRT.

REFERENCES

1. Levey AS, Coresh J, Balk E, et al. National Kidney Foundation practice guidelines for chronic kidney disease: evaluation, classification, and stratification. *Ann Intern Med.* 2003; 139(2):137–147.
2. Chobanian AV, Bakris GL, Black HR, et al. The Seventh Report of the Joint National Committee on Prevention, Detection, Evaluation, and Treatment of High Blood Pressure: the JNC 7 report. *JAMA.* 2003;289(19):2560–2572.
3. Kidney Disease Outcomes Quality Initiative (K/DOQI). K/DOQI clinical practice guidelines on hypertension and antihypertensive agents in chronic kidney disease. *Am J Kidney Dis.* 2004;43(5 suppl 1):S1–S290.
4. KDOQI; National Kidney Foundation II. Clinical practice guidelines and clinical practice recommendations for anemia in chronic kidney disease in adults. *Am J Kidney Dis.* 2006;47(5 suppl 3):S16–S85.
5. K/DOQI clinical practice guidelines for bone metabolism and disease in chronic kidney disease. *Am J Kidney Dis.* 2003;42(4 suppl 3):S1–S201.
6. KDIGO clinical practice guideline for the diagnosis, evaluation, prevention, and treatment of Chronic Kidney Disease-Mineral and Bone Disorder (CKD-MBD). *Kidney Int Suppl.* 2009;(113):S1–S130.
7. Go AS, Chertow GM, Fan D, et al. Chronic kidney disease and the risks of death, cardiovascular events, and hospitalization. *N Engl J Med.* 2004;351(13):1296–1305.
8. Levey AS, Bosch JP, Lewis JB, et al. A more accurate method to estimate glomerular filtration rate from serum creatinine: a new prediction equation. Modification of Diet in Renal Disease Study Group. *Ann Intern Med.* 1999;130(6):461–470.
9. Schold JD, Navaneethan SD, Jolly SE, et al. Implications of the CKD-EPI GFR estimation equation in clinical practice. *Clin J Am Soc Nephrol.* 2011;6(3):497–504.
10. Stevens LA, Claybon MA, Schmid CH, et al. Evaluation of the Chronic Kidney Disease Epidemiology Collaboration equation for estimating the glomerular filtration rate in multiple ethnicities. *Kidney Int.* 2011;79(5):555–562.
11. Stancu S, Barsan L, Stanciu A, et al. Can the response to iron therapy be predicted in anemic nondialysis patients with chronic kidney disease? *Clin J Am Soc Nephrol.* 2010;5(3): 409–416.
12. Wavamunno MD, Harris DC. The need for early nephrology referral. *Kidney Int Suppl.* 2005;(94):S128–S132.
13. Toto RD. Treatment of hypertension in chronic kidney disease. *Semin Nephrol.* 2005;25(6): 435–439.

14. Hou FF, Zhang X, Zhang GH, et al. Efficacy and safety of benazepril for advanced chronic renal insufficiency. *N Engl J Med.* 2006;354(2):131–140.

15. Mann JF, Schmieder RE, McQueen M, et al. Renal outcomes with telmisartan, ramipril, or both, in people at high vascular risk (the ONTARGET study): a multicentre, randomised, double-blind, controlled trial. *Lancet.* 2008;372(9638):547–553.

16. Bianchi S, Bigazzi R, Campese VM. Long-term effects of spironolactone on proteinuria and kidney function in patients with chronic kidney disease. *Kidney Int.* 2006;70(12):2116–2123.

17. Hayat A. Safety issues with intravenous iron products in the management of anemia in chronic kidney disease. *Clin Med Res.* 2008;6(3–4):93–102.

18. Drueke TB, Locatelli F, Clyne N, et al. Normalization of hemoglobin level in patients with chronic kidney disease and anemia. *N Engl J Med.* 2006;355(20):2071–2084.

19. Singh AK, Szczech L, Tang KL, et al. Correction of anemia with epoetin alfa in chronic kidney disease. *N Engl J Med.* 2006;355(20):2085–2098.

20. Pfeffer MA, Burdmann EA, Chen CY, et al. A trial of darbepoetin alfa in type 2 diabetes and chronic kidney disease. *N Engl J Med.* 2009;361(21):2019–2032.

21. KDOQI. KDOQI Clinical Practice Guideline and Clinical Practice Recommendations for anemia in chronic kidney disease: 2007 update of hemoglobin target. *Am J Kidney Dis.* 2007;50(3):471–530.

22. Cheng S, Coyne D. Paricalcitol capsules for the control of secondary hyperparathyroidism in chronic kidney disease. *Expert Opin Pharmacother.* 2006;7(5):617–621.

23. Sprague SM, Coyne D. Control of secondary hyperparathyroidism by vitamin D receptor agonists in chronic kidney disease. *Clin J Am Soc Nephrol.* 2010;5(3):512–518.

24. de Brito-Ashurst I, Varagunam M, Raftery MJ, et al. Bicarbonate supplementation slows progression of CKD and improves nutritional status. *J Am Soc Nephrol.* 2009;20(9): 2075–2084.

25. Grundy SM, Cleeman JI, Merz CN, et al. Implications of recent clinical trials for the National Cholesterol Education Program Adult Treatment Panel III Guidelines. *J Am Coll Cardiol.* 2004;44(3):720–732.

26. Baber U, Toto RD, de Lemos JA. Statins and cardiovascular risk reduction in patients with chronic kidney disease and end-stage renal failure. *Am Heart J.* 2007;153(4):471–477.

27. Madero M, Sarnak MJ, Wang X, et al. Uric acid and long-term outcomes in CKD. *Am J Kidney Dis.* 2009;53(5):796–803.

28. Gaffo AL, Saag KG. Management of hyperuricemia and gout in CKD. *Am J Kidney Dis.* 2008;52(5):994–1009.

29. Goicoechea M, de Vinuesa SG, Verdalles U, et al. Effect of allopurinol in chronic kidney disease progression and cardiovascular risk. *Clin J Am Soc Nephrol.* 2010;5(8):1388–1393.

30. Okusa MD, Chertow GM, Portilla D. The nexus of acute kidney injury, chronic kidney disease, and World Kidney Day 2009. *Clin J Am Soc Nephrol.* 2009;4(3):520–522.

31. Kurella Tamura M, Covinsky KE, Chertow GM, et al. Functional status of elderly adults before and after initiation of dialysis. *N Engl J Med.* 2009;361(16):1539–1547.

32. Centers for Disease Control and Prevention. Recommended adult immunization schedule–United States, 2011. *MMWR Morb Mortal Wkly Rep.* 2011;60(4):1–4.

33. Vascular Access Work Group. Clinical practice guidelines for vascular access. *Am J Kidney Dis.* 2006;48(suppl 1):S176–S247.

34. Cooper BA, Branley P, Bulfone L, et al. A randomized, controlled trial of early versus late initiation of dialysis. *N Engl J Med.* 2010;363(7):609–619.

Hemodialysis

25

Steven Cheng

GENERAL PRINCIPLES

- The loss of kidney function in end-stage renal disease (ESRD) results in uremia and an impairment in the regulation of fluids and electrolytes. Without intervention, ESRD is inevitably fatal.
- Therapeutic options include hemodialysis (HD), peritoneal dialysis, transplantation, and supportive/palliative care. HD is the most commonly utilized form of renal replacement therapy.

Epidemiology
- Of the 490,000 patients with ESRD in the United States, over 300,000 are currently on HD.[1]
  - Like the general ESRD population, the prevalent HD population is predominately white (55% white, 38% black, 4% Asian, 3% Native American/other), with a slightly higher proportion of males (54%).
  - Diabetes is the most common underlying diagnosis, followed by hypertension, glomerulonephritis, and congenital and cystic kidney diseases.
  - The largest age group of HD patients is between 70 and 79 years. This differs from the generalized ESRD population, whose mean age is 58 years, and reflects a younger and generally healthier cohort undergoing transplant and peritoneal dialysis.
- Despite advances in care, the **mortality rate** in HD patients is startling.
  - **Cardiovascular disease is clearly the leading cause of death** among patients on HD, followed by septicemia.
  - The probability of death in the first 5 years after starting HD is 63%.[2]
    - Among diabetics on HD, this probability rises to 71%.
    - Dialysis patients over the age of 65 have a mortality rate seven times higher than the general Medicare population. Dialysis patients between the ages of 20 and 64 have a mortality rate eight times higher.

DIAGNOSIS

Clinical Presentation: Who Requires Dialysis?
- Given the poor outcomes for patients on HD, every effort should be undertaken to preserve residual renal function.
  - Early nephrology referrals, patient education, and serious consideration of transplant options may be helpful in attenuating the progression to ESRD.

- ○ Even with aggressive early medical care, dialysis may become necessary to relieve uremic symptoms, electrolyte imbalances, or fluid accumulation due to declining renal function.
- The vast majority of patients who require HD have chronic kidney diseases with a gradual but progressive loss of renal function over time.
  - ○ Patients usually develop **uremic symptoms** and require dialysis initiation, as their estimated glomerular filtration rate **(GFR) falls below 10 mL/min/1.73 m²**.[3]
  - ○ Patients with **significant comorbidities,** particularly diabetes, may require dialysis initiation at an earlier stage, usually near an estimated **GFR of 15 mL/min/1.73 m²**.
  - ○ **Uremic symptoms** develop due to the accumulation of toxic metabolites, which are no longer adequately cleared by the failing kidney.
    - ▪ This may manifest in a variety of ways, including nausea, vomiting, poor energy levels, decreased appetite, lethargy, pruritus, and a metallic aftertaste.
    - ▪ Motor neuropathies may be elicited on physical exam, while asterixis, tremor, and myoclonus suggest uremic encephalopathy.
    - ▪ Uremic pericarditis manifests as a pericardial friction rub or pericardial effusion, and is a clear indication for urgent initiation of dialytic therapy.
- **Acute kidney injury** may also require dialytic support, particularly in those who develop pulmonary edema, hyperkalemia, or metabolic acidosis.
  - ○ **Acute indications** for the initiation of dialysis can be remembered with the **mnemonic AEIOU:**
    - ▪ Acidosis: life-threatening metabolic acidosis with a pH <7.2, not responsive to conservative treatments.
    - ▪ Electrolyte abnormalities: life-threatening hyperkalemia associated with electrocardiogram (ECG) changes and symptomatic hypermagnesemia and hypercalcemia.
    - ▪ Intoxications: there are a limited number of intoxications for which HD is indicated. It should be considered in patients with deteriorating medical status, those whose measured levels of a substance are indicative of poor outcomes, or those with metabolic derangements (e.g., metabolic acidosis caused by intoxication). Substances that are effectively cleared with dialysis have the following characteristics:
      - ☐ Low molecular weight (<500 Da)
      - ☐ High water solubility
      - ☐ Low degree of protein binding
      - ☐ Small volumes of distribution (<1 L/kg)
      - ☐ High dialysis clearance relative to endogenous clearance
      - ☐ The following substances can be cleared with dialysis: barbiturates, bromides, chloral hydrate, alcohols, lithium, theophylline, procainamide, salicylates, atenolol, and sotalol.
    - ▪ Overload: fluid overload or pulmonary edema not responsive to aggressive diuresis
    - ▪ Uremia: mental status changes attributable to uremia, uremic pericarditis, or neuropathy, bleeding diatheses, or vomiting associated with uremia.

TREATMENT

Dialysis Modalities

- Choosing the appropriate HD modality is an important decision that should be made with the consideration of both patient preference and a practical assessment of patient resources and capabilities.
  - The primary variables that differentiate the various modalities are: location, independence, duration, and cumulative dialysis dose.
- **Intermittent in-center** HD is the most common form of HD.
  - This form of HD typically involves treatments three times per week, with each session averaging between 3 and 4 hours in duration.
  - Patients receive HD at an in-center location, where trained staff are able to set up and supervise each treatment. For patients new to HD, this is often the modality of choice to acclimate patients to a supervised and controlled HD session.
- **Intermittent home** HD is similar to intermittent in-center HD in frequency and duration of treatments.
  - The key difference is location, giving patients the greater freedom of undergoing treatments at their own homes.
  - The home environment must be carefully evaluated, and both water supply and electricity must be able to accommodate the dialysis system. Furthermore, patients need to demonstrate sufficient responsibility over their treatments and the ability to cannulate their own arteriovenous accesses with a safe and sterile technique.
- **Short daily** HD exposes patients to more frequent treatments (usually six times per week), although with a shorter duration of each session.
  - The cumulative weekly dose of dialysis is similar to that obtained on intermittent HD. However, dividing the treatments into frequent, shorter treatments may prevent intradialytic complications, particularly hypotension and cramping.
  - This modality is predominately performed at home, although some in-center locations are able to accommodate the daily treatments.
- **Nocturnal** HD is different, in that it offers a larger cumulative dose of dialysis each week.
  - Patients who undergo nocturnal HD at home typically have longer treatment time periods, averaging 6 to 8 hours, performed six nights per week.
  - This modality does have the added convenience of allowing the patient greater freedom during the day.
  - Like short daily HD, nocturnal HD is predominately done at home, although in-center locations are available. In-center nocturnal HD typically offers 8-hour treatments, three nights per week.
- The decision to dialyze patients with acute renal failure is often performed based on acute indications, and the selection of modalities is often done in consideration of the patient's hemodynamic status. A full description of dialysis options, including continuous dialysis modalities, is addressed in Chapter 15, Renal Replacement Therapy in Acute Kidney Injury.

Dialysis Access

- For HD to be effective, there must first be an effective system of blood delivery from the patient to the machine, and vice versa. This is referred to as a *dialysis access*.

- There are **three types of dialysis access:** arteriovenous fistulas (AVFs), arteriovenous grafts (AVG), and dialysis catheters.
  - Fistulas and grafts are vascular conduits that can support a high flow of blood. They are cannulated at each dialysis treatment with two needles—one through which arterial blood is pumped through the dialyzer, and the other through which blood is returned into the venous system.
  - Catheters are placed in a central venous position, typically in the internal jugular location, with flow through separate luminal ports to simulate arterial output and venous return. Specific characteristics of each type of access are described below.
- The **AVF** is the most desirable form of vascular access. It is created by the surgical manipulation of a patient's native vasculature.
  - Construction is performed under regional anesthesia by an experienced vascular surgeon and can consist of either a side-to-side anastomosis between an artery and vein or a side-of-artery to end-of-vein anastomosis.
  - The goal is to provide an access site that can withstand repeated cannulation with large bore needles, and can sustain the high flow of blood necessary for dialysis. Flow through an AVF averages between 600 and 800 cc/min and may be able to maintain patency at flows of 200 cc/min.
  - Complications with thrombosis, infection, and vascular steal are lower in comparison to the AVG.
  - Placement of an AVF requires foresight, as they can take 3 to 4 months to mature. Furthermore, the construction of an adequate AVF may be impossible if the patient lacks healthy vasculature. In particular, patients with advanced diabetes or peripheral vascular disease may not have vessels that are amenable to the creation of a fistula.
- The **AVG** can be placed in patients for whom an AVF cannot be created.
  - In lieu of the patient's native vasculature, a synthetic graft (frequently created from polytetrafluoroethylene) is placed for the arteriovenous connection.
  - Long-term patency rates are less impressive than those obtained with AVF. However, the AVG does have a few advantages, including a large surface area for cannulation and a shorter maturation time, on the rate of 3 to 4 weeks.
  - Flow rates through an AVG are typically 1000 to 1500 cc/min, with thrombosis occurring at flows less than 600 to 800 cc/min.
- A **catheter is the least desirable form of vascular access** for HD.
  - Cuffed tunneled dialysis catheters are typically placed in the right internal jugular vein, with a tunneled exit site just below the ipsilateral clavicle.
  - These can be placed in patients requiring HD who do not yet have a site for a permanent vascular access. However, given variable success with flows, difficulties with recirculation, catheter dysfunction, and significant risk of infection, the catheter should not be used except as an access of last resort.

BASIC MECHANISM OF HD

- The goal of HD is to replace the basic functions of the failing kidney. To approximate normal kidney function, HD must clear uremic solutes, adjust serum electrolytes, and remove accumulated fluid.

- **Diffusion** and **convection** are the mechanisms responsible for the balance of solutes and electrolytes. **Ultrafiltration** is the mechanism responsible for the removal of fluid.
  - ○ **Diffusion** uses the difference in solute concentration between blood and dialysate to drive the movement of small particles.
    - ■ To maximize the gradient between blood and dialysate, the blood flows through fibers with a semi-permeable membrane in one direction, while the dialysate flows in the opposite direction.
    - ■ Although any molecule smaller than the membrane pore is capable of moving between compartments, diffusion favors the movement of smaller molecules, as they possess a higher particle velocity and a greater likelihood of contact with the membrane surface.
    - ■ The lower concentration of potassium and higher amount of bicarbonate in dialysate are responsible for removal of potassium and correction of metabolic acidosis in the blood.
  - ○ **Ultrafiltration** utilizes a hydrostatic pressure gradient to move fluid from blood to the discarded dialysate.
    - ■ The extent of ultrafiltration can be controlled by the dialysis machine.
  - ○ **Convection** is based on the principle of solute drag.
    - ■ When fluid moves from blood to dialysate, the flow of fluid "drags" particles across the dialysis membrane.
    - ■ Convection moves small and middle-sized molecules across the pores of the dialysis membrane.

Dialysis Prescription

- The dialysis prescription should be tailored to the specific goals of attaining adequate clearance of toxins, maintaining electrolyte balance, and removing excess fluid gains (Table 25-1).

Attaining Dialysis Adequacy: Time, Flow, and Choice of Dialyzer

- **For chronic HD, the adequacy of dialysis dose is modeled by two equations, the Kt/V and the urea reduction ratio.** Both can be measured with dialysis treatments and reflect the clearance of urea.
  - ○ Kt/V is a ratio that relates the volume of cleared plasma (Kt) to the volume of urea distribution (V).
    - ■ The guidelines instituted by the National Kidney Foundation's Kidney Disease Outcomes Quality Initiative (K/DOQI) set the *minimal Kt/V* for a patient dialyzed thrice weekly at 1.2 for each dialysis treatment. However, the *target* goal is 15% higher, that is, a Kt/V of 1.4.[4]
  - ○ The **urea reduction rate (URR)** similarly reflects the removal of urea and is calculated using blood urea nitrogen (BUN) from pre- and postdialysis treatment:
    - ■ $URR = (BUN_{pre} - BUN_{post})/BUN_{pre}$
    - ■ A Kt/V of 1.3 roughly correlates to a URR of 70%. K/DOQI guidelines recommend the attainment of a minimal URR of 65% and a target URR of 70%.
- For the goal of attaining adequate Kt/V and URR values, the principle variables are: duration of treatment, blood flow, dialysate flow, and dialyzer size.
  - ○ A typical dialysis treatment is between 3 and 4 hours in length and is administered thrice weekly. Time on dialysis can be increased if Kt/V and/or URR

TABLE 25-1	GUIDELINES FOR MAINTENANCE HEMODIALYSIS PRESCRIPTION		
Goal	Variable	Typical Prescription	Comments
Dialysis adequacy (Kt/V > 1.2 or URR > 65%)	Time	3–4 hours	Can be adjusted in 15-minute increments
	Frequency	3 times/week	Consider adding weekly treatments for large volumes of distribution.
	Dialyzer	Variable by institution	High-efficiency dialyzers have larger surface areas.
	Blood flow	350–450 mL/minute	AV grafts and fistulas: 400–500 mL/minute Catheters: 350–400 mL/minute
	Dialysate flow	500–800 mL/minute	Little benefit for dialysate flow rates >800 mL/minute
Electrolyte balance	Dialysate [K]	2–3 mEq/L	0 or 1 mEq/L can be used for severe hyperkalemia but requires monitoring of serum [K] at 30- to 60-minute intervals.
	Dialysate [Na]	140–145 mEq/L	Should be no more than 15–20 mEq/L higher than serum [Na] in patients with chronic hyponatremia.
	Dialysate [Ca]	2.5 mEq/L	Consider higher Ca content in ARF or hypocalcemia.
	Dialysate [HCO₃]	35–38 mEq/L	Can be lowered to 28 mEq/L for alkalotic patients.
Volume regulation	Ultrafiltration	Based on EDW; typically 2–3 L	UF >4 L during a single treatment may lead to uncomfortable fluid shifts and hypotension.

ARF, acute renal failure; AV, arteriovenous; EDW, estimated dry weight; Kt/V, volume of cleared plasma (Kt) to the volume of urea distribution (V); UF, ultrafiltration; URR, urea reduction rate.

reflect poor dialysis. However, it is often dependent on the patient's willingness to stay for additional treatment time.

○ Blood flow rate is largely dependent on the access used. Most grafts and fistulas can support blood flow between 400 and 500 cc/min. Catheters are less predictable, and, on average, support flows of 350 to 400 cc/min.

- Maximizing blood flows can be extremely helpful in attaining target goals.
- Patients with decreasing dialysis adequacy and poor blood flows from their access should be evaluated for vascular stenosis or thrombosis.
- Correction of flow-limiting complications or changing the type of access from a catheter to an AVG/AVF permits higher blood flows and improves dialysis adequacy.

○ Dialysate flow rate is generally between 500 and 800 cc/min.

- Titrating the dialysate flow rate is an option, particularly in those with a prescribed dialysate flow under 800 cc/min, but it is unlikely that increasing the rate beyond 800 cc/min will contribute significantly to improved clearance.

○ Dialyzer size refers to the amount of exposed surface area between blood and dialysate.

- A larger exposed surface area can also be used to help improve adequacy.
- The availability of various dialyzers is institution dependent, though most dialysis facilities are stocked with high-efficiency dialyzers.

Attaining Electrolyte Balance: The Dialysate Composition

- The choice of dialysate is the key variable for the balance of serum electrolytes and the correction of conditions such as hyperkalemia.
- Potassium, sodium, calcium, and bicarbonate levels are the primary electrolytes that can be controlled in the choice of a dialysate solution.

○ **Potassium concentration in the dialysate** can vary widely depending on the patient's pre-HD potassium concentration.

- For a patient potassium of ≥5.5 mEq/L, a dialysate potassium concentration of 2 or 3 mEq/L is appropriate.
- In those with a propensity toward arrhythmias, the 3 mEq/L bath is preferred to avoid precipitating hypokalemia.
- A dialysate potassium concentration of 4 mEq/L is appropriate for patients with hypokalemia or persistent serum potassium <3.5 mEq/L.
- In those with a potassium of >6.5 to 7.0 mEq/L or EKG changes concerning for hyperkalemia, a 0 or 1 mEq/L potassium bath may be required for a rapid correction. However, this can cause a rapid fall in potassium levels, and serum potassium levels should be monitored every 30 to 60 minutes.
- It is important to also acknowledge that there is a rebound in potassium levels 1 to 2 hours after dialysis. Further supplementation of potassium based on laboratory results drawn immediately after a dialysis treatment is unwise unless there are extenuating circumstances.

○ A **dialysate sodium concentration** of 140 to 145 mEq/L is appropriate in most circumstances, but can be adjusted in patients with preexisting dysnatremias to prevent overcorrection.

- Low serum sodium levels in dialysis patients are often indicative of excessive free water intake in the context of limited, or absent, capacity for renal water handling.
- The majority of these patients can be managed through the enforcement of a fluid restriction.

- Initiating dialysis on patients with chronic hyponatremia requires caution. When dialyzing patients with a chronic serum sodium of <130 mEq/L, the dialysate sodium concentration should be no more than 15 to 20 mEq/L above the serum levels.
- Patients with hypernatremia should also be corrected slowly. Dialysate sodium should be between 3 and 5 mEq/L lower than serum levels.
○ Most dialysate preparations are available with 2.5, 3, or 3.5 mEq/L **Ca concentrations**.
  - A 2.5 mEq/L calcium concentration is equivalent to an ionized calcium concentration of 5 mg/dL.
  - In chronic HD patients, there are concerns about positive calcium balance contributing to vascular calcification and cardiovascular morbidity and mortality.[5] Because of this, a 2.5 mEq/L Ca bath is generally recommended.
  - In patients with persistent hypocalcemia, as in patients who have had a parathyroidectomy, this may need to be increased to maintain serum calcium levels in a safe range.
  - A higher calcium bath or 3 or 3.5 mEq/L is also used in patients who undergo HD acutely or have a significant concurrent acidosis, as the correction of acidosis on dialysis further lowers the plasma calcium concentrations.
○ Most chronic dialysis centers use dialysate solutions containing **bicarbonate levels** of 35 to 38 mEq/L. This is usually sufficient to correct the metabolic acidosis associated with chronic renal failure.
  - There are patients who are susceptible to alkalosis, particularly those who are receiving total parenteral nutrition (TPN), have vomiting or nasogastric suction, have poor protein intake, or have respiratory alkalosis. To avoid detrimental effects of alkalemia, including arrhythmias, headaches, soft tissue calcifications, a lower bicarbonate bath of 20 to 28 mEq/L can be used.

Attaining Appropriate Volume Status: Prescribing Ultrafiltration
- The goal of volume removal in dialysis patients is to attain the patient's estimated dry weight (EDW).
  ○ The **dry weight** refers to **a weight in which the patient is clinically euvolemic and does not demonstrate symptomatic volume contraction** (particularly cramping).
  ○ Ultrafiltrating to the EDW allows physicians to remove fluid weight that is gained in between dialysis treatments.
  ○ Ideally, dialysis patients should restrict fluid intake to limit intradialytic weight gains to <4 kg, as excessive fluid gains may exceed the capacity to ultrafiltrate during a single treatment.
  ○ Attempts to remove >4 to 5 L of fluid during a standard 3 to 4 hour treatment may cause uncomfortable fluid shifts and intradialytic hypotension.
  ○ In patients who are well over their dry weight with evidence of edema, aggressive volume removal can be paired with additional treatments to continue ultrafiltration.
- It is also important to acknowledge that a patient's dry weight is not a fixed number.
  ○ As a result of improved or worsened nutritional status, a patient's dry weight may increase or decrease. This is a result of true weight that is gained, and not merely fluid retention.

○ Patients with limited intradialytic fluid gains and no edema, who note hypotension, lightheadedness, or severe cramping, should be considered for an increase in their EDW.

○ Patients who are attaining their usual EDW, but develop worsening edema or shortness of breath, should be challenged with fluid removal to a lower EDW to prevent florid volume retention.

Anticoagulation

• Heparinization during HD minimizes clotting of the dialysis circuit during the treatment.

○ Clotting is particularly problematic among patients with a high hemoglobin and hematocrit, a high rate of ultrafiltration, and a low blood flow on dialysis.

○ In the United States, unfractionated heparin is most commonly used to prevent this, although low-molecular-weight heparins can also be used.

○ Heparin may be given as a bolus of 1000 to 2000 units, followed by a constant infusion of 1000 to 1200 units per hour.

○ Alternatively, a bolus can be followed by intermittent re-bolusing as necessary to maintain target clotting times.

COMPLICATIONS

Access Complications

• **Poor flow:**

○ **Stenosis** of an AVG or AVF can affect both arterial and venous flow.[6] It should be suspected in patients with a decreased rate of blood flow on dialysis, declining dialysis adequacy, or elevated venous pressures on dialysis.

○ Prolonged bleeding time periods from the access after needle removal may also indicate vascular congestion as a result of a venous outflow obstruction.

○ Patients with a suspected stenosis should have an evaluation of their access with a fistulogram.

  ▪ A percutaneous transluminal angioplasty or surgical revision is warranted in lesions that are >50% of the lumenal diameter.

  ▪ If angioplasty is required more than two times within a 3-month period, the patient should be referred back to vascular surgery for a possible revision.

  ▪ Stents are sometimes placed for surgically inaccessible lesions, limited access, or patients with surgical contraindications.

○ **Thrombosis** can be detected by the absence of a bruit or thrill, and should be addressed promptly to salvage the access.

  ▪ Evaluation with a fistulogram is necessary to exclude the possibility of stenosis.

  ▪ Thrombectomies can be performed to treat AVG thrombosis, though they have limited success in AVF. Thrombosis of a fistula may require referral to the access surgeon for reevaluation. If extensive surgical revision or new fistula placement is necessary, patient may require a tunneled catheter for access until the new access is ready.

○ Poor flow from a catheter can result from malpositioning, kinking, thrombus formation, and central venous stenosis.

  ▪ Early malfunction, preventing successful use shortly after catheter placement, may require positional adjustments or an exchange over a guide wire.

- Thrombosis and stenosis should be suspected in previously functional catheters that are now unable to sustain flows >300 cc/min.
    - Intralumenal thrombosis is a common complication that can be treated by instilling the catheter with a thrombolytic, such as alteplase.[7]
    - A dwell time of 30 minutes is usually sufficient to restore flow, although a repeated trial for 30 to 60 minutes is warranted if suspected catheter thrombosis does not respond to the initial treatment.
    - Persistent tunneled catheter failure warrants a contrast study to evaluate for a fibrin sheath. These can be removed or disrupted via fibrin sheath stripping or balloon angioplasty.
- The placement of stiff, nonsilicone catheters—particularly in the subclavian position—also increases the risk of central stenosis. Although this may remain clinically silent during catheter use, it can cause dysfunction in subsequent arteriovenous accesses. For this reason, subclavian catheters should be avoided for HD unless absolutely necessary.

- **Recirculation:**
    - Recirculation describes a phenomenon by which blood returning to the patient through the venous needle is taken back up by the arterial needle and recirculated through the dialysis mechanism (Fig. 25-1).
    - Recirculation adversely affects the efficiency and adequacy of dialysis.
    - Recirculation can occur from different mechanisms.
        - Stenosis at the venous end of an access can impair flow and allow the blood to be pulled back through the extracorporeal circuit.
        - Recirculation can also occur if the site of venous return is in close proximity to the arterial outflow.

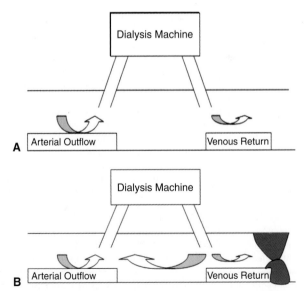

FIGURE 25-1. A: Normal blood flow on dialysis. **B:** Access recirculation.

- Correction of stenosis, proper needle placement, and repositioning of dialysis catheters are all useful in decreasing the likelihood of access recirculation.
- **Infection:**
  - Infections represent the second most common cause of mortality in ESRD patients and are an important part of management in dialysis patients.
  - **Exit site infections** are identified by wound cultures at the site of an erythematous or tender catheter.
    - Infected sites should be cleaned thoroughly and topical antibiotics should be applied.
    - In the presence of an exudate or discharge, wound cultures should be sent and intravenous (IV) antibiotics initiated.
    - If there is discharge from the actual tunnel site, the catheter should be removed.
  - **Catheter-related bacteremia** is identified by constitutional symptoms along with growth from blood cultures and stigmata associated with catheter infection (purulence, erythema, and tenderness).
    - Initial antibiotic coverage should include gram-positive organisms, particularly *Staphylococci*, as well as gram-negative organisms.
    - Dual coverage with vancomycin and gentamicin is recommended as empiric therapy.
    - Blood culture growth, speciation, and antibiotic sensitivities should guide continued therapy.
    - **Removing an infected catheter is more successful than attempts to salvage catheters with antibiotics alone.** However, as dialysis patients require regular access for treatment sessions, some find it impractical to remove all catheters. [8]
      - In a stable patient who demonstrates prompt clinical improvement and has no indications of a tunneled infection, immediate removal of the catheter may not be necessary and the patient should be started on a 3-week course of antibiotics. However, once blood cultures are negative, a catheter exchange is recommended.
      - Patients who demonstrate a poor clinical response after 36 hours of antibiotic therapy or any deterioration of clinical status should have the catheter promptly removed.
      - If dialysis is necessary prior to clinical improvement, a temporary dialysis catheter can be placed for individual treatment sessions.
      - **Catheters should also be removed as soon as possible for all catheter-related infections with *Staphylococcus aureus* or gram-negative organisms.**
  - Infections of grafts or fistulas are less common.
    - Areas of fluctuance should be evaluated with ultrasound for evidence of an abscess.
    - Extensive graft infections may require partial or complete graft excisions.
    - Infections of AVFs are rare and require a course of 6 weeks of antibiotics. There should be a cautious examination for septic emboli or metastatic infections, particularly endocarditis and osteomyelitis. Occasionally, fistula resection is required.
- **Hemodynamic complications:**
  - Limb ischemia as a result of a **steal syndrome** is an important complication of vascular access.[9]
  - Patients with mild symptoms, such as coldness or paresthesias, can be followed conservatively.

- ○ **Pain and poor wound healing require surgical evaluation** and **motor/sensory loss is considered a surgical emergency.**
- ○ The high flows through vascular access may also be problematic for patients with cardiovascular disease. High output failure may be exacerbated due to the placement of an AVG and may require ligation to restore hemodynamic stability.
- **Aneurysms and pseudoaneurysms:**
  - ○ Aneurysms and pseudoaneurysms can develop in fistulas and grafts, stimulated by the trauma of repetitive cannulation. Generally, these can be managed with observation and by avoiding cannulation at the site of aneurysmal dilation.
  - ○ However, in patients who demonstrate rapid growth of the aneurysm, poor eschar formation, or spontaneous bleeding, surgical evaluation should be made urgently. Rupture of an aneurysm or pseudoaneurysm can result in prompt exsanguination and imminent death.

Complications of Urea Clearance

- **Dialysis disequilibrium syndrome** occurs in response to an acute reduction of uremic solutes in patients with chronic kidney disease.
  - ○ This is typically seen after the initiation of dialysis, when aggressive treatment prescriptions result in a rapid reduction of uremic solutes. Cells that have accommodated to the uremic milieu may not be able to rapidly respond to the dramatic osmolal change, resulting in symptoms of dialysis disequilibrium.[10]
  - ○ The syndrome may manifest with nausea, restlessness, confusion, or, in the most serious cases, seizure and coma.
  - ○ Prevention consists of limiting the first dialysis treatment to a reduction in urea of no more than 30% in order to avoid a dramatic shift in solute concentration.
- **Uremia also contributes to nausea, malnutrition, and pruritus.**
  - ○ The differential for these symptoms is broad, but special attention should be paid to the adequacy of dialysis.
  - ○ Pruritus may also result from concurrent disorders of mineral metabolism, particularly the deposition of mineral salts and hyperphosphatemia.
  - ○ Adherence to dietary restriction, compliance with phosphorus binders, and control of the parathyroid–bone–mineral axis are required.
  - ○ Symptoms of pruritus may also be amenable to diphenhydramine or other antihistamines, although oral administration is preferred because of the addictive potential of IV diphenhydramine.

Skin Lesions

- **Calcific uremic arteriolopathy,** previously known as calciphylaxis, is caused by arteriolar mineralization and subsequent tissue ischemia.
  - ○ A number of factors that are thought to promote the underlying process of ectopic mineralization have been reported, including elevated phosphorus and parathyroid hormone levels and the administration of calcium-containing agents and the anticoagulant warfarin.
  - ○ Lesions often begin as erythematous or subcutaneous nodular lesions that can be very painful. Progression to poorly healing ulcerative lesions is associated with a high mortality rate, especially when located centrally.
  - ○ Treatment options are limited, but proper wound care is crucial to avoid infectious sequelae and subsequent amputations.

- Once the diagnosis is made, calcium-based supplements, vitamin D analogs, and warfarin should be stopped, while non–calcium-based phosphorus binders are titrated for aggressive control of serum phosphorus levels.[11]
- Sodium thiosulfate, which improves the solubility of calcium, has been used with variable success.[12]
- In patients with refractory hyperparathyroidism or persistent hypercalcemia and hyperphosphatemia, parathyroidectomy can considered, though this does not guarantee an improvement in wound healing or a survival benefit.

- **Nephrogenic systemic fibrosis:**
  - This is a newly recognized condition characterized by progressive fibrosis and induration of skin, as well as other soft tissues. It tends to progress proximally, resulting in joint contractures and progressive immobility.
  - Lesions typically have a "woody" texture. As of yet, there are no curative options.
  - Cumulative exposure to gadolinium contrast agents have been associated with the development of nephrogenic systemic fibrosis and thus should be avoided, if possible, in patients with ESRD.[13] If such a contrast study is necessary, most agree that immediate HD after contrast exposure is warranted.[14]

Dialyzer Reactions

- **Type A reactions:**
  - Characterized by severe dyspnea, pruritus, abdominal cramping, and angioedema occur in the first 30 min of treatment.
  - They have previously been attributed to ethylene oxide used in device sterilization, contaminated dialysate, latex allergy, and bradykinins, particularly in patients taking angiotensin-converting enzyme inhibitors in conjunction with exposure to the AN69 dialysis membrane.[15]
  - Treatment of suspected type A reactions includes cessation of dialysis, diphenhydramine (25 mg IV for pruritus), oxygen as needed, and 200 mL normal saline if hypotensive. Blood should not be returned.
  - To prevent subsequent reactions, an alternate sterilant may be tried, and dialyzers should be thoroughly rinsed before use.
- **Type B reactions:**
  - These are characterized by mild back pain and chest pain and occur in the first hour of dialysis.
  - One may attempt to treat through symptoms with supplemental oxygen and antihistamine therapy as needed. Symptoms should diminish during the remainder of therapy.
  - As the etiology of type B reactions is uncertain, methods for prevention are also uncertain, although trial of an alternate membrane may help.

Cardiovascular Complications

- Cardiovascular disease is by far the largest cause of mortality in patients with ESRD. As patients are at great cardiovascular risk, chest pain should not be treated lightly in the dialysis units.
  - Although a high suspicion for coronary disease should be maintained, a broad differential should be considered, including musculoskeletal causes, dialyzer reactions, reflux disease, and pulmonary edema.
  - In suspected angina, patients should be placed on nasal oxygen, ultrafiltration should be held, an ECG should be obtained, and nitroglycerin should

be considered if tolerated by the blood pressure. If chest pain persists, dialysis should be discontinued and further work up afforded.

- Both hypotension and hypertension are commonly seen in patients on dialysis.
  - ○ Hypotension may be a product of excessive volume removal, and ultrafiltration should be stopped with saline return administered as necessary to maintain hemodynamic stability. However, it is also important to rule out cardiovascular etiologies as well as infection or sepsis.
  - ○ Febrile patients who develop hypotension during dialysis treatments should have blood cultures drawn and empiric antibiotics dosed after treatment.
  - ○ The management of hypertension in patients with chronic kidney disease is discussed elsewhere in this book.

REFERENCES

1. National Institutes of Health, National Institute of Diabetes and Digestive and Kidney Diseases. U.S. Renal Data System, USRDS 2006 Annual Data Report, Bethesda, MD: National Institutes of Health, National Institute of Diabetes and Digestive and Kidney Diseases, 2006.
2. Bradbury BD, Fissell RB, Albert JM, et al. Predictors of early mortality among incident US hemodialysis patients in the Dialysis Outcomes and Practice Patterns Study (DOPPS). *Clin J Am Soc Nephrol.* 2007;2:89–99.
3. Obrador GT, Arora P, Kausz AT, et al. Level of renal function at the initiation of dialysis in the U.S. end-stage renal disease population. *Kidney Int.* 1999;56(6):2227–2235.
4. NKF – K/DOQI Clinical Practice Guidelines. Available at: http://www.kidney.org/professionals/kdoqi/guidelines.cfm. Accessed on March 4, 2011.
5. Noordzij M, Cranenburg EM, Engelsman LF, et al. Progression of aortic calcification is associated with disorders of mineral metabolism and mortality in chronic dialysis patients. *Nephrol Dial Transplant.* 2011;26(5):1662–1669.
6. Maya ID, Oser R, Saddekni S, et al. Vascular access stenosis: comparison of arteriovenous grafts and fistulas. *Am J Kidney Dis.* 2004;44(5):859–865.
7. Clase CM, Crowther MA, Alistair JI, et al. Thrombolysis for restoration of patency to haemodialysis central venous catheters: a systemic review. *J Thromb Thrombolysis* 2001; 11(2):127–136.
8. Katneni R, Hedayati SS. Central venous catheter-related bacteremia in chronic hemodialysis patients: epidemiology and evidence-based management. *Nat Clin Pract Nephrol.* 2007; 3(5):256–266.
9. Schanzer H, Eisenberg D. Management of steal syndrome resulting from dialysis access. *Semin Vasc Surg.* 2004;17(1):45–49.
10. Patel N, Dalal P, Panesar M. Dialysis disequilibrium syndrome: a narrative review. *Semin Dial.* 2008;21(5):493–498.
11. Rogers NM, Teubner D, Coates TH. Calcific uremic arteriolopathy: advances in pathogenesis and treatment. *Semin Dial.* 2007;20(2):150–157.
12. Sood AR, Wazny LD, Raymond CB, et al. Sodium thiosulfate-based treatment in calcific uremic arteriolopathy: a consecutive case series. *Clin Nephrol.* 2011;75(1):8–15.
13. Cheng S, Abramova L, Saab G, et al. Nephrogenic fibrosing dermopathy associated with exposure to gadolinium-containing contrast agents. *MMWR Morb Mortal Wkly Rep.* 2007;56(7):137–141.
14. Saab G, Cheng S. Nephrogenic systemic fibrosis: a nephrologist's perspective. *Hemodial Int.* 2007;11:S2–S6.
15. Parnes EL, Shapiro WB. Anaphylactoid reactions in hemodialysis patients treated with the AN69 dialyzer. *Kidney Int.* 1991;40:1148.

Peritoneal Dialysis

26

Seth Goldberg

GENERAL PRINCIPLES

- Peritoneal dialysis (PD) is a form of renal replacement therapy that utilizes the patient's natural peritoneum as a semipermeable membrane between the blood and an infused dialysis solution.
- It was observed almost a century ago that solutes equilibrate across the peritoneal membrane, and this discovery paved the way for PD in the treatment of renal failure.
- With technical advancements over the ensuing decades, PD has become a viable option for patients with end-stage renal disease; however, it remains underused in the United States, with only 10% to 15% of dialysis patients on PD as opposed to hemodialysis (HD).
- As compared to HD, actual treatment costs of PD are similar; however, the overall cost of care is higher for HD when vascular access complications are factored.
- Patients on PD require fewer hospitalizations and shorter durations of stay.
- Although neither dialysis modality offers a survival advantage over the other, greater satisfaction and convenience are qualities frequently promoted by patients on PD as compared to those on HD.

Physiology

- **Diffusion:**
  - Most solute removal in PD occurs by diffusion.
  - Substances retained in renal failure (urea, creatinine, potassium, phosphorus) are present in higher concentrations in the blood and thus travel down the gradient into the dialysis solution.
  - Dextrose, which is present in high concentrations in the dialysis solution, diffuses inwardly.
  - The alkaline equivalent, usually lactate, also diffuses inwardly, correcting the metabolic acidosis present in renal failure.
- **Ultrafiltration:**
  - This is the process by which excess water is removed from the body.
  - As opposed to HD, where hydrostatic pressure pulls off excess water, in PD an osmotic gradient causes water to shift from the blood to the relatively hyperosmolar dialysis solution.
  - The hyperosmolar gradient is produced most commonly by the high dextrose concentration in the dialysis solution.
- **Absorption:**
  - Absorption is the reuptake of water and the dissolved solutes in bulk through the lymphatics of the abdominal wall.
  - This counteracts their removal making PD less efficient.
  - Increased abdominal pressure (such as a sitting posture or the standing position) favors absorption.

Patient Selection

- Success of PD depends primarily on appropriate patient selection.
- Patients need to be highly motivated and capable of performing regular treatments within their home environment, without direct supervision of a trained medical specialist.
- Patients who prefer PD over HD tend to be more independent, as the flexible schedule is more conducive to employment and travel as compared to the rigid schedule of in-center HD.
- Some **relative and absolute contraindications for PD** include:
  - The presence of uncorrectable mechanical defects (irreparable abdominal hernia)
  - A recent abdominal operation (including aortic vascular graft)
  - Frequent diverticulitis and/or other intraabdominal infections and pathology
  - Abdominal wall cellulitis
  - A history of repeated abdominal operations with adhesion formation
  - Patients who are physically unable to perform their own exchanges and who lack a suitable caregiver at home.

Apparatus

- **Catheter and setup:**
  - Most centers use a two-cuff silastic Tenckhoff catheter.
  - The intraabdominal portion contains many side-port perforations to maximize fluid flow.
  - Surgically placed, the catheter should have a break-in period of 10 to 14 days prior to initiation to reduce the incidence of early leaks or infection.
  - The deep cuff is stitched to the abdominal wall musculature and secures the catheter in its position.
  - The superficial cuff allows for granulation tissue to form, creating a barrier to infection; however, externalization of this cuff may occur and does not signify catheter migration.
  - Tunneled presternal catheters are associated with reduced infectious complications in obese patients.
  - The Y-set is the standard setup in manual PD (Fig. 26-1).[1]

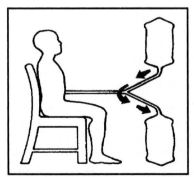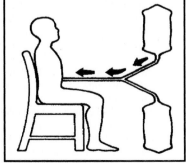

FIGURE 26-1. The Y-set for peritoneal dialysis (PD), with demonstration of the "flush-before-fill" technique.

TABLE 26-1	STANDARD PERITONEAL DIALYSIS SOLUTION COMPONENTS
Sodium	132 mEq/L
Potassium	0 mEq/L
Chloride	Variable (95–105 mEq/L)
Calcium	2.5 mEq/L (1.25 mmol/L) or 3.5 mEq/L (1.75 mmol/L)
Phosphorus	0 mEq/L
Magnesium	1.5 mEq/L or 0.5–0.75 mEq/L
Lactate	35 mEq/L or 40 mEq/L
Dextrose	Variable (1.5%, 2.5%, 4.25%)

○ Infection risk is reduced as there is only one connection point (at the stem emerging from the patient) where sterile technique may accidentally be broken.

○ The flush-before-fill technique is where the patient first flushes air out of the tubing by allowing a small amount of dialysis solution to pass into the drain bag; the drain bag is then clamped and the rest of the dialysis solution is infused into the peritoneal cavity via gravity (10 to 15 minutes).

○ Between exchanges, the bags are disconnected and the stem is capped.

○ When the specified dwell time is complete, a new transfer set is attached and the peritoneal cavity is drained via gravity (20 to 25 minutes) before a new infusion is started, again with the flush-before-fill technique.

○ It is generally recommended that the catheter should not be submerged in water.

• **Dialysis solution:**

○ Standard PD solutions contain sodium, chloride, lactate, magnesium, calcium, and varying concentrations of dextrose (Table 26-1).

○ Most commercial solutions contain a sodium concentration of 132 mEq/L to allow a small amount of sodium to move out from the blood; this protects against hypernatremia that might otherwise occur, particularly with the more hypertonic solutions.

○ Potassium is not present in standard solutions.

○ Phosphorus is also absent, but removal by PD is not efficient and is usually unable to fully remove the daily dietary load.

○ In the present era of wide-spread calcium-containing phosphorus binders, a PD solution with a lower calcium concentration (2.5 mEq/L) is preferred.

○ Lactate has been the primary alkaline equivalent used in PD because of technical difficulty with bicarbonate in the manufacturing process; the resultant acidic pH of 5.5 can cause inflow pain and may be damaging to the mesothelium.

○ Newer dual-chamber bags with bicarbonate are available, allowing for mixing at the time of use, although they have yet to become standard.

○ The hypertonicity that allows for ultrafiltration to occur is typically created by dextrose in the solution.

○ The dextrose concentration can be 1.5%, 2.5%, or 4.25%, with the higher concentrations providing a stronger osmotic force and a greater degree of ultrafiltration.

TABLE 26-2	DEXTROSE-CONTAINING DIALYSIS SOLUTIONS		
Dextrose	Glucose	Osmolarity	Color Code
1.5% (1.5 g/dL)	1.36 g/dL	346 mOsm/L	Yellow
2.5% (2.5 g/dL)	2.27 g/dL	396 mOsm/L	Green
4.25% (4.25 g/dL)	3.86 g/dL	485 mOsm/L	Red

○ Most commercially available solutions have color-coded tabs with which patients may be more familiar rather than the actual percentage of dextrose (Table 26-2).

○ A drawback of dextrose-containing solutions is that 60% to 80% can diffuse inwardly during a dwell, thereby dissipating the osmotic gradient, limiting the achieved ultrafiltration, and leading to the development of metabolic complications.

○ Newer solutions with long-chain glucose polymers (icodextrin) allow for a more sustained osmotic effect, equivalent to a 2.5% dextrose solution over an 18-hour period; the icodextrin can lead to falsely elevated glucose levels on some test strips and such results must be interpreted cautiously.

○ Amino acids can also be used as an osmotic agent, particularly in malnourished patients, although frequent or long-term use may lead to a metabolic acidosis and elevations in the serum urea concentration; ultrafiltration capacity is limited, roughly equivalent to a 1.5% dextrose solution.[2]

• **Peritoneal membrane:**
  ○ The membrane separating the blood in the capillaries from the solution in the peritoneal cavity consists of many layers.
    ▪ Unstirred layer in the blood
    ▪ Capillary endothelium
    ▪ Capillary basement membrane
    ▪ Interstitium
    ▪ Peritoneal basement membrane
    ▪ Peritoneal mesothelium
    ▪ Unstirred layer in the peritoneal solution
  ○ Most resistance to solute movement occurs at the capillary endothelium (via filtration pores) and interstitium (which may be of variable thickness).
  ○ The total surface area in adults is ~2 m², consisting of both the parietal and visceral layers; not all capillaries are readily available to participate in solute exchange, as some may be too far from the cavity under baseline conditions.
  ○ Larger dwell volumes can stretch the membrane, recruiting more capillaries to participate in solute exchange; peritonitis increases the vascularity of the membrane thus making the peritoneum leakier.
  ○ The "three-pore model" describes large pores (>25 nm) through which proteins and other macromolecules pass, small pores (4 to 6 nm) for electrolytes and solutes like urea and creatinine, and ultrasmall pores (0.3 to 0.5 nm), which serve much like aquaporins allowing only solute-free water to pass, acting like a sieve.
  ○ The peritoneal cavity can typically accommodate 2 to 3 L of fluid without discomfort or respiratory compromise.

TABLE 26-3 PERITONEAL MEMBRANE TYPES

Membrane Type	D/P Creatinine Ratio	Characteristics
High	>0.81	Transports solutes quickly, poor ultrafiltration and problems with protein loss
High average	0.65–0.81	Transports solutes well, with adequate ultrafiltration
Low average	0.50–0.64	Transports solutes somewhat slowly, with good ultrafiltration
Low	<0.50	Transports solutes slowly, with excellent ultrafiltration

D/P, dialysate-to-plasma.

○ Not all membranes are alike, and there is considerable amount of patient-to-patient variability in the character of the peritoneal membrane.
○ Four classes of membrane transport characteristics are defined based on ease of creatinine diffusion (Table 26-3).
○ A **peritoneal equilibration test** (PET) allows one to determine the type of membrane a patient possesses and then tailor the PD prescription to maximize efficiency.
  ■ A 2-L infusion of 2.5% dextrose solution is allowed to dwell for 4 hours.
  ■ The dialysate-to-plasma ratio of creatinine is calculated.
○ Higher values correlate with better solute diffusion and clearance; however, the osmotic gradient is also more rapidly lost, limiting ultrafiltration.
○ The Canada–USA (CANUSA) Study Group found a greater risk of technique failure or death in patients with high transport membranes undergoing manual exchanges; the underlying mechanism for this increased risk is thought to involve poor ultrafiltration (with resultant hypertension and left ventricular hypertrophy) and increased protein losses.[3]

Modalities and Prescription
• **Manual exchanges:**
  ○ **Continuous ambulatory peritoneal dialysis** (CAPD) involves patient-operated manual exchanges performed throughout the day.
  ○ Fluid volumes of 2 to 3 L are typical, with dwell times each ranging from 6 to 8 hours.
  ○ Most patients are first educated and trained in CAPD prior to learning other modalities, as this can be used as a backup or emergency modality in the event of a power outage or machine malfunction.
  ○ Patients admitted to the hospital overnight can resort to CAPD if nurse staffing or machine availability is limited.
  ○ A sample prescription would be 2 L of 2.5% dextrose solution with four exchanges of ~6 hours each (or can be unevenly spaced at more convenient times of the day such as awakening, noon, dinner, and bedtime, with the longest dwell overnight).

- **Automated cycler exchanges:**
  - In **continuous cycling peritoneal dialysis** (CCPD), also known as **automated PD**, the patient undergoes automated exchanges overnight, with three or more relatively short cycles.
  - The final exchange remains in the peritoneal cavity on awakening, and the patient disconnects from the machine and is free to go about doing daily activities.
  - The "continuous" label in the name of this modality refers to the retained daytime dwell that allows for solute transfer to occur around the clock.
  - An extra manual exchange is sometimes added during the day if clearance or ultrafiltration targets are not reached.
  - A sample prescription would have four dwells of 2 hours each, with 2.5 L of 2.5% dextrose solution, and a final fill (daytime dwell) of 2 L of icodextrin prior to disconnecting.
- **Prescriptions:**
  - In choosing a PD modality, the patient's membrane type should be known, as determined from the results of the PET.
  - Those with **high transport membranes** dissipate their osmotic gradients more rapidly, and **short repeated dwells** may be required to achieve adequate ultrafiltration (bringing in fresh hypertonic solution); these patients fare better on CCPD.
  - Those with **low transport membranes** have difficulty with solute diffusion and would benefit from the **long, evenly spaced dwells of CAPD.**
  - Patients with either high-average or low-average membranes can usually achieve adequate solute removal and ultrafiltration with either modality; thus selection can generally depend on patient preference.

Adequacy of PD

- **Clearance targets:**
  - The 2006 Kidney Disease Outcomes Quality Initiative (KDOQI) guidelines recommend a **weekly clearance of urea (Kt/V_{urea}) of at least 1.7,** reflecting combined contribution from PD and residual renal function in patients producing >100 mL of urine per day.
  - Clearance adequacy should be **measured within the first month** after initiating therapy, then at **4-month intervals** unless there has been a change in the prescription or in the clinical status of the patient.
  - The clearance is calculated from the 24-hour Kt/V_{urea} shown below, where V_D is the total volume of dialysate used (in L), D_{urea} is the dialysate urea concentration, P_{urea} is the plasma urea concentration, and V_{urea} is the estimated volume (in L) of distribution of urea (total body water or from Watson or Hume formulae).
    - 24-hour $Kt/V_{urea} = (V_D)(D_{urea})/(P_{urea})(V_{urea})$
    - The 24-hour Kt/V_{urea} is then multiplied by 7 for the weekly clearance.
    - Residual renal function is calculated with the same equation, substituting urine values for V_D and D_{urea}, then multiplied by 7 and added to the dialysate clearance.
    - Note the similarity of this equation to the generic UV/P clearance equation.
  - **Protection of residual renal function** is important in the PD population, with avoidance of nephrotoxic medications and contrast as much as possible; the adequacy of PD in Mexico (ADEMEX) study showed a statistically significant association between loss of residual renal function and death.[4]

- Improved clearance can be achieved by increasing the amount of dialysis solution used over the 24-hour period; for example, this can be achieved by adding an extra exchange or by using larger dwell volumes.
- However, there are diminishing returns, as more time is "lost" draining and filling the peritoneal cavity or when larger volumes increase the intraabdominal pressure such that the balance is tilted toward more fluid reabsorption by the lymphatics.

- **Ultrafiltration targets:**
  - Ultrafiltration targets are less clearly defined than clearance, although a minimum of 750 mL of net fluid removal per day has been associated with better outcomes in anuric patients.[5]
  - To enhance ultrafiltration, a higher dextrose concentration can be used (4.25% solution); shorter dwell times (particularly in patients with leaky high transport membranes) can also aid in increasing ultrafiltration.
  - In volume overloaded patients, restricting sodium and water may help, as may administering diuretics in patients making urine.
  - **Ultrafiltration failure** is a term used to describe a condition of fluid overload in association with net ultrafiltration of <400 mL after a 4-hour dwell of 2 L of 4.25% dextrose; this can be the result of rapid loss of the osmotic gradient (high transporters), decreased peritoneal membrane water permeability (peritonitis, fibrosis, adhesions), or from increased reabsorption by the lymphatics.
  - Failure of adequate ultrafiltration may necessitate a switch to HD.

COMPLICATIONS

Infectious Complications

- **Peritonitis:**
  - Table 26-4 describes some of the common signs and symptoms found of peritonitis in PD patients.
  - Peritonitis remains a common and potentially serious complication in the PD population.
  - Although many cases can be treated in the out-patient setting, recurrent episodes threaten the long-term integrity of the peritoneal membrane.
  - Most common causes include **inadvertent breaks in sterile technique,** migration of pathogens from the catheter site, or transvisceral passage of bacteria from gut pathology such as diverticulitis.
  - Presentation can be subtle, but the most common features are cloudy peritoneal fluid, abdominal pain, and/or fever.
  - For diagnosis, the spent dialysis solution should be evaluated by **Gram stain, culture** (preferably prior to antibiotics), and **white blood cell count with differential;** a white blood cell count **>100 cells per mm³, of which at least 50%** are polymorphonuclear neutrophils, is supportive of the diagnosis.
  - The International Society of Peritoneal Dialysis has recommended empiric therapy using a combination of a **first-generation cephalosporin (cefazolin or cephalothin) with ceftazidime.**
  - Routine use of **aminoglycoside therapy is NOT recommended** in PD patients, in order to preserve residual renal function.[6]
  - In most cases, **intraperitoneal dosing** is the preferred route of antibiotic therapy; when patients are bacteremic or overtly septic, intravenous antibiotics should be administered instead.

TABLE 26-4 COMMON SIGNS AND SYMPTOMS IN PD PATIENTS

Sign/Symptom	Character	Causes	Management Issues
Abdominal pain	Inflow pain	Excessively large volume of dwell Low pH of infused solution	Reduce volume of dwell Add bicarbonate to solution (10 mEq/L)
	Diffuse/rebound	Peritonitis Bowel obstruction GI tract pathology (appendicitis, mesenteric ischemia) Abdominal hernia	Check fluid cell count and differential, culture, Gram stain, empiric antibiotics Abdominal or vascular imaging Surgical correction
	Focal/localized	Constipation	Trial of stool softener or enema
Change in dialysate	Cloudy fluid	Peritonitis Allergic reaction to solution or dialysis equipment Chylous leak/superior vena cava syndrome Pancreatitis GI tract pathology (appendicitis, mesenteric ischemia) Fibrin strands	Check fluid cell count and differential (eosinophils for allergic process), culture, Gram stain, empiric antibiotics Check triglyceride level Check amylase level Abdominal or vascular imaging Add heparin (200–500 units/L) into dialysis solution for fibrin strands
	Bloody fluid	Malignancy Sclerosing encapsulating peritonitis Gynecologic source (retrograde menstruation, cyst rupture) Tuberculous peritonitis	Check dialysate fluid cytology Abdominal imaging, with possible need for biopsy *Mycobacterium tuberculosis* polymerase chain reaction
Fever	Temperature >38°C	Peritonitis Allergic reaction to solution or dialysis equipment GI tract pathology (appendicitis, mesenteric ischemia) Exit-site or tunnel infection Non-abdominal infectious source	Check fluid cell count and differential (eosinophils for allergic process), culture, Gram stain, empiric antibiotics Abdominal or vascular imaging General fever workup as in nondialysis patients

GI, gastrointestinal.

TABLE 26-5   INTRAPERITONEAL DOSES OF SELECTED ANTIBIOTICS

Antibiotic	Intraperitoneal Dose
Cefazolin, cephalothin	15–20 mg/kg per bag once a day
Ceftazidime	15–20 mg/kg per bag once a day
Cefepime	1000 mg once a day
Gentamicin, tobramycin	0.6 mg/kg per bag once a day
Amikacin	2 mg/kg per bag once a day
Vancomycin	15–30 mg/kg (1000–3000 mg) every 5–7 days
Fluconazole	200 mg every 24–48 h
Ampicillin	125 mg/L in ALL exchanges
Aztreonam	1 g/L loading, then 250 mg/L in ALL exchanges

○ Suggested intraperitoneal doses for selected antibiotics are listed in Table 26-5; the intermittent dosing schedule refers to the antibiotic being added only to the longest dwell (nighttime fill for CAPD, daytime dwell for CCPD).

○ Treatment strategies that are available after the results of the Gram stain and culture are obtained are outlined in Table 26-6.

○ Gram-positive infections can frequently be treated with a single antibiotic agent, tailored once the sensitivities are known.

○ Infections with *Pseudomonas* species are particularly difficult to eradicate and a second antibiotic to which it is sensitive is recommended; in up to two-thirds of cases, **catheter removal** may become necessary.

○ **Fungal peritonitis** can lead to rapid deterioration and immediate catheter removal is almost always mandatory along with anti-fungal agents; close monitoring in the in-patient setting is typically recommended for this situation.

○ A polymicrobial or anaerobic infection suggests an abdominal abscess or perforation, requiring urgent imaging or surgical exploration.

• **Exit-site and tunnel infection:**

○ Catheter site infections are suspected if **erythema or exudates are present externally;** crust formation at the exit site, however, does not necessarily indicate infection, and positive wound cultures in the absence of other symptoms may simply indicate colonization.

○ *Staphylococcus aureus* is the most common cause of exit-site infections.

○ As with peritonitis, the Gram stain and culture are helpful in guiding antibiotic therapy.

○ Gram-positive organisms can be treated with an **oral cephalosporin or penicillinase-resistant antibiotic;** resistant strains may require vancomycin and rifampin.

○ Gram-negative organisms can usually be treated with **oral ciprofloxacin (500 mg bid);** with *Pseudomonas aeruginosa,* addition of ceftazidime or an aminoglycoside may become necessary, as well as catheter removal.

○ For infections that respond to therapy, antibiotics can be discontinued after 2 weeks; relapsing infections or those that progress to tunnel infections or peritonitis may necessitate catheter removal.

TABLE 26-6 TREATMENT OF PERITONITIS

Type	Organism	Antibiotic	Choices	Duration
Gram positive	Enterococcus	IP vancomycin or ampicillin	Can add aminoglycoside; if VRE, consider daptomycin or quinupristin/dalfopristin	21 days
	Staphylococcus aureus	IP vancomycin or first-generation cephalosporin	Can add oral rifampin 450–600 mg/d for 5–7 days	21 days
	Other gram positive	IP first-generation cephalosporin	IP vancomycin if resistant	14 days
Gram negative	Pseudomonas/Stenotrophomonas	IP ceftazidime with aminoglycoside if urine <100 mL/d	If urine >100 mL/d, substitute aminoglycoside with oral ciprofloxacin (500 mg bid), or IV piperacillin (4 g bid), or oral TMP/SMX (double strength per day), or IP aztreonam	21–28 days
	Other single gram negative	IP aminoglycoside if urine <100 mL/d	IP ceftazidime if urine >100 mL/d	14 days
	Multiple gram negatives or anaerobes	IP cefazolin, IP ceftazidime, and oral metronidazole (500 mg tid)	Abdominal imaging and/or surgical intervention	14–21 days
Fungal	Yeasts or other fungi	Immediate catheter removal; IV amphotericin B and flucytosine until sensitivities available	Continue oral flucytosine (1000 mg daily) and fluconazole (100–200 mg daily) an additional 10 days after catheter removal if patient is stable	Variable

IP, intraperitoneal; IV, intravenous; TMP/SMX, trimethoprim–sulfamethoxazole; VRE, vancomycin-resistant Enterococcus.

○ Meticulous **exit-site care** is essential to prevent such infections, with hand washing for 2 minutes before manipulating the catheter dressings; daily application of **0.1% gentamicin cream** has been shown to be effective in reducing the incidence of exit-site infections with *Staphylococcus aureus* and *Pseudomonas aeruginosa.*

○ Catheter anchorage with tape and gauze dressings helps to prevent exit-site trauma.

○ **Vigorous scrubbing at the exit-site or prolonged submersion into water should be avoided.**

Mechanical Complications

- **Outflow failure:**
  ○ Outflow failure is defined as a drain volume that is consistently and substantially less than the volume being infused in the absence of an obvious fluid leak.
  ○ Common causes include **kinking** of the catheter, **constipation, adhesion formation, or fibrin plugging.**
  ○ Tracking of fluid along the abdominal wall can cause an apparent outflow failure and may manifest as scrotal edema.
  ○ A systematic approach can be used to investigate and correct the problem:
    ■ Check a plain film of the abdomen to evaluate the course of the catheter, which should ideally be directed toward the pelvis to avoid contact with the omentum.
    ■ **Constipation should be treated aggressively** and can resolve ~50% of cases of outflow failure (mechanism unclear); **magnesium and phosphate products should be avoided** in the treatment of constipation in end-stage renal disease. Lactulose is an acceptable choice.
    ■ Heparin can be added to the PD solution (250 to 500 units/L), especially if fibrin strands are evident in the discarded fluid; heparin is not systemically absorbed from the peritoneal cavity, thus minimizing the risk of anticoagulation.
    ■ Thrombolytic agents (tissue plasminogen activator, 1 mg/mL for 1 hour) may also help break up fibrin strands.
  ○ If these conservative measures fail to correct the problem, surgical consultation with catheter repositioning or replacement may be necessary.

- **Back pain:**
  ○ In the PD population, the infused solution causes a shift in the center of gravity, producing excess stress on the lumbar spine.
  ○ Management includes bed rest in the acute situation, along with decreasing the volume of the dwells.
  ○ A concomitant increase in the number of exchanges may be needed to maintain adequate solute clearance.
  ○ When applicable, physical therapy with muscle-strengthening exercises may help alleviate symptoms.

- **Hernias:**
  ○ Abdominal hernias develop in **10% to 20%** of PD patients, resulting from the increased intraabdominal pressure created by the infused fluid.
  ○ Risk factors include large-volume dwells, a sitting position during dwell carriage, obesity, and multiparity; any condition that weakens the abdominal musculature, such as deconditioning, can also pose a risk for hernia formation.

- Diagnosis is clinical and treatment is typically with surgical repair.
- Small abdominal hernias carry the greatest risk of bowel incarceration, which can present with worsening abdominal pain and loss of reducibility at the hernia site.
- After surgical repair, intraabdominal pressures must be kept as low as possible to facilitate healing; patients with good residual renal function may be able to discontinue PD for 1 week, then gradually reinitiate with small volumes (1 L exchanges) for another week.
- Supine dialysis also helps to reduce the intraabdominal pressure.
- Patients with little residual renal function may need to temporarily switch to HD until the wound is completely healed.
- **Fluid leakage:**
  - Risk factors for fluid leakage are similar to those for hernia formation.
  - Early leaks are those that occur within 1 month of catheter placement and typically occur at the exit site.
  - Late leaks can extend into the subcutaneous tissue or into the pleural space (hydrothorax), presenting more subtly with weight gain, shortness of breath, or apparent outflow failure.
  - Hydrothoraces are almost exclusively found on the right side, as the left hemidiaphragm has additional coverage by the heart and pericardium; diagnostic thoracentesis reveals markedly elevated glucose levels when the pleural fluid originates from the peritoneal solution.
  - Treatment of fluid leakage entails draining the peritoneal cavity dry for 24 to 48 hours; if the leak recurs, longer periods off PD may be needed with temporary support on HD.
  - A hydrothorax that is symptomatic requires medical or surgical pleurodesis.
  - Genital edema is a specific form of fluid leakage that can occur via a patent processus vaginalis that results in a hydrocele; this can also occur through a defect in the abdominal wall at the catheter site, allowing fluid to track down through subcutaneous tissue.
  - As with abdominal hernias, reduction in the intraabdominal pressure with small-volume or supine PD may alleviate the symptoms; anatomical defects, however, may need to be corrected surgically.
- **Sclerosing encapsulating peritonitis:**
  - Sclerosing encapsulating peritonitis is an uncommon clinical entity where a **fibrous transformation of the peritoneal membrane entraps loops of bowel** causing symptoms of intestinal obstruction, with nausea, vomiting, and anorexia.
  - A **bloody dialysis fluid** drainage may alert the physician to this problem.
  - The incidence is ~2.5% and is more common in patients receiving long-term PD (>5 to 8 years); it can even occur after patients have previously discontinued PD.
  - Although the mechanism is not clearly defined, chemical irritation of the peritoneal membrane is suspected as the inciting event. Recurrent bouts of peritonitis have also been implicated as a risk factor.
  - Treatment options are limited, consisting of **bowel rest and surgical** lysis of adhesions when obstruction occurs.
  - Immunosuppression with prednisone in doses ranging from 10 to 40 mg/d have shown modest benefit and case series using tamoxifen (20 mg bid) have shown success.[7,8]
  - The overall prognosis of patients with sclerosing encapsulating peritonitis is poor, with a **1-year mortality rate >50%.**

Metabolic Complications

- **Hyperglycemia:**
  - As much as 75% of the dextrose in the dialysis solution may diffuse inwardly to the blood, particularly in patients with leaky high transport membranes.
  - Patients with underlying diabetes mellitus or glucose intolerance are most susceptible to this complication.
  - The calories provided by the dextrose account for much of the 5% to 10% weight gain frequently observed in the first year on PD.
- **Hyperlipidemia:**
  - An atherogenic lipid profile is frequently encountered in patients on PD.
  - The inward diffusion of dextrose results in **elevated triglycerides,** as well as the elevation in total cholesterol and **low-density lipoprotein (LDL);** smaller proteins, such as high-density lipoprotein, are lost in the spent dialysate further increasing cardiovascular risk.
  - Treatment is focused on dietary modification, exercise, and HMG-coenzyme A reductase inhibitors as first-line medical therapy.
  - Specific LDL cholesterol targets in PD patients have not been defined, and in the absence of established coronary disease or coronary disease equivalents, the accepted target is <100 mg/dL.
- **Protein loss and malnutrition:**
  - Protein loss of ~0.5 g/L of drainage occurs in PD, and the rate of loss may be even greater in patients with high transport membranes.
  - The major protein lost is albumin.
  - Factors that increase membrane permeability, such as peritonitis, can significantly magnify the rate of protein loss.
  - The KDOQI guidelines recommend a **dietary protein intake of 1.2 to 1.3 g/kg/d** for PD patients.
- **Hypokalemia:**
  - Approximately **one-third** of PD patients experience hypokalemia.
  - Patients are typically in a negative potassium balance, as standard PD solutions lack this electrolyte, and increased endogenous insulin release (stimulated by the sugar load) leads to an intracellular potassium shift.
  - Poor nutritional status in hospitalized patients (particularly when placed on a low-potassium "renal diet") may further exacerbate hypokalemia.
  - With mild hypokalemia, it is recommended that patients liberalize their potassium intake, or oral supplements are initiated.
  - In severe hypokalemia, addition of potassium to the PD solution may be required.

Indications for Change to HD

- Despite the safety and effectiveness of PD, patients are sometimes required to switch to HD temporarily or permanently.
- **Common reasons for a permanent switch** include:
  - Consistent failure to achieve adequacy targets (Kt/V_{urea} <1.7)
  - Inadequate fluid removal (ultrafiltration failure)
  - Severe hypertriglyceridemia that is resistant to therapy
  - Frequent peritonitis or other infectious complications
  - Irreparable mechanical problems, including sclerosis encapsulating peritonitis
  - Severe protein malnutrition resistant to aggressive management

- Patients may occasionally require a **temporary switch** to HD for the following reasons:
  - Surgical operations involving the peritoneal cavity (e.g., perforated ulcer, bowel obstruction, rarely renal cell cancers)
  - Peritoneal fluid leaks
  - Infectious complications requiring temporary catheter removal
- The presence of a PD catheter does not preclude renal transplantation, and the catheter can be surgically removed at the time of transplantation or at a later date.
- As with other forms of renal replacement therapy, the leading causes of death for patients on PD are cardiovascular disease and infections.
- A statistically significant association between the loss of residual renal function and mortality has been described, stressing the importance of preserving kidney function whenever possible.

REFERENCES

1. Daugirdas JT, Blake PG, Ing TS. *Handbook of Dialysis*. 4th ed. Philadelphia, PA: Lippincott Williams & Wilkins; 2007.
2. Le Poole CY, Welten AGA, Weijmer MC, et al. Initiating CAPD with a regimen low in glucose and glucose degradation products, with icodextrin and amino acids (NEPP) is safe and efficacious. *Perit Dial Int*. 2005;25:S64–S68.
3. Churchill DN, Thorpe KE, Nolph KD, et al. Increased peritoneal membrane transport is associated with decreased patient and technique survival for continuous peritoneal dialysis patients: the Canada-USA (CANUSA) peritoneal dialysis study group. *J Am Soc Nephrol*. 1998;9:1285–1292.
4. Paniagua R, Amato D, Vonesh E, et al. Effects of increased peritoneal clearances on mortality rates in peritoneal dialysis: ADEMEX, a prospective, randomized, controlled trial. *J Am Soc Nephrol*. 2002;13:1307–1320.
5. Brown EA, Davies SJ, Rutherford P, et al. Survival of functionally anuric patients on automated peritoneal dialysis: the European APD outcome study. *J Am Soc Nephrol*. 2003; 14:2948–2957.
6. Li PK, Szeto CC, Piraino B, et al. ISPD guideline/recommendations. *Perit Dial Int*. 2010; 30:393–423.
7. Kawanishi H, Kawaguchi Y, Fukui H, et al. Encapsulating peritoneal sclerosis in Japan: a prospective, controlled, multicenter study. *Am J Kidney Dis*. 2004;44:729–737.
8. Moustafellos P, Hadjianastassiou V, Roy D, et al. Tamoxifen therapy in encapsulating sclerosing peritonitis in patients after kidney transplantation. *Transplant Proc*. 2006;38:2913–2914.

Principles of Drug Dosing in Renal Impairment

27

Lyndsey Bowman and Jennifer Iuppa

GENERAL PRINCIPLES

- Deciding on the appropriate dosing strategy of medications in patients with chronic kidney disease (CKD) or acute kidney injury (AKI) require an understanding of the basic principles of pharmacokinetics, including absorption, protein binding, metabolism, and elimination.
- Many drugs and their metabolites are renally eliminated and require special consideration when prescribed to patients with impaired renal function.[1]
- Renal impairment affects glomerular blood flow and filtration, tubular secretion, reabsorption, renal bioactivation, and metabolism. Both pharmacokinetic and pharmacodynamic properties of medications are altered.
- One of the most important drug-related problems in patients with renal impairment is inappropriate medication dosing. Errors are common, often overlooked, and may lead to toxicity or ineffective therapy. These errors are preventable. One study estimated that as many as 40% of patients with CKD stages 3 to 5, received dosages on average 2.5 times higher than the recommended upper limit of the dosing range.[2]
- Dosing for medications that undergo renal elimination is based primarily on an estimate of glomerular filtration rate (GFR). Kidney Disease Outcomes Quality Initiative (KDOQI) recommends the Modification of Diet in Renal Disease (MDRD) study equation.
- Caution should be used when estimating GFR in older patients, as decreased creatinine production and excretion as a function of old age may lead to overestimation of GFR.
- Patient-specific dosages calculated using these equations should only be conducted in the presence of stable renal function.
- Drugs that can further impair renal function in high-risk patients (underlying CKD, heart failure (HF), liver disease, hypoperfusion) should be used with caution or avoided altogether in preference for safer alternatives. Appendices A and B lists medications that are potentially nephrotoxic and suggests safer alternatives in the setting of renal impairment.

PHARMACOKINETICS

- Pharmacokinetics refers to the action of drugs in the body over time, and is used to understand drug handling as a means to optimize efficacy and minimize toxicity. It is based on **four parameters** of drug activity: **absorption, distribution, metabolism, and clearance.**
- In patients with renal impairment, the pharmacokinetic profile of many commonly prescribed medications is altered. To optimize drug usage and preserve patient safety, it is necessary to understand these effects.[3,4]

Absorption

- Intestinal absorption and bioavailability (the fraction of medication that reaches systemic circulation) are influenced by many variables and are the result of numerous physiologic processes.
- Patients with CKD and AKI exhibit changes in the gastrointestinal tract that affect bioavailability.

Renal Failure-Induced Changes

- **Gastroparesis:** Patients with CKD often suffer from gastroparesis. This results in delayed gastric emptying and prolongs the time to maximum drug concentrations (C_{max}). The overall extent of absorption is not commonly affected, but delayed C_{max} can be important when rapid onset of action is desired.
- **Gastric alkalinization:** As a result of the common use of medications, including phosphate binders, antacids, H_2-receptor antagonists, and proton pump inhibitors, the absorption of many medications requiring an acidic environment (e.g., furosemide and ferrous sulfate) is reduced.
- **Cationic chelation:** Ingestion of cation-containing antacids (e.g., calcium, magnesium, aluminum hydroxide, sodium polystyrene sulfonate) decreases the absorption of many coadministered medications because of chelation (quinolone antibiotics, warfarin, levothyroxine, tetracycline, and so forth).
- Alterations to intestinal first-pass metabolism and p-glycoprotein efflux system:
  - Many medications are subject to intestinal metabolism by the cytochrome P450 enzyme system.
  - In CKD, reductions in metabolism occur and, in animal studies, they have been estimated to result in a 30% decrease in function.
  - p-Glycoprotein, an efflux transport protein in the intestinal tract, also exhibits decreased activity.
  - Increased medication bioavailability occurs as a result of both of these changes.
  - Two medications with narrow therapeutic index (TI) affected by these variations are cyclosporine and tacrolimus.

Distribution

- Drug distribution or volume of distribution (V_d) is the total amount of drug present in the body, divided by the plasma concentration, expressed in liters.
- The V_d determines peak concentrations. Plasma protein binding, tissue binding, active transport, and body composition can all impact the V_d.
- Alterations in protein binding can affect drug concentrations by changing the ratio of free to bound medication.
- Plasma drug concentrations are representative of both bound and unbound drug, but only free drug is capable of crossing cellular membranes and exerting pharmacologic effects.

Renal Failure-Induced Changes

- **Altered protein binding:**
  - Hypoalbuminemia due to the nephrotic syndrome often leads to an increase in the free drug fraction of medications that are highly bound to albumin.
  - **Acidic drugs** (e.g., penicillins, cephalosporins, phenytoin, furosemide, salicylates) are those that **are predominantly affected** and **can lead to drug-related toxicities.**

- Alternatively, an increase in α1-glycoprotein (an acute phase protein) associated with renal dysfunction will lead to increase in protein binding of medications bound to nonalbumin proteins.
  - **Alkaline drugs** (e.g., propranolol, morphine, oxazepam, vancomycin, and so forth) are affected by this phenomenon and thus plasma drug **concentrations are decreased.**
  - In addition, accumulation of metabolites and endogenous substances increase competition for binding sites (e.g., digoxin, warfarin, phenytoin, valproic acid, dihydropyridine calcium channel blockers, nonsteroidal anti-inflammatory drugs [NSAIDs]).
  - A classic example is **phenytoin.**
    - Traditionally, total plasma phenytoin levels were followed.
    - In uremia, many toxins accumulate and can displace phenytoin from albumin.
    - Therefore, although the total drug level could still be therapeutic, the free (unbound) or effective drug level may exceed the therapeutic range.
    - The unbound or free plasma concentration should always be measured in addition to total concentrations.
  - Qualitative changes to these binding sites can also occur, resulting in decreased drug-binding affinity.
- **Altered tissue binding:** Changes in tissue binding are most often irrelevant except for digoxin, in which the V_d is reduced by 50% in stage 5 CKD.
  - **Changes in body composition: Fluid retention** can increase the V_d of hydrophilic drugs (e.g., pravastatin, fluvastatin, morphine, codeine) and may cause decreased serum concentrations; whereas **increased adipose tissue and muscle wasting** would be expected to increase serum concentrations secondary to a reduced V_d.

Metabolism

- The majority of drugs in the clinical setting undergo first-order kinetics (drug concentrations decline logarithmically over time) and rates are proportional to the total body concentration of drug present.[5]
- There are numerous sites in the body in which metabolism occurs, primarily intestine, liver, and kidneys.
- Biotransformation at these sites happens through one of two phases of reactions:
  - **Phase I reactions** (more common) include hydrolysis, reduction, and oxidation. These serve to increase drug hydrophilicity to prepare for excretion or further phase II metabolism.
  - **Phase II reactions** or conjugation reactions include glucuronidation, sulfation, glutathione conjugation, acetylation, and methylation.

Renal Failure-Induced Changes

- **Altered biotransformation:**
  - Renal insufficiency significantly slows both phase I and phase II reactions.
  - Changes to oxidation reactions result in reduced activity of several of the CYP450 isoenzymes (2C9, 2C19, 2D6, 3A4).
  - All phase II reactions are slowed affecting **acetylation** (dapsone, hydralazine, isoniazid, procainamide), **glucuronidation** (acetaminophen, morphine, lorazepam, oxazepam, naproxen), **sulfation** (acetaminophen, minoxidil, dopamine, albuterol), and **methylation** (dobutamine, dopamine, 6-mercaptopurine).
  - The resultant effect is increased serum drug concentrations.

- **Accumulation of renally excreted active metabolites:** Dosage adjustments may be necessary for certain medications in order to prevent toxicity from active metabolites.[6] (See Appendix C: Common Medications with Active Metabolites.)

Elimination

- Elimination is typically reported as a **half-life (T½)**, or the time needed to reduce medication plasma concentrations by 50%.
- **Approximately five half-lives are required to eliminate 97% of drug from the body.**
- This parameter is especially useful for estimation of the time required to achieve steady state (approximately four to five half-lives), and to estimate appropriate drug dosing intervals.
- The rate of renal elimination is dependent on GFR, renal tubular secretion, and reabsorption.
- Medication-specific characteristics (e.g., molecular weight and protein binding) determine glomerular filtration with filtration rate dependent on free fraction.
- Drugs that are highly protein bound are not filtered, but instead actively secreted into the proximal convoluted tubule through a saturable process. In the distal portion of the nephron, substantial passive reabsorption occurs.
- This process is affected by urine concentrating activities, pH, lipophilicity, and protein binding.

Renal Failure-Induced Changes

- **Reduced glomerular filtration:** Decreased GFR results in prolonged free drug elimination T½.
- **Reduced secretion by active transport** (e.g., ampicillin, furosemide, penicillin G, dopamine, trimethoprim).
- **Reduced passive reabsorption** (e.g., aspirin, lithium).

DOSAGE ADJUSTMENTS OF COMMONLY USED DRUGS

- In general, renal insufficiency makes it difficult to predict whether a medication dose will produce an adequate, supratherapeutic, or subtherapeutic effect.[7]
- **Loading doses,** used to rapidly achieve a therapeutic drug concentration, do not typically need to be altered.
  - An important exception to this rule is **digoxin.** In the presence of renal impairment, the V_d of digoxin is dramatically reduced, requiring on average a 50% dose reduction. Physiologic determinants affecting loading doses, such as an increase in total body water (in the case of edema or ascites), may warrant a higher than normal loading dose to account for change in V_d, whereas dehydration may require a loading dose reduction. The following equation can be used to estimate the dose required to achieve a specific serum concentration:

$$\text{Loading dose} = V_d \times \text{IBW} \times \text{Cp}$$

  (V_d [L/kg]; IBW [ideal body weight; kg]; Cp [desired plasma concentration; mg/L])
- **Maintenance doses** are used to achieve steady-state concentrations.
  - Dose reduction, increasing the interval, or both can be used to avoid the accumulation of renally eliminated drugs or their metabolites.

○ A strategy of dose reduction achieves more constant drug concentrations with a higher risk of toxicity (inadequate time for drug elimination).

○ Extending the interval allows time for drug elimination between doses, but is associated with a higher risk of subtherapeutic drug concentrations.

Anticoagulants

- **Warfarin** metabolism is not significantly altered in renal insufficiency.
  ○ One study, however, has shown that compared to patients with no/mild kidney impairment, those with moderate kidney impairment required 9.5% lower doses (P <0.001) and those with severe kidney impairment required 19% lower doses (P <0.001).[8]
  ○ In addition, renal dysfunction puts patients at a higher risk of hemorrhage, likely due to platelet dysfunction and drug interactions.
- **Low-molecular-weight heparins** primarily undergo renal clearance and require dose adjustment in renal failure.
  ○ Anti-Xa monitoring has been recommended in this population for GFRs <30 mL/min (peak level to be drawn 4 hours postdose).
  ○ Similar to warfarin, the risk of hemorrhage is higher in patients with renal insufficiency.
- **Bivalirudin, desirudin, and lepirudin** are direct thrombin inhibitors that are all renally eliminated and require dose adjustment.
- **Argatroban** is not renally cleared and is the preferred agent in a patient with renal insufficiency but without hepatic dysfunction.

Antihypertensive Agents and Diuretics

- **Thiazide diuretics,** considered first-line therapy for uncomplicated hypertension, are not recommended with serum creatinine (SCr) levels that exceed 2.5 mg/dL or GFRs below 30 mL/min.
  ○ These agents require activity in the lumen of the nephron to produce a natriuretic effect, which is not achieved with advanced renal impairment.
- **Acetazolamide** should be avoided in stage 4 or 5 CKD because of increased risk of metabolic acidosis.
- **Loop diuretics** are the most commonly prescribed diuretics in patients with renal impairment.
  ○ Their clearance is often decreased, but patients require higher doses to achieve similar intraluminal concentrations.
  ○ This can lead to a higher risk of ototoxicity.
  ○ Drug resistance often occurs as a result of decreased drug delivery to the nephron lumen, increased sodium reabsorption between dosages, and increased distal sodium reabsorption.
  ○ Increasing the dose, switching to a continuous infusion, or adding a thiazide diuretic to alter distal sodium absorption are strategies that can be used to overcome resistance.

Potassium-Sparing Diuretics

- The **aldosterone antagonist, spironolactone,** has been shown to reduce mortality in patients with severe HF and is commonly used for this indication.
  ○ This agent should be used with caution in renal insufficiency after several reports have documented severe life-threatening hyperkalemia that can occur in patients treated with spironolactone for HF.

- ○ Risk factors for hyperkalemia include advanced age, diabetes, advanced CKD, and worsening left ventricular ejection fraction.
- ○ In the Randomized Aldactone Evaluation Study (RALES), there was a 2% incidence of severe hyperkalemia in the treatment arm, but this study excluded patients with SCr values >2.5 mg/dL or a history of hyperkalemia.
- **Amiloride and triamterene** inhibit the epithelial sodium channel, thereby increasing natriuresis with a potassium-sparing action.
  - ○ They lack the indication for HF, but place patients at a similar risk of hyperkalemia.

Angiotensin-Converting Enzyme Inhibitors/Angiotensin-2 Receptor Blockers

- They are considered first-line therapy for patients with diabetes mellitus and proteinuria or early CKD.
- These agents have been shown to reduce proteinuria, slow progression of kidney disease, and provide long-term cardiovascular protection.
- They exert their effects through inhibition of the renin–angiotensin–aldosterone system, and cause efferent arteriolar dilation.
- Many patients experience an acute decline in GFR >15% from baseline with proportional elevations in SCr in the first week.
- If the rise in SCr is <30%, these medications can be continued safely in most patients, and can be expected to return to baseline in 4 to 6 weeks.
- Common practice includes discontinuation of the angiotensin-converting enzyme inhibitors (ACEIs)/angiotensin-2 receptor blockers (ARBs) if the SCr rises >30% or serum potassium is >5.6 mEq/L.
- These agents may also be associated with a minor drop in hemoglobin, which may become significant in the presence of anemia due to other causes.
- Few patients require discontinuation, and anemia is usually responsive to erythropoietin therapy.
- ACEIs in general require renal dose adjustment, whereas the ARBs are all hepatically eliminated and no adjustment is necessary.
- Patients with renal impairment are at an increased risk of developing severe hyperkalemia or acute renal failure (<5% overall), with the highest risk being in patients with diabetes or a history of hyperkalemia.
- Electrolytes and renal function should be evaluated in the first 4 to 7 days after initiation or adjustment, and caution should be used with concomitant agents that can cause nephrotoxicity or hyperkalemia (i.e., potassium-sparing diuretics, NSAIDs).

β-Blockers

- Hydrophilic β-blockers such as atenolol, bisoprolol, nadolol, acebutolol are renally eliminated and require dose reduction with renal impairment.
- There is no need for dose adjustment of metoprolol, propranolol, or labetalol.
- However, propranolol exhibits increased protein binding in CKD, leading to less free drug and decreased effectiveness.

Calcium Channel Blockers

- These are not renally cleared and there is no alteration of half-life with renal insufficiency.
- Nondihydropyridines (e.g., verapamil, diltiazem) may be superior because of their ability to limit proteinuria.

Hypoglycemic Agents

Metformin
- This is 90% to 100% renally excreted and its use is not recommended with:
  ○ Elevation of SCr >1.5 mg/dL in men or 1.4 mg/dL in women
  ○ Patients aged >80 years
  ○ Patients with severe congestive HF
  ○ Any scenario that can affect renal perfusion
- These conditions increase the risk of severe, life-threatening lactic acidosis.

Sulfonylureas
- Several sulfonylureas, including **glyburide,** should be avoided in patients with stage 3 to 5 CKD. Glyburide has an active metabolite that is renally eliminated and accumulation can cause prolonged hypoglycemia.
- **Glipizide** does not have an active metabolite and is safe for use in renal insufficiency.

Insulin
- **Insulin** is **renally eliminated** and all preparations require dose reduction in renal failure.

Antimicrobials
- Many antimicrobial agents are renally eliminated and require dose adjustment.
- Errors are common and place patients at increased risk of toxicity or ineffectiveness.
- Dose adjustments are complex and vary based on individual medication and degree of renal dysfunction.
- Appendices D and E lists common antimicrobial and antiretroviral agents that require dose adjustment.
- In-depth recommendations to dosing aminoglycosides and vancomycin (two of the most common antimicrobials affecting renal function) are discussed below.

Aminoglycosides
- Aminoglycosides are one of the most common medications associated with AKI. It has a very low TI.
- It is completely filtered by the glomerulus and taken up by the proximal tubular cells. The toxicity leads to acute tubular necrosis in the proximal tubules. There are additional toxic effects as well.[9]
- There are **two available dosing strategies:** traditional and extended-interval (EI) dosing.
  ○ **Traditional dosing:**
    ■ **Step 1: Calculate dosing weight.** To calculate dosing weight (DW), the patient's actual body weight (ABW) must be compared with the patient's ideal body weight (IBW). Corrections need to be made if the patient is obese. The following can be used to calculate these weights:

      IBW male = 50 kg + 2.3 [height (in.) − 60]
      IBW female = 45.5 kg + 2.3 [height (in.) − 60]
      Obese DW = IBW + 0.4 (ABW − IBW)
      The DW can now be calculated as follows:
      If ABW >1.2 (IBW), then DW = obese DW
      If IBW <ABW <1.2 (IBW), then DW = IBW
      If IBW >ABW, then DW = ABW

- **Step 2: Calculate loading dose.** Calculation of the loading dose is based on DW. The dose may be lowered in patients with volume depletion. Gentamicin dosing can vary based on the site of infection.
- **Step 3: Estimate creatinine clearance.** Creatinine clearance can be estimated using the Cockroft–Gault equation:

$$\text{Est. creatinine clearance} = \frac{(140 - \text{age}) \times \text{weight} \times (\text{if female})}{72 \times \text{SCr}}$$

- **Step 4: Calculate maintenance dose.** The maintenance dose is a percentage of the loading dose (Table 27-1).
- **Step 5: Therapeutic drug monitoring.** Obtain peak and trough concentrations with the third maintenance dose. The preferred peak and trough can be selected clinically, with **consideration given to the site and severity of infection,** causative microorganism, minimum inhibitory concentration, immunocompetency of the patient, and intent of therapy (Table 27-2). Recheck the level whenever there is a change in dosing regimen or change in renal function; recheck every 1 to 2 weeks if duration of therapy is >2 weeks.
- **EI dosing:**
  - EI dosing is equally effective and may be less toxic compared with traditional, every 8 hour, dosing.
  - EI aminoglycosides take advantage of concentration-dependent killing through high peak levels and the postantibiotic effect.
  - EI dosing is **NOT recommended** in the following situations, wherein there might be alterations to renal perfusion and drug pharmacokinetics.
    - Pregnancy
    - Anasarca/severe congestive HF/liver failure
    - End-stage renal disease (ESRD) patients on hemodialysis and peritoneal dialysis

TABLE 27-1   **CALCULATION OF THE MAINTENANCE DOSE**

Creatinine Clearance (mL/min)	Half-Life (h)	q8h (%)	q12h (%)	q24h (%)
>90	3.1	84	100	—
80–89	3.4	80	91	—
70–79	3.9	76	88	—
60–69	4.5	—	84	—
50–59	5.3	—	79	—
40–49	6.5	—	—	92
30–39	8.4	—	—	86
25–29	9.9	—	—	81
20–24	11.9	—	—	75
<20	>12	Give loading dose, follow-up levels, and redose when level drops to <2 µg/mL		

TABLE 27-2	TRADITIONAL DOSING: TARGET AMINOGLYCOSIDE CONCENTRATIONS			
Aminoglycoside	Site of Infection	Loading Dose (mg/kg dosing weight)	Peak (µg/mL)	Trough (µg/mL)
Gentamicin/ tobramycin	General	—	4–8	<2
	Gynecologic, eye, soft tissue	1–1.5	5–7	<2
	Lung	2	8–10	<2
	Cystic fibrosis lung	2–2.5	10–12	<2
	Urinary tract	1–1.5	3–5	<2
	CNS	2.5	8–10	<2
	Blood	2	6–8	<2
	Sepsis	2.5	6–8	<2
	Endocarditis/synergy	1–1.5	3–5	<2
Amikacin	General	—	25–35	4–10

CNS, central nervous system.

- CKD or AKI with GFR <30 mL/min
- Endocarditis
- Cystic fibrosis
- Mycobacterial infection
- Extremes of age—elderly and infants
- Burns covering >20% body surface area
- Critically ill patients with hemodynamic instability

○ EI dosing protocol: Calculate the patient's DW as outlined above. The initial intravenous dosing regimen is as follows:
  - Gentamicin, 5 mg/kg DW (round to nearest 50 mg)
  - Tobramycin, 5 mg/kg DW (round to nearest 50 mg)
  - Amikacin, 15 mg/kg DW (round to nearest 100 mg)

○ For therapeutic drug monitoring, obtain a single, random drug level 8 to 12 hours after the initial dose. Determine the appropriate maintenance dose according to Figure 27-1.[10]

○ Repeat drug level as necessary. For patients with impaired renal function, estimated dosing intervals are provided in Table 27-3.

- **Dialysis patients:**
  ○ Patients on **dialysis should be dosed according to traditional method** for aminoglycosides.
  ○ Doses for gentamicin/tobramycin are 1.5 to 2 mg/kg (or 1 mg/kg if using for synergy, for a gram-positive bacteremia, or a urinary tract infection) and the amikacin dose is 7.5 mg/kg.
  ○ **Monitoring random levels** in dialysis patients is absolutely necessary, and is strongly recommended to prevent potential toxicity and to avoid inadequate treatment.
  ○ Random levels should be drawn **immediately prior** to the next dialysis session.

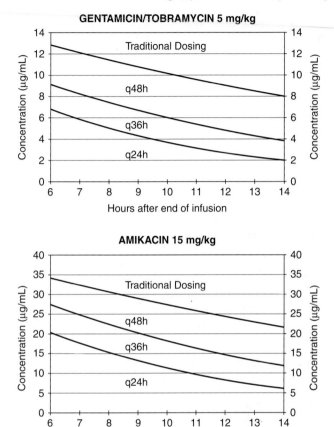

FIGURE 27-1. Nomograms depicting maintenance dose schedules for gentamicin, tobramycin, and amikacin.

○ Patients are given another dose when the trough level falls to <2 µg/mL for gentamicin/tobramycin and <10 µg/mL for amikacin.
○ Usually, dosing can be scheduled every 48 hours for peritoneal dialysis, every 24 to 48 hours for patients on continuous renal replacement therapy (CRRT), and three times weekly for intermittent hemodialysis (IHD).

Vancomycin
- The typical dosing regimen is **10 to 15 mg/kg, every 12 hours,** based on actual body weight and renal function.
- For patients with impaired renal function, estimate dosing intervals according to Table 27-4. Patients on dialysis need specialized dosing regimens as described below.

TABLE 27-3	ONCE-DAILY DOSING: AMINOGLYCOSIDE INTERVALS IN PATIENTS WITH IMPAIRED RENAL FUNCTION

Creatinine Clearance (mL/min)	Usual Dosing Interval
>60	q24h
40–59	q36h
30–39	q48h
<30	Not recommended (see the section "Traditional dosing")

- **Frequent monitoring** of vancomycin levels is indicated if concomitant nephrotoxic or ototoxic agents are being used, if there is changing renal function, suboptimal response to therapy, hemodynamic instability, or extremes of body weight.
- **Trough levels** (every 4 to 7 days) are recommended in patients receiving longer courses of therapy (>5 days) to ensure that concentrations are adequate but not excessive.
  - Vancomycin levels are not recommended for patients receiving a short course of therapy (<5 days).
  - Levels should be obtained at steady state or immediately before administration of the third maintenance dose.
  - Desired trough levels are three times the minimum inhibitory concentration, with 10 to 15 mg/L for skin and soft tissue infections.
  - Higher trough levels of 15 to 20 mg/L are recommended for bloodstream, bone, lung, or central nervous system infections.
- **Peak levels should not be routinely obtained.**
- **Dialysis patients:**
  - Dosing frequency depends on the clearance of the dialyzer being used and residual renal function.
  - With the **newer high-clearance dialyzers,** a significant amount of the drug may be cleared after a dialysis session, leading to **suboptimal drug levels** until the next scheduled dose.
  - Traditional concepts of "dose and forget" regimens for vancomycin are not applicable with the newer dialyzers, and patients may need to be **dosed as frequently as every third to fifth day.**

TABLE 27-4	VANCOMYCIN DOSING IN PATIENTS WITH IMPAIRED RENAL FUNCTION

Body Weight (kg)	Dose (mg)	Creatinine Clearance (mL/min)	Suggested Interval (h)
<45	500	>60	12
45–60	750	35–60	24
60–90	1000	15–34	48
>90	1250–1500	<15	Random dosing

○ Thus, at least initially, attention must be directed toward ensuring that trough levels define a dosage interval if prolonged therapy is planned.

○ The usual practice is to redose at a level of <15 mg/L (random or predialysis).

○ A common regimen for vancomycin in hemodialysis patients using high-flux membrane dialyzers is to give a 1 g loading dose at initiation of therapy, followed by supplementary doses of 500 to 1000 mg after each subsequent dialysis.

○ One should check a predialysis vancomycin level before the third or fourth dialysis treatment on this regimen or sooner in critically ill patients.

○ Patients on CRRT need frequent monitoring of drug level (daily or every other day) and doses should be given every 12 hours.

Analgesics

NSAIDs and COX-2 Inhibitors

- NSAIDs are used daily by one in five Americans and are generally safe with a small risk of mild complications (e.g., peripheral edema or increased blood pressure).
- Patients with renal insufficiency, however, are **at higher risk of development of more serious side effects** such as:
  ○ Worsening fluid overload and HF
  ○ Uncontrolled hypertension
  ○ AKI
  ○ Hyponatremia
  ○ Hyperkalemia
- Renal side effects are a result of prostaglandin inhibition, leading to excessive vasoconstriction and decreased renal blood flow.
- These agents should either be used extremely cautiously or, preferably, completely avoided in this patient population.

Narcotic Analgesics

- These agents should be used cautiously in patients with renal insufficiency because of the risk associated with accumulation of toxic metabolites common to many of these agents.
- Metabolites of meperidine, dextropropoxyphene, morphine, tramadol, and codeine can accumulate causing central nervous system and respiratory side effects.
- One of the safest opioid analgesics to use in the setting of renal failure in hospitalized patients is **hydromorphone,** which is primarily metabolized via glucuronidation in the liver.

DOSE ADJUSTMENTS DURING RENAL REPLACEMENT THERAPY

- There are different modalities used for renal replacement therapy (RRT) in the setting of AKI or ESRD. These modalities are described elsewhere in this book.
- These procedures remove nitrogenous and other waste products that accumulate in renal failure; however, they also remove drugs and active metabolites.
- The efficiency with which each procedure removes drugs from the body depends on many factors:
  ○ Drug characteristics (molecular weight, plasma protein binding, volume of distribution)

- ○ The dialyzer (membrane type, surface area, thickness)
- ○ Geometry of the dialysis system (countercurrent or concurrent blood and dialysate flow)
- ○ Dialysis conditions (blood and dialysate flow rates, duration of dialysis treatment).
- ○ Types of RRT—IHD, CRRT, sustained low-efficiency dialysis
- • Careful consideration needs to be taken to replace drug lost, based on an estimation of the amount removed.

REFERENCES

1. Bennett WM. Guide to drug dosage in renal failure. *Clin Pharmacokinet.* 1988;15(5): 326–354.
2. Cantu TG, Ellerbeck EF, Yun SW, et al. Drug prescribing for patients with changing renal function. *Am J Hosp Pharm.* 1992;49(12):2944–2948.
3. Keller F, Giehl M, Frankewitsch T, et al. Pharmacokinetics and drug dosage adjustment to renal impairment. *Nephrol Dial Transplant.* 1995;10(9):1516–1520.
4. Boxenbaum H, Tannenbaum S, Mayersohn M, et al. Pharmacokinetics tricks and traps: drug dosage adjustment in renal failure. *J Pharm Pharm Sci.* 1999;2(1):2–4.
5. Dreisbach AW. The influence of chronic renal failure on drug metabolism and transport. *Clin Pharmacol Ther.* 2009;86(5):553–556.
6. Gabardi S, Abramson S. Drug dosing in chronic kidney disease. *Med Clin North Am.* 2005;89(3):649–687.
7. Matzke GR, Frye RF. Drug administration in patients with renal insufficiency. Minimising renal and extrarenal toxicity. *Drug Saf.* 1997;16(3):205–231.
8. Nolin TD. On warfarin use in kidney disease: a therapeutic window of opportunity? *Am J Kidney Dis.* 2010;56(5):805–808.
9. Lopez-Novoa JM, Quiros Y, Vicente L, et al. New insights into the mechanism of aminoglycoside nephrotoxicity: an integrative point of view. *Kidney Int.* 2011;79(1):33–45.
10. Bailey TC, Little JR, Littenberg B, et al. A meta-analysis of extended-interval dosing versus multiple daily dosing of aminoglycosides. *Clin Infect Dis.* 1997;24(5):786–795.

Care of the Renal Transplant Patient

28

Christina L. Klein

GENERAL PRINCIPLES

- Approximately a **half-million patients in the United States have end-stage renal disease (ESRD)**, and prevalence continues to increase annually.[1,2]
- **Renal transplantation is the preferred treatment** for ESRD in appropriate candidates, as survival, quality of life, and cost savings are enjoyed compared with chronic dialysis.
- Owing to limited organ donor availability, <20% of candidates on the transplant waitlist will receive a transplant annually; 16,000 transplants were done in the United States in 2009.[2]
- Many ESRD patients projected to benefit from transplantation are not referred to or complete a transplant evaluation.
- Approximately **65% of the renal transplants** done annually in the United States are from **deceased donors (DDs)** and the remainder are from living donors (LDs), either related or unrelated.[2]
- Allograft survival time for a DD kidney transplant averages >8 years, whereas that of an LD kidney averages >12 years. Improved patient survival is also observed in recipients of LD compared to DD kidneys.
- Death with a functioning allograft is the leading cause of graft loss; the majority of deaths are due to **cardio- and cerebrovascular disease, malignancy, and infection.**
- There are ~**150,000 kidney transplant recipients** actively cared for in the United States health care system. Transplantation is a treatment, not a cure, for ESRD and requires continued follow-up and surveillance throughout the life of the patient or graft. Improved understanding of posttransplant complications can maximize graft and patient survival.[2]

TRANSPLANT EVALUATION

Objective

- Education regarding the potential risks and benefits of transplant as an option for ESRD treatment is provided.[2–7]
- Potential kidney transplant recipients are carefully evaluated in order to detect and treat coexisting illnesses that impact transplant candidacy, perioperative risk, and survival after transplantation.
- In general, candidates should have a projected life expectancy exceeding 5 years.
- Patients should be referred if **GFR <30 mL/min,** with evidence of progressive irreversible renal disease. Points for time on waitlist accrue once GFR ≤20 mL/min. Depending on blood type, age, region, race, and degree of sensitization (panel reactive antibody), **average wait time** for a DD organ can exceed **5 to 10 years.**[2]

- **Preemptive transplant** (before dialysis) is encouraged, as patient and graft survival are inversely correlated with duration of time on dialysis.

Studies

- In addition to a complete blood count, chemistry panel, and coagulation studies, blood type, serologic testing for HIV, cytomegalovirus (CMV), varicella zoster virus, herpes simplex virus (HSV), Epstein–Barr virus (EBV), Hepatitis B and C, and rapid plasma reagin is done.[3,4]
- **Electrocardiogram and chest x ray** are done for each candidate; depending on cardiopulmonary history, further testing may include cardiac stress test, echocardiogram, cardiac catheterization, pulmonary function tests, chest computed tomography (CT).
- **Cancer screening** is done as per general population guidelines for Papanicolaou smear, mammogram, prostate exam, prostate-specific antigen, and colonscopy.
- Urinalysis, urine culture and **imaging of the kidneys (ultrasound/CT)** are routinely performed; candidates with a urologic history may need further studies (e.g., voiding cystourethrogram) as appropriate.
- Immunologic testing is done to assess "sensitization" or presence of preformed anti-human leukocyte antigen (HLA) antibodies resulting from prior transplant, pregnancy, and blood transfusions.
  - **HLA:** Major histocompatibility complex in humans, which are essential components of immune function. HLA antigens not shared by the donor and recipient can stimulate rejection. The six HLA antigens considered in kidney transplantation "matching" are the two alleles at the A, B, and DR loci.
  - **Panel reactive antibody:** Quantification of preexisting anti-HLA antibodies. Expressed as a percentage, reflecting the degree of sensitization to a *potential donor pool.*
  - **Donor-specific antibodies:** Preexisting antibodies in the recipient against *specific donor HLA antigens;* may preclude transplantation depending on crossmatch results.
  - **Cross match:** Complement-dependent cytotoxicity (CDC) testing uses recipient cells and donor serum to detect presence of antidonor cytotoxic antibody. A positive CDC crossmatch is a contraindication to transplantation. Flow crossmatch is more sensitive than the CDC crossmatch, but can detect non-HLA or noncytotoxic antibody. Transplant with a positive flow crossmatch but negative CDC crossmatch should be done with caution and appropriate posttransplant monitoring.

Absolute/Relative Contraindications

- **Absolute:** Kidney transplantation should not be pursued in cases where limited life expectancy minimizes potential benefit of transplant or insurmountable psychosocial barriers to posttransplant compliance exist.[3–5] **Reversible renal disease, current infection, active immunologic disease that led to renal failure, active or metastatic malignancy, high operative risk, active substance abuse, noncompliance, and poorly controlled psychosis** are accepted absolute contraindications.
- **Relative:** Coronary artery disease, congestive heart failure, obesity, active hepatitis or chronic liver disease, peripheral vascular disease, cerebrovascular disease, malnutrition, and history of malignancy (excluding basal cell skin cancer) necessitate careful pretransplant assessment to determine candidacy.

- Kidney transplant is done at select centers for patients **with HIV infection** having an undetectable viral load and CD4 count >200 cells per µL on antiviral therapy. History of opportunistic infection and malignancy must be reviewed.
- Patients with ESRD and other end-stage organ failure may be candidates for **combined organ transplantation** (e.g., kidney–liver, if cirrhosis or primary oxalosis; kidney–pancreas, if Type 1 diabetes; kidney–heart, if severe irreversible cardiomyopathy).
- Attention is given to cause of ESRD and **likelihood of recurrence,** although no disease has a recurrence and graft failure rate that precludes initial kidney transplantation other than primary oxalosis. Retransplant must be carefully considered in cases of graft loss due to recurrent disease.

Waitlist Management

- Periodic review of waitlisted patients should include review of medical history, interim illnesses and hospitalizations, and current functional status. In addition, testing should be updated per center protocol.[3–5] Review may be indicated **every 1 to 2 years,** depending on patient comorbidities.
- **Blood transfusions should be avoided** because of risk of HLA sensitization; if required, leukocyte-depleted blood should be administered.
- **Immunizations** for pneumococcus, influenza, Hepatitis B, and varicella (if antibody negative) should be administered prior to transplant.

Donor Options

- **LD:** Similar graft outcomes are observed in the current era of immunosuppression between living related and living unrelated donors.[5,7,8] The exception to this is a two haplotype match from a sibling, which has superior survival.
- **DD:** Majority of cadaveric kidneys in the United States are obtained from *donors after brain death;* kidneys from *donors after cardiac death* are increasingly used and have higher rates of delayed graft function (DGF), but acceptable long-term graft survival.
- *Expanded criteria donors* are aged >60 years or between 50 and 59 with two of the following: hypertension, stroke as cause of death, terminal creatinine >1.5. These kidneys have poorer long-term graft survival, but may be appropriate for patients with high waitlist mortality such as the older candidates, select diabetics, those with limited dialysis access options or intolerant of dialysis.
- **Hepatitis C virus (HCV)-positive candidates** may opt to receive a kidney from a Hepatitis C-positive donor; studies suggest comparable graft and patient survival rates compared to kidneys from Hepatitis C-negative donors.[7]
- Options for patients with an HLA or ABO incompatible, but otherwise medically acceptable donor, include **desensitization and ABO-incompatible** transplant protocols or local/national **kidney exchange programs.**[8]

TRANSPLANT IMMUNOSUPPRESSION

General Principles

- Immunosuppression is used for **induction** at the time of transplant to promote graft acceptance, to prevent rejection (maintenance), and for the treatment of acute rejection (AR).[5,8]

- Adverse effects of immunosuppression are both immune-mediated (e.g., increased risk of infection and malignancy) and nonimmune effects.
- Immunosuppressive protocols tend to be center and organ specific, but can be individualized based on immunologic or side-effect profile. At present, the most commonly used **maintenance** immunosuppressive combination in the United States is prednisone, tacrolimus, and mycophenolate.

Antibody Therapies

- Antibody therapies have many applications in transplant, including induction, treatment of acute cellular- and antibody-mediated rejection, and treatment of select recurrent diseases.
- **Polyclonal:**
  - **Antithymocyte globulin:** This is produced by injecting human thymocytes into animals and collecting sera containing cytotoxic antibodies against a variety of T-cell markers. The available preparations are horse antithymocyte globulin (ATGAM) and rabbit antithymocyte globulin (Thymoglobulin). They cause T-lymphocyte depletion, and are used for **induction as well as for treatment of rejection.** Common side effects include fever, chills, arthralgias, and myelosuppression; serum sickness and anaphylaxis (rare) can also occur.
- **Monoclonal:**
  - **Basiliximab** (Simulect®): This is a humanized monoclonal antibody inhibiting the alpha subunit of the interleukin-2 receptor (CD25), thereby inhibiting IL-2 activation of T cells. **It is used for induction only.** There are few side effects, although rare cases of anaphylaxis are reported. Another IL-2R antagonist, Daclizumab (Zenapax), is no longer available.
  - **Alemtuzumab** (Campath 1H): This is a humanized monoclonal antibody against CD52 approved for use in CLL. It causes rapid and profound B- and T-cell depletion and is used off-label in transplantation, in desensitization protocols, for **induction and treatment of rejection.**
  - **Rituximab** (Rituxan®): This is a monoclonal antibody directed against CD20 on B lymphocytes, causing rapid and sustained B-cell depletion. It is used off-label in transplantation **for densensitization** and ABO-incompatible kidney transplant protocols,[8] **for treatment of acute humoral rejection,** for certain **recurrent diseases** (e.g., focal segmental glomerulosclerosis [FSGS]), and for CD20+ posttransplant **lymphoproliferative disorders.**

Maintenance Immunosuppression

- Available immunosuppressive agents for maintenance immunosuppression include glucocorticoids, calcineurin inhibitors (CNIs), antimetabolites, and mammalian target of rapamycin inhibitors (mTORi).
- Owing to the different mechanisms of action, along with the renal and nonrenal toxicities of each drug, combination therapy is used to achieve desired immunosuppressive effect while minimizing other side effects.
- **Glucocorticoid (prednisone, prednisolone):** This is an anti-inflammatory agent, which inhibits cytokine and chemokine production and induces lymphopenia. **Adverse side effects** are well known and include development of posttransplant diabetes mellitus, bone disease, poor wound healing, infections, cataracts, bruising, dyslipidemia, psychopathologic effects, and steroid myopathy. **Maintenance doses are generally ≤0.1 mg/kg;** steroid-free or minimization protocols are offered at select centers, but higher AR rates and lack of

long-term data limit general acceptance of steroid withdrawal. "Stress dose" increases in steroids are generally not needed for routine surgery or illness, and may only increase risk of infection, poor wound healing, or hyperglycemia.

- **CNIs (cyclosporine, tacrolimus):** These inhibit calcineurin, thereby preventing cytokine gene expression and subsequent T-cell activation. Cyclosporine and tacrolimus have similar side effects, including **renal vasoconstriction**, development of chronic interstitial fibrosis, hypertension, hyperkalemia, hypomagnesemia, hyperuricemia, and risk of drug-induced thrombotic microangiopathy. Hirsutism, hyperlipidemia, hypertension, and gingival hyperplasia are associated with cyclosporine, while **tacrolimus is more neurotoxic and diabetogenic.**
  - ○ Cyclosporine formulations include Sandimmune® (dependent on bile for absorption), microemulsion formula (Neoral®), and generic (Gengraf®). **Formulations are not interchangeable;** if changes are made, then close monitoring of drug levels needed with dose adjustment should be carried out as necessary. Typical **starting dose** of **6 to 8 mg/kg/d** divided bid is tapered to achieve long-term maintenance **troughs of 75 to 200 ng/mL.**
  - ○ Tacrolimus, also available in generic formulation; as with cyclosporine, a change of formulation necessitates monitoring of drug levels and allograft function. Typical **starting dose of 0.15 to 0.3 mg/kg/d** divided bid is tapered to achieve maintenance **trough levels of 3 to 7 ng/mL.**
  - ○ **Intravenous** administration of CNIs is almost **never indicated,** as tacrolimus is readily absorbed and can be given via a nasogastric tube or sublingually. For patients on cyclosporine, temporary conversion to tacrolimus is preferable to intravenous administration.
- **mTORi (sirolimus, everolimus):** These prevent cytokine- and growth factor-mediated T-cell proliferation. Adverse effects include **potentiation of CNI-induced nephrotoxicity,** hypertriglyceridemia, hyperlipidemia, anemia, thrombocytopenia, leukopenia, poor wound healing, proteinuria, interstitial pneumonia, oral ulcers, acne, pericardial/pleural effusion (rare). **Typical dose of 2 to 5 mg** daily is administered to achieve target **trough levels of 5 to 12 ng/dL.**
- **Antimetabolites (azathioprine, mycophenolate mofetil [Cellcept®, MMF], mycophenolic acid [Myfortic®, MPA]):** Azathioprine is a purine analog, whereas mycophenolate is converted to an active metabolite (mycophenolic acid), which inhibits the *de novo* pathway of purine synthesis. Both inhibit gene replication and lymphocyte proliferation.
  - ○ **Azathioprine is dosed at 1 to 2 mg/kg/d.** Side effects include bone marrow suppression (especially with concomitant use of allopurinol), neoplasias, hepatotoxicity (rare).
  - ○ Typical doses are **500 to 1000 mg bid for MMF,** and **360 to 720 mg bid for MPA.** Drug levels are not routinely followed. Generic formulations are available, but should be used only for financial necessity as relative clinical effectiveness is unknown. Important side effects include diarrhea, nausea, gastroesophageal reflux, myelosuppression, and increased risk of CMV.

Infectious Prophylaxis

- **Immunizations:** Pneumococcal, hepatitis B, and varicella (if antibody negative) vaccinations should be given prior to transplant. Live vaccines should be avoided posttransplant. Inactivated influenza vaccination is recommended yearly.
- Prophylaxis is given per center protocol at the time of transplant and reinstituted following augmentation of immunosuppression (e.g., treatment of rejection).

- **Trimethoprim/sulfamethoxazole** prevents *Pneumocystis jiroveci,* urinary tract infections, listeria, and nocardia.
- **Valganciclovir** or oral **ganciclovir** prevents CMV infection and is administered if recipient and/or donor are seropositive pretransplant. Choice of agent and duration are dictated per center protocol and dependent on donor/recipient serostatus.
- **Acyclovir** prevents reactivation of HSV, and is also administered lifelong to EBV seronegative recipients of an EBV seropositive organ, given the associated risk of posttransplant lymphoproliferative disease (PTLD).
- **Fluconazole, clotrimazole troche,** or **nystatin suspension** is used to prevent oropharyngeal candidiasis.

Pharmacology and Drug–Drug Interactions

- Patients are instructed to **notify their transplant center with any medication changes made by other providers to ensure no potential drug–drug interactions** or effect on immunosuppressant drug levels may occur. The following are commonly encountered interactions, but is not meant to be all-inclusive. A transplant pharmacist is an invaluable resource for medication dosing and safety issues.
- Both CNI and mTORi are metabolized by the cytochrome P450 IIIA microsomal enzyme systems, and therefore several potential drug–drug interactions exist that place patients at risk for either drug toxicities or rejection.
  - **Drugs than INCREASE levels:** diltiazem, verapamil, nicardipine, azole antifungals, erythromycin, clarithromycin
  - **Drugs that DECREASE levels:** rifampin, rifabutin, antiepileptics (phenytoin, barbiturates, carbamazepine)
- **Tacrolimus and cyclosporine** should **not be used together.**
- CNIs have synergistic nephrotoxicity with amphotericin, aminoglycosides, nonsteroidal anti-inflammatory drugs, angiotensin-converting enzyme inhibitor/angiotensin receptor blocker (ACEI/ARB; potentiate hemodynamic effects), and mTORi (increased nephrotoxicity).
- Additionally, use of CNIs with HMG-CoA reductase inhibitors, fibric acids, nicotinic acid increases risk of **myopathy.**
- **Azathioprine:** If initiating febuxostat or allopurinol, the dose of azathioprine must be reduced by 25–50% or allopurinol should be completely avoided. There is a high risk for bone marrow suppression as these drugs prevent the metabolism of azathioprine by inhibiting xanthine oxidase.

CAUSES OF ALLOGRAFT DYSFUNCTION

- Differential diagnosis for posttransplant allograft dysfunction depends on many factors; importantly, **the timing after transplantation** (Table 28-1).[5,9–11]
- DGF is commonly defined need for dialysis during the first posttransplant week. This is usually secondary to acute tubular necrosis (ATN) related to donor hypovolemia, hypotension, or prolonged ischemia time, but can be due to surgical or medical complications. It affects 10% to 30% of DD transplants and is uncommon after LD transplant.
- For allograft dysfunction in the early perioperative period, urologic and vascular surgical complications should be investigated and the possibility of rejection considered; other common etiologies include hypovolemia, hyperglycemia, drug toxicity (commonly CNI toxicity), and infection.
- AR, recurrent disease, chronic allograft nephropathy, CNI toxicity, BK virus nephropathy, and transplant renal artery stenosis are transplant-specific causes

TABLE 28-1	DIFFERENTIAL DIAGNOSIS OF RENAL ALLOGRAFT DYSFUNCTION	
First Week Posttransplant	**<3 Months Posttransplant**	**>3 Months Posttransplant**
ATN	Acute rejection	Acute rejection
Accelerated rejection	Calcineurin inhibitor toxicity	Chronic rejection
Hypovolemia	Hypovolemia	Calcineurin inhibitor toxicity
Obstruction	Hyperglycemia, hypercalcemia	Hypovolemia
	Obstruction	Obstruction
Urinary leak	Infection	Recurrent or *de novo* renal disease
Vascular thrombosis	Infectious (e.g., BKVN) or drug-induced interstitial nephritis	Infection
Atheroemboli	Recurrent renal disease	Transplant renal artery or iliac stenosis
Infections	Malignancy (allograft PTLD)	Malignancy
Thrombotic microangiopathy	Thrombotic microangiopathy	Thrombotic microangiopathy

ATN, acute tubular necrosis; BKVN, BK virus nephropathy; PTLD, posttransplant lymphoproliferative disease.

of renal dysfunction. However, it is important to recognize that renal failure can also ensue from all causes affecting nontransplant patients.

Surgical Complications
- Urologic causes of graft dysfunction include **urine leak and obstruction.**
  - **Urine leak** can result from ureteral necrosis due to inadequate blood supply or mechanical disruption of the ureteral implantation into the bladder. Diagnosis can be confirmed by **nuclear scan** or, if Jackson Pratt (JP) drain is present, a **JP fluid creatinine,** which is significantly greater than serum creatinine, clinches the diagnosis. Management options are continued foley catheterization, diverting nephrostomy, or surgical revision.
  - **Obstruction** can result from perinephric fluid collections causing ureteral compression, ureteral stenosis (ischemic), or ureteral obstruction by nephrolithiasis or a blood clot. Bladder obstruction can also occur due to catheter obstruction or, commonly in males, due to prostatic hypertrophy.
    - Perinephric fluid collections are commonly **lymphoceles,** although seromas and urinomas also occur. If causing obstruction, percutaneous drainage or surgical correction can be performed.
    - Ureteral stenosis and obstruction are managed with stenting, nephrostomy, or surgical repair.

- Bladder obstruction is managed by foley catheter placement and urologic consultation, with surgical treatment for benign prostatic hyperplasia if necessary.
- Vascular: **Renal artery or vein thrombosis** is an uncommon and often irreversible cause of graft dysfunction. Occurrence is associated with hyperacute or accelerated rejection, hypercoagulable disorders, and technical issues. Anticoagulation and surgical thrombectomy can occasionally be successful, although graft loss remains high.

Renal Complications

- **AR:** This affects 10% to 15% of transplants within the first year using present immunosuppressive protocols. AR is more common if induction immunosuppression is not administered.[5,9–11]
  - ○ **Accelerated rejection** rarely occurs due to the use of the pretransplant crossmatch, and is caused by preformed antibodies against donor antigens. **Hyperacute rejection** leads to rapid postperfusion graft thrombosis and loss, whereas **delayed hyperacute rejection** occurs within the first few days after transplant. The risk for **acute cellular rejection** is greatest in the first weeks-to-months after transplant. Signs and symptoms include elevated serum creatinine, decreased urine output, edema, worsening hypertension. Fever, anuria, pain over allograft, or swollen allograft are often not observed.
  - ○ Banff criteria are applied to biopsy findings to grade presence and severity of rejection and rule out other etiologies. Presence of interstitial infiltrates, tubulitis, and/or arteritis is consistent with acute cellular rejection. Important differential diagnoses include infectious and drug-induced interstitial nephritis causing similar interstitial findings. Pathologic features consistent with **acute humoral rejection** can range from ATN, peritubular capillaritis, glomerulitis to necrotizing arteritis and mural fibrinoid necrosis in severe cases. Positive C4d stain on immunofluorescence and/or concurrent circulating antidonor antibodies are needed to diagnose humoral rejection. Mixed cellular and antibody-mediated rejection can occur. Treatment strategies are guided by Banff classification, timing (early vs. late), clinical factors, and underlying renal function.
- **Chronic allograft failure (CAF)** is **second to death with a functioning graft** (DWFG) as the most common cause of graft loss. Characteristic histologic features include interstitial fibrosis and tubular atrophy.[10]
  - ○ Both **immunologic and nonimmunologic factors** can contribute to CAF, causing slow, progressive decline in allograft function, commonly with proteinuria. Previously used terms including *chronic allograft nephropathy* and *chronic rejection* have fallen out of favor because of lack of a specific nephropathy and the contributions of nonimmunologic causes to CAF.
  - ○ Immunologic risks include rejection, poor HLA matching, and CNI use. Nonimmunologic risks include donor source (cadaveric), prolonged ischemia time periods, donor age, size mismatching, and recipient factors including hypertension, hyperlipidemia, and tobacco use.
- **Recurrent disease:** In patients with glomerulonephritis, recurrent disease is **the third** most common cause of graft loss. Recurrent disease may present with elevated serum creatinine, proteinuria, and/or hematuria, with the diagnosis generally confirmed on allograft biopsy. Both risk for recurrence and risk of graft loss due to recurrence should be considered. For example, primary FSGS

recurs in 20% to 40% of first transplants, but close to 100% in retransplants, if the first allograft was lost because of recurrence. Early recurrence of FSGS is associated with a poorer prognosis than late, insidious recurrence.[11]

TRANSPLANT RECIPIENT OUTCOMES

- The primary cause of graft loss is patient death with a functioning graft.[5,12–14]
- Immunosuppressive effects contribute to posttransplant mortality, including cardiovascular and cerebrovascular risk factors, malignancy, and infection.
- **Cardiovascular disease is the most common cause of death** in patients with a functional allograft. Coronary artery disease, congestive heart failure, and left ventricular hypertrophy are more frequent in ESRD and transplant patients because of traditional risk factors (age, sex, diabetes, hypertension, dyslipidemia, tobacco use) and nontraditional risk factors (dialysis duration, proteinuria, inflammation, vascular calcification, altered coagulation profiles).

HYPERTENSION

- This affects 60% to 80% of transplant recipients. Etiology is often multifactorial, including medications (CNI, steroids, others), rejection, or other causes of acute/chronic graft dysfunction, transplant renal artery stenosis, obstructive sleep apnea.[12]
- Treatment goal is to achieve blood pressure <130/80 mm Hg.
- Transplant-specific considerations influence antihypertensive choices. ACEI/ARBs are associated with anemia, hyperkalemia, and are generally avoided in the immediate perioperative period because of hemodynamic effects, although they may be renoprotective in the long term. Verapamil and diltiazem lead to increased CNI levels, and alternative dihydropyridine calcium channel blockers (e.g., amlodipine) are preferred. Hypovolemia can ensue with diuretic use.

ENDOCRINE AND METABOLIC COMPLICATIONS

- **Hyperlipidemia** occurs in over half of transplant recipients. Causes include medication-induced (mTORi > corticosteroids > CNI; also thiazides) renal dysfunction, proteinuria, obesity, age, diabetes, and genetic factors.[12–14] It is essential to control hyperlipidemia with appropriate medications
  - A randomized study demonstrated a 29% reduction in major adverse cardiac events comparing fluvastatin versus placebo in renal transplant patients. Treatment was according to the National Cholesterol Education Program guidelines.
  - There are some pharmacologic concerns regarding the use of statins and fibrates. There is increased risk for myopathy with CNI + HMG-CoA reductase inhibitors, fibric acids, nicotinic acid.
  - Close monitoring for side effects and laboratory abnormalities should be done.
  - Bile acid sequestrants may decrease immunosuppressive medication absorption.

- **Posttransplant diabetes mellitus** (PTDM) is also termed new-onset diabetes after transplant:
  - A total of 30% to 40% of patients have pretransplant diabetes, with an additional 25% of patients without pretransplant diabetes developing PTDM by 3 years.
  - Hyperglycemia may worsen posttransplant because of corticosteroids, as well as decreased half-life of endogenous and exogenous insulin because of improved kidney function.
  - Risk factors for PTDM include age, obesity and weight gain posttranpslant, race/ethnicity (more common in African Americans and Hispanics), CNI use, Hepatitis C infection, and male gender.
  - Diagnostic criteria for PTDM are controversial, but the current American Diabetes Association guidelines may be utilized.
- **Obesity:** Average BMI is increasing in transplant candidates as well as in the general population, prompting BMI cutoffs of 35 to 40 kg/m^2 at most centers.
  - Although obese patients have overall improved mortality after transplant compared with maintenance dialysis, obesity causes increased risk of DGF, treatment for AR, graft loss, prolonged wound healing, and infectious complications.
  - Treatment includes dietary modification, exercise and lifestyle counseling, consideration for bariatric surgery.
  - Studies suggest little impact of steroid withdrawal versus continuation on posttransplant weight gain, emphasizing the importance of lifestyle modifications.
- **Bone disease:** Unlike the general population, causes of bone disease in ESRD patients are multifactorial.
  - They include osteitis fibrosa related to secondary hyperparathyroidism, as well as adynamic (low-turnover) bone disease, β2-microglobulin-associated arthropathies, and less commonly aluminum-related osteomalacia.
  - This is compounded by the use of corticosteroids pre- and posttransplant, causing bone loss and osteoporosis.
  - Bisphosphonates may worsen adynamic bone disease. Therefore, routine use of bone densitometry screening as well as the use of bisphosphonates is controversial in transplant recipients.
  - Monitoring of hyperparathyroidism posttransplant and correction of vitamin D deficiency is presently advised, with consideration for parathyroidectomy in patients with persistent hypercalcemia and secondary hyperparathyroidism posttransplant.

HEMATOLOGIC COMPLICATIONS

- **Anemia** is relatively common and multifactorial.[5,14]
  - It can be caused by perioperative or other sources of blood loss, iron, vitamin B12, or folate deficiency.
  - Decreased renal erythropoietin production is seen in the presence of renal allograft dysfunction and medications such as ACEI, ARB, and mTORi.
  - Hemolytic anemia can result from recurrent, *de novo* or drug-induced thrombotic microangiopathy.
  - Parvovirus infection should be considered in cases of refractory anemia and may respond to intravenous immunoglobulin infusion therapy.

- **Posttransplant erythrocytosis,** defined by a hematocrit exceeding 50% to 52%, occurs in 10% to 20% of renal transplant recipients.
  ○ Secondary causes should be excluded, including transplant renal artery stenosis, smoking, renal cell, hepatocellular or breast cancers, native polycystic kidney disease, or inappropriate erythropoietin use.
  ○ Treat if hematocrit >55% to avoid thrombotic complications.
  ○ ACEI therapy is effective if tolerated.
  ○ Refractory cases or those intolerant of ACEI/ARB may require phlebotomy and hematology referral.

MALIGNANCY

- Posttransplant malignancy can be **recurrent,** *de novo,* **or donor transmitted (rare).**[5,15]
- Immunosuppression inhibits normal immune surveillance, causes direct DNA damage, and promotes viral-mediated oncogenesis. Many transplant recipients have a history of pretransplant immunosuppression exposure (e.g., cytoxan for systemic lupus erythematosus nephritis), and cumulative exposure should be considered in assessing malignancy risk.
- Important viral/malignancy associations include Hepatitis B and C (**hepatocellular carcinoma**), EBV (PTLD), human herpes virus 8 (**Kaposi sarcoma**), and human papilloma virus (squamous cell skin cancer, vulvar, vaginal, and cervical cancer).
- **Overall risk is three to four fold** that of age-matched general population. Greatest risks are for nonmelanoma skin and lip cancer, PTLD, Kaposi sarcoma, renal cell carcinoma, as well as bladder, cervical, vulvar, perineal, anogenital, and liver cancers.
  ○ Patients with toxic or obstructive nephropathies have the highest risk of **renal and bladder cancers.**
  ○ PTLD accounts for one-fifth of malignancies posttransplantation, with an incidence of 1% to 2%. Development is associated with the use of antilymphocyte therapy for induction or rejection. Majority are non-Hodgkin lymphomas of B-cell origin, resulting from EBV-induced B-cell proliferation. Treatment options include immunosuppression reduction and possibly chemotherapy. Rituximab is utilized for CD20+ PTLD.
- General population guidelines are followed for breast, cervical, prostate, and colon cancer screening. **Annual skin exam** and use of sunscreen are advised for all recipients. Other screening is patient specific; for example, alpha fetoprotein (AFP) and liver ultrasound in HCV-positive recipients for hepatocellular carcinoma screening.
- Life-threatening malignancies may warrant significant or total withdrawal of immunosuppression.

INFECTIONS

- Immediately posttransplant, patients should be monitored for common postoperative infections such as **wound, line, urinary infections, and pneumonia.**[5,16]
- Intensive immunosuppression used at time of transplant increases the risk of **opportunistic infections in the first 6 months,** including CMV and other viral pathogens, *Pneumocystis jiroveci, Aspergillus, Cryptococcus,* other fungal infections, mycobacterial disease, *Listeria monocytogenes, Nocardia.*

- After 6 months, the risk of opportunistic infections persists but to a lesser degree, with infections more commonly due to community-acquired pathogens, particularly in those with successful graft function posttransplant.
- Factors to consider in the differential diagnosis of infection include time from transplant, cumulative immunosuppression history, other immunodeficiency states, donor and recipient exposure/infection history, recent hospitalizations, foreign bodies (stents, catheters, valves), open wounds, fluid collections, comorbidities (HIV, diabetes, liver disease), nutritional status, occupational and environmental exposures.
- For mild or moderate infections, maintenance of immunosuppression with appropriate antimicrobial administration is advised. More severe or certain viral infections (CMV, polyoma virus) warrant **immunosuppression reduction** commonly achieved by discontinuation of the antimetabolite and possible reduction in CNI doses.

Specific Viral Pathogens

- **CMV:** This is the most common viral pathogen postkidney transplant, affecting 10% to 30% of recipients (75% if no prophylaxis).[5,16,17] Prophylaxis type and duration (3 to 12 months) are dependent on pretransplant donor and recipient serologies. CMV-seronegative patients receiving a CMV-seropositive organ are at greatest risk.
  - ○ **Symptoms:** Fever, malaise, leukopenia, thrombocytopenia. It can involve the intestine (40%), liver (20%), lung (10%), kidney, eye, central nervous system (rare).
  - ○ **Diagnosis:** Seroconversion with a positive IgM titer, blood polymerase chain reaction demonstrating viral replication, or by histopathology of infected tissue. A high index of suspicion is required, given the vague presentation.
  - ○ **Treatment:** Oral valganciclovir (450 to 900 mg PO bid) or intravenous ganciclovir (2.5 to 5.0 mg/kg bid [adjusted as per renal function]) for 3 to 4 weeks; foscarnet and cidofovir reserved for ganciclovir-resistant cases only due to significant drug toxicities.
- **BK (polyoma virus):** BK virus is present as a latent infection in 60% to 80% of transplant recipients, with reactivation driven by immunosuppression. Manifestations include interstitial nephritis and ureteral stenosis; graft loss can occur due to BK virus nephropathy.
  - ○ BK virus nephropathy can be confirmed by the presence **of viral inclusions on allograft biopsy;** intersitital nephritis can otherwise mimic acute cellular rejection.
  - ○ As viremia precedes nephropathy, **preemptive reduction or withdrawl of antimetabolite,** if viremia is present, can prevent nephropathy development.
- **EBV:** This is associated with PTLD. In EBV-seronegative recipients from an EBV-seropositive donor, lifelong acyclovir prophylaxis is recommended. However, a benefit of antiviral therapy in treatment of PTLD has not been established. Rather, PTLD is treated with reduction or withdrawl of immunosuppression and often with chemotherapy with Rituximab.
- **Hepatitis B and C:** The incidence of Hepatitis B is declining in the ESRD population because of immunization. Approximately 5% of transplant recipients have Hepatitis C.
  - ○ Candidates who are Hepatitis BsAg- or Hepatitis C-positive require hepatology evaluation prior to transplant to determine renal transplant candidacy.

Renal transplant is **contraindicated if cirrhosis is present,** unless combined liver–kidney transplant is pursued.

○ Antiviral therapy should be used in Hepatitis BsAg-positive transplant candidates pre- and posttransplant, particularly if evidence of viral replication (HBeAg, HBV DNA) is present.

○ Antiviral therapy for Hepatitis C should be considered pretransplantation, as the posttransplant administration of interferon is associated with an increased risk of AR.

○ Studies demonstrate **inferior patient and graft outcomes in HCV-positive** compared to HCV-negative recipients. However, for the HCV-positive patient, transplant is associated with improved survival compared with maintenance dialysis and is the treatment of choice.

SPECIAL CONSIDERATIONS

Pregnancy

- Female transplant recipients of childbearing age must be counseled regarding increased fertility and likelihood of pregnancy following successful transplant, to include contraception if desired, and medication counseling.[18]
- Improved outcomes are seen if pregnancy occurs **>12 to 24 months** after a successful transplant in a recipient with **serum creatinine <1.5 to 2.0 mg/dL,** minimal proteinuria, no history of rejection, requiring minimal/no hypertensive therapy, with minimal comorbid conditions, and with appropriate preconception medication counseling.
- Immunosuppressive practice in transplantation has arisen from clinical experience. All immunosuppressive drugs are **Food and Drug Administration pregnancy safety class C** (risk cannot be ruled out) **or D** (positive evidence of risk), driven by both human data and animal studies. However, **MMF has been clearly demonstrated to be teratogenic,** causing facial and ear structural malformations, and should be substituted with Azathioprine. **mTORi are avoided** due to embryotoxicity and fetotoxicity in animal models. Prednisone, CNIs, and azathiprine are used during pregnancy.
- CNI levels may fall during pregnancy because of increases in maternal blood volume, and **close monitoring of drug levels** is needed to avoid precipitation of rejection.
- Common complications include preeclampsia, preterm delivery, and small for gestational age infants. Additionally, urinary tract infections are common and should be treated promptly in the transplant recipient with culture documentation of clearance.

REFERENCES

1. United States Renal Data System. http://www.usrds.org. Accessed December 12, 2010.
2. Scientific Registry of Transplant Recipients. http://www.srtr.org. Accessed December 12, 2010.
3. Kasiske BL, Cangro CB, Hariharan S, et al. The evaluation of renal transplant candidates: clinical practice guidelines. *Am J Transplant.* 2001;2:5–95.
4. Knoll G, Cockfield S, Blydt-Hansen T, et al. Canadian society of transplantation consensus guidelines on eligibility for kidney transplantation. *CMAJ.* 2005;173:1181–1184.
5. Danovitch G, ed. *Handbook of Kidney Transplantation.* Philadelphia, PA: Lippincott Williams & Wilkins; 2010.

6. Stock PG, Barin B, Murphy B, et al. Outcomes of kidney transplantation in HIV-infected recipients. *N Engl J Med.* 2010;363(21):2004–2014.

7. Terrault NA, Adey DB. The kidney transplant recipient with hepatitis C infection: pre and posttransplant treatment. *Clin J Am Soc Nephrol.* 2007;2(3):563–575.

8. Montgomery RA. Renal transplantation across HLA and ABO barriers: integrating paired donation into desensitization protocols. *Am J Transplant.* 2010;10(3):449–457.

9. Sis B, Mengel M, Haas M, et al. Banff '09 meeting report: antibody mediated graft deterioration and implementation of Banff working groups. *Am J Transplant.* 2010;10(3):464–471.

10. Najafian B, Kasiske BL. Chronic allograft nephropathy. *Curr Opin Nephrol Hypertens.* 2008;17(2):149–155.

11. Ponticelli C, Glassock RJ. Posttransplant recurrence of primary glomerulonephritis. *Clin J Am Soc Nephrol.* 2010;5(12):2363–2372.

12. Ojo AO. Cardiovascular complications after renal transplantation and their prevention. *Transplantation.* 2006;82(5):603–611.

13. Bloom RD, Crutchlow MF. New-onset diabetes mellitus in the kidney recipient: diagnosis and management strategies. *Clin J Am Soc Nephrol.* 2008;3(2):S38–S48.

14. Djamali A, Samaniego M, Muth B, et al. Medical care of kidney transplant recipients after the first posttransplant year. *Clin J Am Soc Nephrol.* 2006;1(4):623–640.

15. Vajdic C, McDonald S, McCredie M, et al. Cancer incidence before and after kidney transplantation. *JAMA.* 2006;296:2823–2831.

16. Fishman JA. Infections in organ-transplant recipients. *N Engl J Med.* 2007;357:2601–2614.

17. Bohl DL, Brennan DC. BK virus nephropathy and kidney transplantation. *Clin J Am Soc Nephrol.* 2007;2(1):S36–S46.

18. Josephson MA, McKay DB. Considerations in the medical management of pregnancy in transplant recipients. *Adv Chronic Kidney Dis.* 2007;14(2):156–167.

Red Flag Drugs That May Cause Renal Impairment

Antimicrobials
  Acyclovir
  Aminoglycosides
  Amphotericin
  Cephalosporins
  Cidofovir
  Ciprofloxacin
  Foscarnet
  Methicillin
  Pentamidine (IV)
  Sulfonamides
  TMP
  Vancomycin
Analgesics
  Acetaminophen
  NSAIDs

Chemotherapy
  Carboplatin
  Cisplatin
  Methotrexate (high dose)
  Mitomycin
  Nitrosoureas
Diuretics
  Loop diuretics
  Mannitol (high dose)
  Thiazide
Cardiovascular drugs
  ACE inhibitors
  Dopamine (high dose)
  Hydralazine
  Norepinephrine

Immunosuppressive drugs
  Cyclosporine
  Tacrolimus
Neurologic drugs
  Lithium
  Phenobarbital
  Phenytoin
Rheumatologic drugs
  Penicillamine
  Gold
Drugs of abuse
  Amphetamine
  Cocaine
  Heroin
  Phencyclidine

Mechanisms of Nephrotoxicity and Alternatives to Some Common Drugs

B

Drug	Mechanism	Alternatives/Comments
ACE inhibitors	Hemodynamic	Beta blockers, calcium channel blockers
Acetaminophen	ATN	Avoid doses >4 g/day
Acyclovir	ATN	Hydration, dose adjustment
Aminoglycosides	ATN	Monitor serum concentration, nontoxic substitutes
Amphotericin	ATN	Saline loading, lipid products, continuous infusion
Carboplatin	ATN	Hydration
Cephalosporins	Interstitial nephritis	Alternative antibiotics
Cimetidine	Interstitial nephritis	Proton pump inhibitor
Ciprofloxacin	Interstitial nephritis	Alternative antibiotics
Cisplatin	Tubular necrosis	Hydration, carboplatin
Cyclosporine	Hemodynamic, chronic interstitial nephritis	Monitor levels, sirolimus
Foscarnet	ATN	Dose adjust, ganciclovir
Ketorolac	Hemodynamic	Acetaminophen, opiate analgesic
Gold	Glomerulopathy	Methotrexate, hydroxychloroquine
High-dose mannitol	Hemodynamic	Avoid doses >200 g/day
Hydralazine	Glomerulopathy	ACE inhibitors
Lithium	Glomerulopathy, interstitial nephritis	Monitor levels, valproic acid
Loop diuretics	Interstitial nephritis	Non–sulfa-containing diuretics

Drug	Mechanism	Alternatives/Comments
Methicillin	Interstitial nephritis	Vancomycin
Methotrexate	Tubular obstruction	Adjust dosage, urinary alkalinization, allopurinol
NSAIDs	Hemodynamic, interstitial nephritis	Acetaminophen, tramadol, opiate analgesics
Penicillamine	Glomerulopathy	Methotrexate, hydroxychloroquine
Pentamidine	Tubular necrosis	TMP-SMX, dapsone
Phenytoin	Interstitial nephritis, glomerulopathy	Alternative anticonvulsant
Phenobarbital	Interstitial nephritis	Alternative anticonvulsant
Sulfonamides	Tubular obstruction, interstitial nephritis	Non–sulfa-containing antibiotic
Tacrolimus	Hemody namic, interstitial nephritis	Monitor levels, sirolimus
Thiazides	Interstitial nephritis	Alternative diuretics

ATN, acute tubular necrosis.

Common Medications with Active Metabolites

Drug	Metabolite	Cumulative Toxicity
Acetaminophen	N-acetyl-p-benzoquinoneimine	Hepatotoxicity, acute tubular necrosis
Allopurinol	Oxypurinol	Bone marrow suppression
Chlorpropamide	2-Hydroxychloropropramide	Hypoglycemia
Meperidine	Normeperidine	Seizures
Primidone	Phenobarbital	Oversedation, coma
Procainamide	N-acetyl-procainamide	Arrhythmia, hypotension, respiratory failure
Nitroprusside	Thiocyanate	Lactic acidosis, hallucinations, coma, tinnitus
Morphine	6-Morphine glucuronide	Oversedation, coma

Dosing Adjustments for Antimicrobials

D

Name	Usual Dose	Creatinine Clearance (mL/min)			Dialysis
		>50	10–50	<10	
Antibiotics					
Amoxicillin	250–500 mg q8h	No change	q8–12h	q24h	HD: dose after HD CAPD: 250 mg q12h
Ampicillin	250 mg–2 g q6h	No change	q8–12h	q24h	HD: dose after HD CAPD: 250 mg q12h
Ampicillin/ sulbactam	1.5–3 g q6h	No change	q8–12h	q24h	HD: dose after HD CAPD: q24h
Aztreonam	2 g q8h	No change	50–75%	25%	HD: extra 0.5 g after HD CAPD: 25%
Cefazolin	1–2 g IV q8h	No change	q12h	q24h	HD: 1 g after HD CAPD: 0.5 g q12h
Cefepime	1–2 g IV q8h	No change	q12–24h	q24h	HD: 1–1.5 g after HD CAPD: 1–2 g q48h
Cefotaxime	1–2 g q8h	q8–12h	q12–24h	q24h	HD: 1 g after HD CAPD: 0.5–1 g qd
Cefotetan	1–2 g q12h	No change	50%	25%	HD: 1 g after HD CAPD: 1 g qd
Ceftazidime	1–2 g q8h	q8–12h	q24–48h	q48h	HD: 1 g after HD CAPD: 0.5 g qd
Cefuroxime	0.75–1.50 g q8h	q8h	q8–12h	q24h	HD: dose after HD CAPD: q24h
Ciprofloxacin PO	250–750 mg q12h	No change	(<30) q24h	q24h	HD, CAPD: 250–500 mg after dialysis
Ciprofloxacin IV	200–400 mg q12h	No change	(<30) q24h	q24h	HD, CAPD: 200–400 mg after dialysis

369

Creatinine Clearance (mL/min)

Name	Usual Dose	>50	10–50	<10	Dialysis
Levofloxacin PO, IV	250–500 mg qd	No change	250 mg q24–48h	250 mg q48h	HD, CAPD: 250 mg q48h
Gatifloxacin PO, IV	400 mg q24h	No change	200 mg q24h	200 mg q24h	HD, CAPD: 200 mg after dialysis
Gemifloxacin	320 mg q24h	No change	160 mg q24h	160 mg q24h	HD: dose after dialysis; CAPD: 160 mg q24h
Clarithromycin	500 mg q12h	No change	75%	50%	HD: dose after dialysis; CAPD: no change
Erythromycin	250–500 mg q6h	No change	No change	50%	No change
TMP-SMX IV	5 mg/kg TMP component q6–8h	No change	(<30) 50% q12h	Not recommended	HD: 50%
TMP-SMX PO	1 tab b.i.d.	No change	(<30) 50%	Not recommended	HD: 50%
Telithromycin	800 mg q24h	No change	(<30): 600 mg q24h	600 mg q24h	HD: Give after HD
Daptomycin	4–6 mg/kg q24h	No change	(<30): 4–6 mg/kg q48h	4–6 mg/kg q48h	HD: 4–6 mg/kg q48h, give after HD CAPD: 4–6 mg/kg q48h
Imipenem	500 mg IV q6h	No change	250 mg q6–12h	125–250 mg q12h	HD: dose after HD CAPD: 125–250 mg q12h
Meropenem	1 g IV q8h	No change	1 g q12h	0.5 g q12h	HD: dose after HD CAPD: 0.5 g q12h
Ertapenem	1 g q24h	No change	(<30) 500 mg q24h	500 mg q24h	HD: 500 mg q24h
PCN G	0.5–4 mU q4h	No change	75%	25–50%	HD: dose after HD CAPD: 25–50%

Drug					
Piperacillin	3–4 g q4–6h	No change	q6–8h	q8h	HD: dose after HD CAPD: q8h
Piperacillin/ tazobactam	3.375 g q6h	No change	2.25 g q6h	2.25 g q8h	HD: 2.25 g q8h + 0.75 g after HD; CAPD: 2.25 g q8h
Ticarcillin/ clavulanate	3.1 g q4h	No change	2 g q4–8h	2 g q12h	HD: extra 3.1 g after HD CAPD: 2 g q12h
Tetracycline	250–500 mg q6h	q8–12h	q12–24h	q24h	Avoid
Antifungals					
Amphotericin	0.4–1 mg/kg/day	No change	No change	q24–48h	HD: no change CAPD: q24–48h
Fluconazole	200–400 mg qd	No change	50%	50%	HD: extra 200 mg after HD CAPD: 50%
Itraconazole	100–200 mg q12h	No change	No change	50%	HD, CAPD: 100 mg q12–24h
Voriconazole IV	6 mg/kg q12h × 2 then 4 mg/kg IV q12h	No change	Not recommended (toxic vehicle may accumulate, use PO route)	Not recommended (toxic vehicle may accumulate, use PO route)	Not recommended (toxic vehicle may accumulate, use PO route)
Voriconazole PO	200 mg PO b.i.d. (if >40 kg); 100 mg PO b.i.d. (if <40 kg)	No change	No change	No change	No change

(continued)

Name	Usual Dose	Creatinine Clearance (mL/min)			Dialysis
		>50	10–50	<10	
Antivirals					
Acyclovir PO	200–800 mg q4–6h	No change	(<25) q8h	q12h	HD: after HD
Acyclovir IV	5–12.4 mg/kg q8h	No change	q12–24h	2.5 mg/kg q24h	HD: after HD CAPD: 2.5 mg/kg q24h
Amantadine PO	100 mg b.i.d.	q24–48h	q48–72h	q7d	No change
Cidofovir induction	5 mg/kg q1wk	No change	0.5–2 mg/kg q1wk	0.5 mg/kg q1wk	Limited data
Cidofovir maintenance	5 mg/kg q2wk	No change	0.5–2 mg/kg q2wk	0.5 mg/kg q2wk	Limited data
Entecavir	0.5–1 mg q24h	No change	(CrCl 30–49): 50% of usual dose (CrCl 10–29): 30% of usual dose	10% of regular dose	HD: Give 10% of regular dose after HD
Famciclovir	500 mg q8h	No change	q12–24h	250 mg q24h	HD: after HD CAPD: no data
Ganciclovir IV	5 mg/kg q24h	2.5–5 mg/kg q24h	0.6–1.25 mg/kg q24h	0.625 mg/kg 3×/wk	HD: 0.6 mg/kg after HD CAPD: 0.625 mg/kg 3×/wk
Ganciclovir PO	1 g t.i.d.	0.5–1 g t.i.d.	0.5–1 g qd	0.5 g 3×/wk	HD: 0.5 g after HD
Valacyclovir	1 g q8h	No change	q12–24h	0.5 g q24h	HD: after HD CAPD: 0.5 g q24h
Valganciclovir	900 mg q12–24h	No change	450 mg q24–48h	Not recommended	—

CAPD, continuous ambulatory peritoneal dialysis; HD, hemodialysis

Name	Usual Oral Dose	Creatinine Clearance (mL/min)			Dialysis
		>50	10–50	<10	
Didanosine (ddI, Videx)	>60 kg, 400 mg qd <60 kg, 250 mg qd	No change	50% of usual dose	25% of usual dose	HD, CAPD: 25%
Lamivudine (3TC, Epivir)	150 mg b.i.d.	No change	150 qd	50 mg qd	HD: 25–50 mg qd CAPD: no data
Stavudine (d4T, Zerit)	>60 kg, 40 mg b.i.d. <60 kg, 30 mg b.i.d.	No change	50% q12–24h	50% q24h	HD, CAPD: 25%
Zidovudine (AZT, Retrovir)	300 mg b.i.d.	No change	No change	300 mg qd	HD: 300 mg qd CAPD: 300 mg qd
Zalcitabine (ddC, Hivid)	0.75 mg t.i.d.	No change	0.75 mg b.i.d.	0.75 mg qd	HD: 0.75 mg qd CAPD: no change
Tenofovir (Viread)	300 mg q24h	No change	Not recommended <60 mL/min	Not recommended	Not recommended

CAPD, continuous ambulatory peritoneal dialysis; HD, hemodialysis.

Note:

Combination products: use separate products and adjust each as necessary. Combivir (AZT + 3TC), Trizivir (Abacavir + AZT + 3TC).

No recommendation or no dosing adjustment necessary:

Nucleoside reverse transcriptase inhibitors (NRTI): abacavir (Ziagen), emtricitabine (Emtriva)

Non-nucleoside reverse transcriptase inhibitors (NNRTI): nevirapine (Viramune), delavirdine (Rescriptor), efavirenz (Sustiva)

Protease inhibitors: atazanavir (Reyataz), amprenavir (Agenerase), indinavir (Crixivan), saquinavir (Invirase, Fortovase), ritonavir (Norvir), nelfinavir (Viracept), lopinavir + ritonavir (Kaletra), tipranavir (Aptivus), darunavir (Prezista)

Fusion inhibitor: enfuvirtide (Fuzeon)

Index

Page numbers followed by *f* refer to figures; page numbers followed by *t* refer to tables.